W9-ASB-797

WEBSTER'S
MEDICAL SPELLER

Webster's
MEDICAL SPELLER

A Merriam-Webster®

G. & C. MERRIAM COMPANY

Springfield, Massachusetts

Library of Congress Cataloging in Publication Data

Main entry under title:

Webster's medical speller

1. Medicine—Terminology. 2. Spellers.
[DNLM: 1. Nomenclature. W15 W385]
R123.W35 610'.1'4 75-22454

ISBN 0-87779-037-x

MADE IN THE U.S.A.

5 6 VH 79 78 77

CONTENTS

PREFACE

Webster's Medical Speller is a pocket-sized guide to the spelling and division of 35,000 medical words and words with special medical meanings. The divisions shown are based on the principles of end-of-line division followed in Webster's New Collegiate Dictionary, the eighth in the Merriam-Webster series of Collegiate dictionaries.

The medical specialist who prepares or processes written matter frequently needs to know such things as whether a word is spelled with one *l* or two, whether a compound word is written with a hyphen, which of several variant spellings or plurals is most widely used, and where a word is divided at the end of a line of print or writing. Webster's Medical Speller provides a ready and authoritative answer to such questions.

Among the special features of Webster's Medical Speller is the entry of inflected forms. Entry has been decided according to the criteria used for Webster's New Collegiate Dictionary except that no cutback forms are shown. In general inflected forms are entered when they are irregular, as in the plural **lice**; when a letter is changed, as in the plural **sensitivities**, or dropped, as in the present participle **operating** or doubled, as in the past participle **embedded**; and when the user might have reasonable doubts or erroneous expectations about the choice of suffixes, as in the plural **helminths** or the Latinized variant plural **carcinomata**. Not only are base words such as **physiology** entered but their derivatives such as **physiologic**, **physiological**, **physiologically**, and **physiologist** also appear in alphabetical sequence. If a verbal noun does not appear at its own alphabetical place, one should look for it at the parent verb; for example, **teething** will be found at **teethe**. Frequently confused words (as **perineal**, **peritoneal**, and **peroneal**) are given short definitions. In addition there is a list of Latin words and abbreviations used in writing prescriptions, along with their full Latin forms and English equivalents. Finally, the speller contains 1500 medical abbreviations, a list of medical symbols, and a table of weights and measures.

The 35,000 word corpus was selected by comparing Webster's Third New International Dictionary with standard medical sources and by comparing one medical source with another. Additional vocabulary was drawn from a computer printout of words in Webster's New Collegiate Dictionary in the twelve subject fields of anatomy, biochemistry, cytology, dentistry, embryology, genetics, medicine, microbiology, neuroscience, pharmacology, physiology, and psychology. Finally, new words were selected from manuscript entries proposed for a forthcoming Addenda to Webster's Third New International Dictionary. The basic word corpus was edited by making word divisions conform to the principles used in Webster's New Collegiate Dictionary and by adding appropriate inflected forms.

Usage is the final arbiter of the form entered in this book. When there was a doubt about current practice, the Merriam vocabulary citation files were consulted for the latest evidence on the form of a word. For example, review of the citational evidence for use of an apostrophe indicates that **Golgi apparatus** and **Golgi complex** are the forms invariably found in print and not **Golgi's apparatus** and **Golgi's complex** but that **Saint Vitus' dance** and **Saint Vitus's dance** occur with equal frequency. At the time of editing *Webster's Medical Speller* the vocabulary files contained about 12 million citations on 3 × 5 slips.

Scientific names of genera and higher taxonomic categories in biological nomenclature are included if they are of medical significance. Names of genera (as *Neisseria*) begin with a capital letter and are written in italics while the names of families (as Babesiidae) and higher taxonomic categories (as Cestoda) begin with a capital letter but are not italicized. Many genus names (*Bacterium*, *Clostridium*, *Penicillium*) are also used as common names which take a plural (bacteria, clostridia, penicillia), and when used in this way they are not capitalized or italicized in either the singular or plural forms. For example, if the context reads "a sample of members of the genus *Clostridium*," both a capital letter and italic type are used. On the other hand, in such a context as "a sample of clostridia," a lowercase initial letter and roman type are used. In this book, only the common name is given when there is evidence in the Merriam citation files for use of the same word as both a genus and a common name. Therefore, when the writer wants to use a genus name and only the common name is given in the speller, he should take particular care to use the singular form, to begin with a capital letter, and to indicate italics.

The word divisions indicated by centered dots do not necessarily separate words into syllables. They are intended only to show points at which words may be divided at the end of a line of type or writing. While considerable time and effort have been expended in achieving consistency of end-of-line divisions, we should point out that alternative divisions may be equally acceptable. The notion of correctness is, perhaps, too strong to be applied to end-of-line division, where respectable publishers differ in both theory and practice. When one is reading a printed page, end-of-line divisions are noticed for the most part only when a division might lead to misunderstanding.

Commonsense and the appearance of the printed page are important considerations in end-of-line division. The easiest principle to remember is that a single letter of a word should not end or begin a line. This principle is extended in the speller to include words that occur as part of a solid compound. For example, **cat·e·chol·amine** is not divided **cat·e·chol·a·mine** because the element **amine** is a word in its own right and the initial letter *a* should not stand alone even when **amine** is part of a larger word. Although many people prefer not to divide a hyphenated compound (as **glucose-6-phosphate**) anywhere but at the hyphen, divisions are indicated for the benefit of those who wish to divide elsewhere. One should avoid dividing at the end of consecutive lines, and the last word in a paragraph or on a page should not be divided.

Several people have contributed to the editing of *Webster's Medical Speller.* Ervina E. Foss and Doris N. Sherwood, retired members of the Merriam-Webster editorial department, helped compile the corpus of 35,000 words. Laverne W. King, another retired editor, collected words, edited copy, and read final proof. Raymond R. Wilson, assistant editor, helped edit copy. John K. Bollard, assistant editor, codified the principles of end-of-line division and made the final decision in difficult cases. The Merriam clerical and typing staff under the supervision of Mrs. Evelyn G. Summers assisted in the preparation of the manuscript.

Roger W. Pease, Jr.
Editor

A

ab•a•ca
abac•te•ri•al
ab•alien•ation
ab•ar•thro•sis
pl ab•ar•thro•ses
aba•sia
ab•ax•i•al
ab•ax•ile
Ab•der•hal•den re•ac•tion
ab•de•rite
ab•do•men
pl ab•do•mens
or ab•dom•i•na
ab•dom•i•nal
ab•dom•i•nal•ly
ab•dom•i•no•an•te•ri•or
ab•dom•i•no•cen•te•sis
pl ab•dom•i•no•cen•te•ses
ab•dom•i•no•hys•ter•ot•o•my
pl ab•dom•i•no•hys•ter•ot•o•mies
ab•dom•i•no•per•i•ne•al
ab•dom•i•no•pos•te•ri•or
ab•dom•i•nous
ab•dom•i•no•ves•i•cal
ab•duce
ab•duced
ab•duc•ing
ab•du•cens
pl ab•du•cen•tes
ab•du•cent
ab•duct
ab•duc•tion
ab•duc•tor
pl ab•duc•to•res
or ab•duc•tors
Abegg's rule
ab•em•bry•on•ic
ab•er•ran•cy
pl ab•er•ran•cies
ab•er•rant
ab•er•ra•tion
abey•ance
ab•i•ent
ab•ies
ab•i•e•tate
ab•i•et•ic
abio•gen•e•sis
pl abio•gen•e•ses
abio•gen•e•tic
abi•o•sis
pl abi•o•ses
abi•ot•ic
abio•tro•phic
abi•ot•ro•phy
pl abi•ot•ro•phies
ab•ir•ri•tant
ab•lac•ta•tion
ablas•te•mic
ablas•tin
ab•late
ab•lat•ed
ab•lat•ing
ab•la•tio
ab•la•tion
ab•lu•tion
ab•nor•mal
ab•nor•mal•i•ty
pl ab•nor•mal•i•ties
ab•nor•mi•ty
pl ab•nor•mi•ties
ab•oma•sal
ab•oma•sum
pl ab•oma•sa
ab•oma•sus
pl ab•oma•si
ab•orad
ab•oral
abort
abor•ti•fa•cient
abor•tion
abor•tion•ist
abor•tive
abor•tus
ABO sys•tem
abou•lia
var of abulia
abrade
abrad•ed
abrad•ing
abra•sion
abra•sive
ab•re•act
ab•re•ac•tion
ab•rup•tio pla•cen•tae
pl ab•rup•tio pla•cen•ta•rum
or ab•rup•ti•o•nes pla•cen•ta•rum

Abrus
ab•scess
ab•scis•sion
also ab•sci•sion

ab•sence
ab•sinthe
or ab•sinth

ab•sin•thin
also ab•sin•thi•in

ab•sin•thism
ab•sin•thi•um
ab•sin•thol
ab•so•lute
ab•sorb
ab•sorb•able
ab•sor•bance
ab•sor•be•fa•cient
ab•sor•ben•cy
pl ab•sor•ben•cies

ab•sor•bent
ab•sorp•ti•om•e•ter
ab•sorp•tion
ab•sorp•tive
ab•ster•gent
ab•sti•nence
ab•stract
ab•strac•tion
abu•lia
or abou•lia

abu•lic
abuse
abused
abus•ing
abut•ment
aca•cia
acal•cu•lia
Ac•a•ly•pha
acamp•sia
acan•tha
acan•thes•the•sia
acan•thi•on
Acan•tho•ceph•a•la
acan•tho•ceph•a•lan
Acan•tho•chei•lo•ne•ma
acan•tho•chei•lo•ne•mi•a•sis
pl acan•tho•chei•lo ne•mi•a•ses

acan•thoid
acan•tho•ker•a•to•der•mia
ac•an•thol•y•sis
pl ac•an•thol•y•ses

ac•an•tho•ma
pl ac•an•tho•mas
or ac•an•tho•ma•ta

ac•an•tho•sis
pl ac•an•tho•ses

ac•an•thot•ic
acap•nia
acar•dia
ac•a•ri•a•sis
pl ac•a•ri•a•ses

acar•i•cid•al
acar•i•cide
also acar•a•cide

acar•id
Acar•i•dae
acar•i•dan
Ac•a•ri•na
ac•a•ri•no•sis
pl ac•a•ri•no•ses

ac•a•ro•der•ma•ti•tis
pl ac•a•ro•der•ma•ti•tis•es
or ac•a•ro•der•ma•tit•i•des

ac•a•roid
ac•a•rol•o•gy
pl ac•a•rol•o•gies

ac•a•ro•pho•bia
ac•a•rus
pl ac•a•ri

acat•a•lep•sy
pl acat•a•lep•sies

acat•a•lep•tic
acau•dal
acau•date
ac•cel•er•ant
ac•cel•er•a•tion
ac•cel•er•a•tor
ac•cel•er•om•e•ter
ac•cen•tu•a•tor
ac•cep•tor
ac•ces•so•ri•us
pl ac•ces•so•rii

ac•ces•so•ry
also ac•ces•sa•ry
pl ac•ces•so•ries
or ac•ces•sa•ries

ac•ci•dent
ac•ci•dent-prone
ac•cip•i•ter
ac•cli•mate
ac•cli•mat•ed
ac•cli•mat•ing

ac·cli·ma·tion
ac·cli·ma·ti·za·tion
ac·cli·ma·tize
ac·cli·ma·tized
ac·cli·ma·tiz·ing
ac·com·mo·date
ac·com·mo·dat·ed
ac·com·mo·dat·ing
ac·com·mo·da·tion
ac·com·mo·da·tive
ac·couche·ment
ac·cou·cheur
ac·cre·tion
ace·dia
acel·lu·lar
ace·nes·the·sia
acen·tric
ace·pha·lia
aceph·a·lo·cyst
aceph·a·lous
aceph·a·lus
pl aceph·a·li
ac·er·o·la
acer·vu·line
acer·vu·lus
pl acer·vu·li
aces·cent
aces·o·dyne
ace·ta
pl of acetum
ac·e·tab·u·lar
ac·e·tab·u·lum
pl ac·e·tab·u·lums *or* ac·e·tab·u·la
ac·e·tal
ac·et·al·de·hyde
acet·amide
ac·et·am·i·dine
ac·et·amin·o·phen
ac·et·an·i·lide
or ac·et·an·i·lid
ac·et·ar·sone
ac·e·tate
ac·et·azol·amide
ac·et·e·nyl
ace·tic
ace·ti·fy
ace·ti·fied
ace·ti·fy·ing
ac·e·tim·e·ter
ac·e·tin
ac·ti·no·spec·ta·cin
ace·to·ac·e·tate
ace·to·ace·tic
ace·to·ace·tyl
ace·to·hex·amide
acet·o·in
ace·to·ki·nase
ac·e·tol
ac·e·tol·y·sis
pl ac·e·tol·y·ses
ace·to·me·roc·tol
ac·e·tom·e·ter
ace·to·mor·phine
ace·to·naph·thone
ac·e·tone
ace·to·ne·mia
also ace·to·nae·mia
ace·to·ne·mic
also ace·to·nae·mic
ace·to·ni·trile
ac·e·ton·uria
ace·to·phe·net·i·din
also ac·et·phe·net·i·din
ace·to·phe·none
ace·to·sol·u·ble
ace·to·to·lu·i·dide
also ace·to·tol·u·ide
ace·tous
ac·e·tract
ace·tum
pl ace·ta
ace·tyl
acet·y·lase
acet·y·la·tion
ace·tyl·cho·line
ace·tyl·cho·lin·es·ter·ase
ace·tyl-coA
ace·tyl co·en·zyme A
acet·y·lene
ace·tyl·meth·yl·car·bi·nol
ace·tyl·sa·lic·y·late
ace·tyl·sal·i·cyl·ic

ach·a·la·sia
ache
  ached
  ach·ing
ach·i·le·ine
Ach·il·lea
Achil·les' ten·don
achil·lo·bur·si·tis
ach·il·lot·o·my
  pl ach·il·lot·o·mies
achlor·hy·dria
achol·ic
achol·uria
achon·dro·pla·sia
achor·dal
achor·date
Acho·ri·on
achroa·cyte
achroi·o·cy·the·mia
achro·ma·cyte
achro·mal
achro·ma·sia
ach·ro·mat·ic
achro·ma·tin
achro·ma·tin·ic
achro·ma·tism
achro·mat·o·cyte
achro·ma·tol·y·sis
  pl achro·ma·tol·y·ses
achro·mat·o·phil
achro·mat·o·phil·ia
achro·ma·top·sia
achro·ma·to·sis
  pl achro·ma·to·ses
achro·mia
  also achro·ma
achro·mic
achro·mo·trich·ia
ach·roö·dex·trin
  also ach·ro·dex·trin
achy
  ach·i·er
  ach·i·est
achy·lia
achy·lia gas·tri·ca
acic·u·lar
ac·id
ac·i·de·mia
ac·id-fast
acid·i·fy
  acid·i·fied
  acid·i·fy·ing
ac·i·dim·e·ter
ac·i·dim·e·try
  pl ac·i·dim·e·tries
acid·i·ty
  pl acid·i·ties
acid·o·phile
  or acid·o·phil
ac·i·do·phil·ic
ac·i·doph·i·lus milk
ac·i·do·sis
  pl ac·i·do·ses
ac·i·dot·ic
acid·u·late
acid·u·lous
ac·id·uria
ac·i·du·ric
ac·id·yl
ac·i·nar
acin·ic
acin·i·form
ac·i·nose
ac·i·nous
ac·i·nus
  pl ac·i·ni
ack·ee
acla·sis
  pl acla·ses
ac·me
ac·mes·the·sia
  also ac·maes·the·sia
ac·ne
ac·ne·form
  or ac·ne·iform
ac·ne ro·sa·cea
  pl ac·nae ro·sa·ce·ae
ac·ne vul·gar·is
  pl ac·nae vul·gar·es
Ac·o·can·thera
acoe·nes·the·sia
aco·ine
  also aco·in
a·con·i·tase
ac·o·nite
ac·o·nit·ic
acon·i·tine
ac·o·ni·tum
acou·me·ter
acous·ma
  pl acous·mas
  or acous·ma·ta
acous·tic

acous·tics
ac·quire
  ac·quired
  ac·quir·ing
ac·ral
acra·nia
  absence of the skull (see Acrania)
Acra·nia
  a division of the chordates (see acrania)
acra·ni·al
ac·rid
ac·ri·dine
acrid·i·ty
  pl ac·rid·i·ties
ac·ri·fla·vine
ac·ri·mo·ny
  pl ac·ri·mo·nies
ac·ro·atax·ia
ac·ro·blast
ac·ro·cen·tric
ac·ro·ce·phal·ic
ac·ro·ceph·a·ly
  also ac·ro·ce·pha·lia
  pl ac·ro·ceph·a·lies
  also ac·ro·ce·pha·lias
ac·ro·cy·a·no·sis
  pl ac·ro·cy·a·no·ses
ac·ro·cy·a·not·ic
ac·ro·der·ma·ti·tis
  pl ac·ro·der·ma·ti·tis·es
  or ac·ro·der·ma·tit·i·des
ac·ro·dont
ac·ro·dyn·ia
ac·ro·ede·ma
ac·ro·ker·a·to·sis
  pl ac·ro·ker·a·to·ses
ac·ro·le·in
ac·ro·me·gal·ic
ac·ro·meg·a·ly
  also ac·ro·me·ga·lia
  pl ac·ro·meg·a·lies
  also ac·ro·me·ga·lias
ac·ro·mi·al
ac·ro·mic·ria
ac·ro·mio·cla·vic·u·lar
ac·ro·mi·on
ac·ro·nyx
ac·ro·pachy
  pl ac·ro·pach·ies
ac·ro·par·es·the·sia
ac·ro·pa·thol·o·gy
  pl ac·ro·pa·thol·o·gies
acrop·a·thy
  pl acrop·a·thies
acrop·e·tal
ac·ro·pho·bia
ac·ro·scle·ro·sis
  pl ac·ro·scle·ro·ses
ac·rose
ac·ro·some
ac·ro·ste·al·gia
ac·ro·te·ric
acrot·ic
ac·ry·late
a·cryl·ic
ac·ry·lo·ni·trile
act
Ac·taea
ac·tin
ac·tin·ic
ac·ti·nism
ac·tin·i·um
ac·ti·no·bac·il·lo·sis
  pl ac·ti·no·bac·il·lo·ses
ac·ti·no·ba·cil·lus
  pl ac·ti·no·ba·cil·li
ac·ti·no·chem·is·try
  pl ac·ti·no·chem·is·tries
ac·tin·o·graph
ac·ti·nog·ra·phy
  pl ac·ti·nog·ra·phies
ac·tin·o·lite
ac·ti·nol·o·gy
  pl ac·ti·nol·o·gies
ac·ti·nom·e·ter
ac·ti·nom·e·try
  pl ac·ti·nom·e·tries
ac·ti·no·my·ces
Ac·ti·no·my·ce·ta·ce·ae
Ac·ti·no·my·ce·ta·les
ac·ti·no·my·cete
ac·ti·no·my·ce·tin
ac·ti·no·my·ce·tous
ac·ti·no·my·cin
ac·ti·no·my·co·ma
  pl ac·ti·no·my·co·mas
  or ac·ti·no·my·co·ma·ta

ac·ti·no·my·co·sis
pl ac·ti·no·my·co·ses
ac·ti·no·my·cot·ic
Ac·ti·no·myx·id·ia
ac·ti·non
ac·tin·o·phage
ac·tin·o·phore
ac·ti·no·phy·to·sis
pl ac·ti·no·phy·to·ses
Ac·ti·nop·o·da
ac·ti·no·ther·a·py
pl ac·ti·no·ther·a·pies
ac·tion
ac·ti·vate
ac·ti·vat·ed
ac·ti·vat·ing
ac·ti·va·tion
ac·ti·va·tor
ac·tive
ac·tive·ly
ac·tiv·i·ty
pl ac·tiv·i·ties
ac·to·my·o·sin
Ac·u·ar·ia
acu·i·ty
pl acu·i·ties
acu·le·ate
acu·mi·nate
acu·mi·nat·ed
acu·mi·nat·ing
ac·u·punc·ture
acute
acy·clic
ac·yl
ac·yl·am·i·no
ac·yl·ase
ac·yl·a·tion
adac·tyl·ia
adac·tyl·ous
ad·a·man·tine
ad·a·man·ti·no·ma
pl ad·a·man·ti·no·mas
or ad·a·man·ti·no·ma·ta
ad·a·man·to·blast
ad·a·man·to·blas·to·ma
pl ad·a·man·to·blas·to·mas
or ad·a·man·to·blas·to·ma·ta
Ad·am's ap·ple
Ad·an·so·nia
adapt
ad·ap·ta·tion
adapt·er
also adap·tor
ad·ap·tom·e·ter
ad·ax·i·al
ad·der
ad·dict
ad·dic·tion
ad·dic·tive
Ad·di·so·ni·an
Ad·di·son's dis·ease
ad·di·tive
ad·du·cent
ad·duct
ad·duc·tion
ad·duc·tor
ad·en·al·gia
ad·e·nase
ad·en·ec·to·my
pl ad·en·ec·to·mies
ad·en·ec·to·pia
aden·i·form
ad·e·nine
ad·e·ni·tis
pl ad·e·nit·i·des
or ad·e·ni·tis·es
ad·e·no·car·ci·no·ma
pl ad·e·no·car·ci·no·mas
also ad·e·no·car·ci·no·ma·ta
ad·e·no·cele
ad·e·no·cys·to·ma
pl ad·e·no·cys·to·mas
or ad·e·no·cys·to·ma·ta
ad·e·no·fi·bro·ma
pl ad·e·no·fi·bro·mas
or ad·e·no·fi·bro·ma·ta
ad·e·no·hy·poph·y·sis
pl ad·e·no·hy·poph·y·ses
ad·e·noid
ad·e·noi·dal
ad·e·noid·ec·to·my
pl ad·e·noid·ec·to·mies
ad·e·noid·ism
ad·e·noid·itis
ad·e·no·ma
pl ad·e·no·mas
or ad·e·no·ma·ta
ad·e·no·ma·to·sis
pl ad·e·no·ma·to·ses

ad•e•no•my•o•ma
pl ad•e•no•my•o•mas
or ad•e•no•my•o•ma•ta

ad•e•no•my•o•sis
pl ad•e•no•my•o•ses

ad•e•no•neu•ral

ad•e•nop•a•thy
pl ad•e•nop•a•thies

ad•e•no•phar•yn•gi•tis
pl ad•e•no•phar•yn•gi•tis•es
or ad•e•no•phar•yn•git•i•des

ad•e•no•sar•co•ma
pl ad•e•no•sar•co•mas
or ad•e•no•sar•co•ma•ta

ad•e•nose

aden•o•sine

aden•o•sine mo•no•phos•phate

ad•e•no•tome

ad•e•not•o•my
pl ad•e•not•o•mies

ad•e•nous

ad•e•no•vi•rus

ad•e•nyl

ad•e•nyl•ate cy•clase

ad•e•nyl cy•clase

ad•e•nyl•ic

adeps
pl adi•pes

adeps la•nae
pl adi•pes la•nae

ad•he•sion

ad•he•si•ot•o•my
pl ad•he•si•ot•o•mies

ad•he•sive

adi•ac•tin•ic

Ad•i•an•tum

adi•a•ther•man•cy
pl adi•a•ther•man•cies

ad•i•ent

Adin•i•da

adip•ic

ad•i•po•cere

ad•i•po•gen•e•sis
pl ad•i•po•gen•e•ses

ad•i•po•ge•net•ic
or ad•i•pog•e•nous

ad•i•pose

ad•i•po•sis
pl ad•i•po•ses

ad•i•pos•i•ty
pl ad•i•pos•i•ties

adip•sia

ad•i•tus
pl ad•i•tus
or ad•i•tus•es

ad•junct

ad•ju•vant

Ad•le•ri•an

ad lib

ad li•bi•tum

ad•max•il•lary

ad•me•di•al

ad•me•di•an

ad•nexa

ad•nex•al

ad•nex•i•tis

ad•o•les•cence

ad•o•les•cent

ado•nis

adon•i•tol

ad•oral

ad•re•nal

ad•re•nal•cor•ti•cal

ad•re•nal•ec•to•mize
ad•re•nal•ec•to•mized
ad•re•nal•ec•to•miz•ing

ad•re•nal•ec•to•my
pl ad•re•nal•ec•to•mies

adren•a•line

ad•re•nal•ism

adren•a•lone

adren•er•gen

ad•ren•er•gic

ad•re•no•chrome

ad•re•no•cor•ti•cal

ad•re•no•cor•ti•co•mi•met•ic

ad•re•no•cor•ti•co•ste•roid

ad•re•no•cor•ti•co•tro•phic
or ad•re•no•cor•ti•co•trop•ic

ad•re•no•cor•ti•co•tro•phin
or ad•re•no•cor•ti•co•tro•pin

ad•re•no•lyt•ic
ad•re•no•ste•rone
ad•re•no•tro•phic
or ad•re•no•trop•ic
ad•sorb
ad•sor•bate
ad•sor•bent
ad•sorp•tion
adul•ter•ant
adul•ter•ate
adul•ter•at•ed
adul•ter•at•ing
adul•ter•a•tion
ad•ven•ti•tia
ad•ven•ti•tial
ad•ven•ti•tious
ady•nam•ia
ady•nam•ic
aë•des
ae•goph•o•ny
var of egophony
ae•lu•ro•pho•bia
aer•ate
aer•at•ed
aer•at•ing
aer•a•tion
aer•if•er•ous
aer•i•form
aero•bac•ter
aer•obe
aer•o•bic
aer•o•bics
aero•bi•ol•o•gy
pl aero•bi•ol•o•gies
aero•bio•scope
aero•bi•o•sis
pl aero•bi•o•ses
aero•bi•ot•ic
aer•odon•tal•gia
aer•odon•tia
aero•dy•nam•ics
aero•em•bo•lism
aero•gel
aero•gen•ic
aer•og•e•nous
aero•gram
aero•med•i•cine
aer•om•e•ter
aero•neu•ro•sis
pl aero•neu•ro•ses
aero-oti•tis me•dia
also aero-oti•tis
or aer•oti•tis
aero•pause
aero•pha•gia
aer•oph•a•gy
pl aer•oph•a•gies
aero•pho•bia
aero•phore
aero•plank•ton
aero•si•nus•i•tis
aero•sol
aero•sol•iza•tion
aero•sol•ize
aero•sol•ized
aero•sol•iz•ing
aero•tax•is
pl aero•tax•es
aero•ther•a•peu•tics
aero•ther•a•py
pl aero•ther•a•pies
aer•oti•tis
var of aero•otitis media
aer•ot•ro•pism
ae•ru•go
pl ae•ru•gos
Aes•cu•la•pi•an
Aes•cu•la•pi•us
aes•cu•le•tin
var of esculetin
aes•cu•lin
var of esculin
aes•the•sia
var of esthesia
aes•thet•ics
or es•thet•ics
aes•ti•vate
aes•ti•vat•ed
aes•ti•vat•ing
aes•ti•va•tion
ae•ti•ol•o•gy
var of etiology
ae•tio•por•phy•rin
var of etioporphyrin
afe•brile
af•fect
af•fec•tion
af•fec•tive
af•fec•tiv•i•ty
pl af•fec•tiv•i•ties
af•fer•ent
conducting toward a nerve center (*see* efferent)
af•fin•i•ty
pl af•fin•i•ties
af•fir•ma•tion
af•flux
af•flux•ion
af•fri•cate

af·fu·sion
afi·brin·o·gen·emia
af·la·tox·in
af·ter·birth
af·ter·brain
af·ter·care
af·ter·damp
af·ter·dis·charge
af·ter·ef·fect
af·ter·im·age
af·ter·im·pres·sion
af·ter·pain
af·ter·po·ten·tial
af·ter·sen·sa·tion
af·ter·taste
af·to·sa
aga·lac·tia
aga·lac·tous
agam·ete
agam·ic
agam·ma·glob·u·lin·emia
aga·mo·gen·e·sis
pl aga·mo·gen·e·ses
aga·mo·ge·net·ic
aga·mog·o·ny
pl aga·mog·o·nies
Ag·a·mo·mer·mis
agam·ont
ag·a·mous
agan·gli·on·ic
agar
agar-agar
aga·ric
agar·i·cin
Agar·i·cus
agas·tric
aga·ve
agen·e·sis
pl agen·e·ses
age·net·ic
ageu·sia
ag·ger
ag·glom·er·ate
ag·glom·er·at·ed
ag·glom·er·at·ing
ag·glom·er·a·tion
ag·glu·ti·na·bil·i·ty
pl ag·glu·ti·na·bil·i·ties
ag·glu·ti·nant
ag·glu·ti·nate
ag·glu·ti·nat·ed
ag·glu·ti·nat·ing
ag·glu·ti·na·tion
ag·glu·ti·na·tive
ag·glu·ti·nin
ag·glu·ti·no·gen
ag·glu·ti·no·gen·ic
ag·glu·ti·noid
ag·gre·gate
ag·gre·gat·ed
ag·gre·gat·ing
ag·gres·sin
ag·gres·sion
aglo·mer·u·lar
aglos·sia
aglu·con
or aglu·cone
agly·con
or agly·cone
ag·ma·tine
ag·mi·nate
ag·mi·nat·ed
ag·nail
Ag·nath·ia
ag·na·thous
ag·no·gen·ic
ag·no·sia
ag·nos·te·rol
ag·o·nal
ag·o·nist
ag·o·nis·tic
ag·o·ny
pl ag·o·nies
ag·o·ra·pho·bia
agou·ti
also agou·ty
pl agou·tis
also agou·ties
agraffe
agram·ma·tism
agran·u·lo·cyte
agran·u·lo·cy·to·sis
pl agran·u·lo·cy·to·ses
agraph·ia
agraph·ic
ag·ro·ma·nia
Ag·ro·py·ron
agryp·nia
pl agryp·ni·ai
ague

aid·man
pl aid·men

ai·lan·thus
ai·le·ron
ail·ment
ai·lu·ro·phobe
ai·lu·ro·pho·bia
ai·nhum
air·bra·sive
air·sick
air·sick·ness
air·way
aitch·bone
ai·ti·ol·o·gy
var of etiology

aj·o·wan
also ai·wain

akary·ote
aki·ne·sia
aki·ne·sis
also aky·ne·sis
pl aki·ne·ses
also aky·ne·ses

aki·net·ic
ala
pl alae

ala·lia
al·a·nine
alan·tin
al·a·nyl
alar
alas·trim
alate
also alat·ed

ala·tion
al·bas·pi·din
al·be·do
pl al·be·dos

al·bi·nism
al·bi·no
pl al·bi·nos

al·bi·no·ism
al·bi·not·ic
al·bo·ci·ne·re·ous
al·bu·gin·ea
Al·bu·go
al·bu·men
al·bu·min
al·bu·mi·nate
al·bu·mi·noid
al·bu·mi·nous
al·bu·min·uria
al·bu·min·uric
al·bu·mose
Al·ca·lig·e·nes
al·cap·ton
al·cap·ton·uria
var of alkaptonuria

Al·cock's ca·nal
al·co·gel
al·co·hol
al·co·hol·ate
al·co·hol·ic
al·co·hol·ism
al·co·hol·ist
al·co·hol·iza·tion
al·co·hol·ize
al·co·hol·ized
al·co·hol·iz·ing
al·co·hol·om·e·ter
al·co·hol·y·sis
pl al·co·hol·y·ses

al·de·hyde
al·do·bi·uron·ic

al·do·hex·ose
al·dol
al·dol·ase
al·don·ic
al·dose
al·do·side
al·do·ste·rone
al·do·ste·ron·ism
al·dox·ime
al·drin
alec·i·thal
alem·bic
alem·mal
Al·e·tris
aleu·ke·mia
aleu·ke·mic
al·eu·rone
also al·eu·ron

alex·ia
alex·in
alex·i·phar·mac
alex·i·phar·mic
alex·i·phar·mi·cal
al·ga
pl al·gae
also al·gas

al·gal
al·ge·do·nic
al·ge·sia
al·ge·sic
al·ge·sim·e·ter
al·get·ic
al·gi·cide
al·gid
al·gin
al·gi·nate

al•gin•ic
al•go•gen•ic
al•go•lag•nia
al•gom•e•ter
al•gom•e•try
pl al•gom•e•tries

al•go•phil•ia
al•go•pho•bia
al•gor
ali•cy•clic
alien•ation
alien•ism
alien•ist
ali•es•ter•ase
ali•form
al•i•ment
al•i•men•ta•ry
al•i•men•ta•tion
al•i•men•to•ther•a•py
pl al•i•men•to•ther•a•pies

ali•na•sal
al•i•phat•ic
al•i•quot
ali•sphe•noid
or ali•sphe•noi•dal

aliz•a•rin
also aliz•a•rine

al•ka•di•ene
al•ka•le•mia
al•ka•les•cence
al•ka•les•cent
al•ka•li
pl al•ka•lies
or al•ka•lis

al•ka•lim•e•ter
al•ka•lim•e•try
pl al•ka•lim•e•tries

al•ka•line
al•ka•lin•i•ty
pl al•ka•lin•i•ties

al•ka•lin•i•za•tion
al•ka•lin•ize
al•ka•lin•ized
al•ka•lin•iz•ing
al•ka•li•za•tion
al•ka•lize
al•ka•lized
al•ka•liz•ing
al•ka•loid
al•ka•lom•e•try
pl al•ka•lom•e•tries

al•ka•lo•sis
pl al•ka•lo•ses

al•ka•lot•ic
al•ka•mine
al•kane
al•ka•net
al•kan•nin
al•kap•ton
al•kap•ton•uria
or al•cap•ton•uria

al•ka•ver•vir
al•kene
al•kide
al•kyl
al•kyl•amine
al•kyl•a•tion
al•kyl•o•gen
al•lan•to•ic
al•lan•toid
al•lan•to•in•ase
al•lan•to•is
pl al•lan•to•i•des

al•lele
al•lel•ic
al•lel•ism
al•le•lo•ca•tal•y•sis
pl al•le•lo•ca•tal•y•ses

al•le•lo•cat•a•lyt•ic
al•le•lo•morph
al•le•lo•mor•phic
al•le•lo•mor•phism
al•ler•gen
al•ler•gen•ic
al•ler•gic
al•ler•gin
al•ler•gist
al•ler•gol•o•gy
pl al•ler•gol•o•gies

al•ler•gy
pl al•ler•gies

al•le•thrin
al•le•vi•ate
al•le•vi•at•ed
al•le•vi•at•ing
al•le•vi•a•tion
al•le•vi•a•tive
or al•le•vi•a•to•ry

al•li•cin
al•li•ga•tion
al•li•in
al•lit•er•a•tion
al•li•um
al•lo•bar
al•lo•bar•bi•tal
al•lo•bar•bi•tone

al·lo·chi·ria
also al·lo·chei·ria

al·lo·cor·tex
al·lo·erot·ic
al·lo·erot·i·cism
al·lo·er·o·tism
al·log·a·my
pl al·log·a·mies

al·lo·ge·ne·ic
al·lo·gen·ic
al·lo·graft
al·lo·ki·ne·sis
pl al·lo·ki·ne·ses

al·lom·er·ism
al·lo·me·tric
al·lom·e·tron
al·lom·e·try
pl al·lom·e·tries

al·lo·mor·phism
al·lo·path
al·lo·path·ic
al·lop·a·thy
pl al·lop·a·thies

al·lo·phan·amide
al·lo·phan·ic
al·lo·phore
al·lo·psy·chic
al·lo·pu·ri·nol
all-or-none
or all-or-noth·ing

al·lose
al·lo·some
al·lo·ste·ric
al·lo·ste·ri·cal·ly
al·lo·tet·ra·ploid
al·lo·trans·plant
al·lo·trans·plan·ta·tion
al·lot·ri·oph·a·gy
pl al·lot·ri·oph·a·gies

al·lo·trope
al·lo·tro·phic
al·lo·trop·ic
al·lot·ro·pism
al·lot·ro·py
pl al·lot·ro·pies

al·lo·type
al·lo·typ·ic
al·lo·typ·i·cal·ly
al·lo·typy
pl al·lo·typ·ies

al·lox·an
al·lox·an·tin
al·lox·a·zine
al·loy
all·spice
al·lu·lose
al·lyl
al·lyl·amine
al·lyl·nor·mor·phine
al·mond
al·oe
al·oe-em·o·din
alo·gia
al·o·in
al·o·pe·cia
al·o·pe·cia ar·e·a·ta
al·o·pe·cic
al·pha
al·pha-ad·ren·er·gic
al·pha glob·u·lin
al·pha-he·li·cal
al·pha-he·lix
al·pha-re·cep·tor
Al·sto·nia
al·sto·nine
al·ter·ant
al·ter·a·tion
al·ter·ative
Al·ter·nar·ia
al·ter·na·tion
al·thaea
or al·thea

Alt·mann's gran·ules
al·tri·cial
al·tri·gen·der·ism
al·tro·hep·tu·lose
al·trose
al·um
alu·mi·na
alu·mi·no·sis
pl alu·mi·no·ses

alu·mi·num
al·ve·o·lar
al·ve·o·lar·ly
al·ve·o·late
al·ve·o·la·tion
al·ve·o·lec·to·my
pl al·ve·o·lec·to·mies

al·ve·o·lo·plas·ty
pl al·ve·o·lo·plas·ties

al·ve·o·lot·o·my
pl al·ve·o·lot·o·mies

al·ve·o·lus
pl al·ve·o·li

al·ve·us
pl al·vei

Alz·hei·mer's dis·ease
amaas
am·a·crine
amal·gam
amal·ga·mate
amal·ga·mat·ed
amal·ga·mat·ing
amal·ga·ma·tion
amal·ga·ma·tor
am·an·din
am·a·ni·ta
aman·ta·dine
am·a·roid
am·a·roi·dal
amas·tia
am·a·tho·pho·bia
am·au·ro·sis
pl am·au·ro·ses

am·au·rot·ic
amaxo·pho·bia
Am·a·zo·na
am·ber·gris
also am·ber·grease

am·bi·dex·ter
am·bi·dex·ter·i·ty
pl am·bi·dex·ter·i·ties

am·bi·dex·trous
am·bi·ent
am·bi·lat·er·al
am·bi·sex·u·al
am·bi·sex·u·al·i·ty
pl am·bi·sex·u·al·i·ties

am·biv·a·lence
am·biv·a·lent
am·bi·ver·sion
am·bi·vert
am·bly·chro·mat·ic
Am·bly·om·ma
am·bly·opia
am·blyo·scope
am·bo·cep·tor
am·bo·mal·le·al
am·bon
also am·bo
pl am·bo·nes

am·bos
am·bo·sex·u·al
am·bro·sin
am·bu·lance
am·bu·lant
am·bu·la·to·ry
ame·ba
var of amoeba

am·e·bi·a·sis
also am·oe·bi·a·sis
pl am·e·bi·a·ses
also am·oe·bi·a·ses

ame·bic
var of amoebic

ame·bo·cyte
var of amoebocyte

ame·boid
var of amoeboid

amei·o·sis
pl amei·o·ses

ame·lio·ra·tion
am·e·lo·blast
am·e·lo·blas·to·ma
am·e·lo·gen·e·sis
pl am·e·lo·gen·e·ses

am·e·lus
pl am·e·li

amen·or·rhea
also amen·or·rhoea

amen·or·rhe·al
also amen·or·rhoe·al

amen·or·rhe·ic
or amen·or·rhoe·ic

amen·tia
am·er·i·ci·um
am·er·ism
am·er·is·tic
ameth·o·caine
am·e·thop·ter·in
am·e·tro·pia
am·e·tro·pic
am·i·dase
am·ide
ami·do·gen
Am·i·dos·to·mum
am·i·dox·ime
amim·ia
am·i·nate
am·i·nat·ed
am·i·nat·ing
amine
ami·no
ami·no·ace·tic
ami·no·ac·id·uria
ami·no·ben·zo·ic

am·i·nol·y·sis
pl ami·nol·y·ses

ami·no·pep·ti·dase
am·i·noph·er·ase
ami·no·phyl·line
am·i·nop·ter·in
ami·no·py·rine
ami·no·sal·i·cyl·ic
ami·no·thi·a·zole
ami·no·trans·fer·ase
ami·to·sis
pl ami·to·ses

ami·tot·ic
am·i·trip·ty·line
amix·ia
am·me·ter
am·mo·nia
am·mo·ni·a·cal
or am·mo·ni·ac

am·mo·ni·ate
am·mo·ni·at·ed
am·mo·ni·at·ing
am·mo·ni·fi·ca·tion
am·mo·ni·um
am·mo·nol·y·sis
pl am·mo·nol·y·ses

am·ne·sia
am·ne·si·ac
am·ne·sic
am·nes·tic
am·nio·cen·te·sis
pl am·nio·cen·te·ses

am·nio·gen·e·sis
pl am·nio·gen·e·ses

am·ni·og·ra·phy
pl am·ni·og·ra·phies

am·ni·on
pl am·ni·ons
or am·nia

am·nio·scope
am·ni·os·co·py
pl am·ni·os·co·pies

Am·ni·o·ta
am·ni·ote
am·ni·ot·ic
am·ni·o·tome
amo·bar·bi·tal
amo·di·a·quin
also amo·di·a·quine

amoe·ba
or ame·ba
pl amoe·bas
or amoe·bae
or ame·bas

am·oe·bi·a·sis
var of amebiasis

amoe·bic
or ame·bic

amoe·bo·cyte
or ame·bo·cyte

amoe·boid
or ame·boid

Amoe·bo·tae·nia
amoe·bous
amok
or amuck

amor·phin·ism
amor·phism
amor·phous
amor·phus
pl amor·phi
or amor·phus·es
am·per·age
am·pere
Am·pere's law
am·phet·a·mine
am·phi·ar·thro·di·al
am·phi·ar·thro·sis
pl am·phi·ar·thro·ses

am·phi·as·ter
am·phi·blas·tic
am·phi·bol·ic
am·phi·cen·tric
am·phi·chrome
am·phi·cra·nia
am·phi·dip·loid
am·phi·ge·net·ic
am·phi·kary·on
am·phi·mic·tic
am·phi·mic·ti·cal·ly
am·phi·mix·is
pl am·phi·mix·es

am·phi·ox·us
pl am·phi·oxi
or am·phi·ox·us·es

am·phi·ploid
am·phi·ploi·dy
pl am·phi·ploi·dies

am·phi·tene
am·phit·ri·chous
am·phi·dip·loi·dy
pl am·phi·dip·loi·dies

am·pho·lyte
am·pho·phil
am·pho·phil·ic

am·phoph·i·lous
am·phor·ic
am·pho·ric·i·ty
pl am·pho·ric·i·ties
am·pho·ter·ic
am·pho·ter·i·cin
am·phot·er·ism
am·pi·cil·lin
am·plex·us
pl am·plex·us
am·pli·tude
am·pul
also am·pule
or am·poule
am·pul·la
pl am·pul·lae
am·pul·lar
am·pul·lu·la
pl am·pul·lu·lae
am·pu·tate
am·pu·tat·ed
am·pu·tat·ing
am·pu·ta·tion
am·pu·tee
amuck
var of amok
amu·sia
amy·e·lin·ic
amy·e·lon·ic
amyg·da·la
pl amyg·da·lae
amyg·da·lin
amyg·da·line
amyg·da·loid
am·yl
am·y·la·ceous
am·y·lase
am·yl·ene
am·y·lo·dex·trin
am·y·loid
am·y·loi·do·sis
pl am·y·loi·do·ses
am·y·lol·y·sis
pl am·y·lol·y·ses
am·y·lo·pec·tin
am·y·lo·plast
am·y·lop·sin
am·y·lose
am·y·lum
am·yl·uria
amyo·to·nia
amyo·tro·phia
amyo·tro·phic
amy·ot·ro·phy
pl amy·ot·ro·phies
ana
an·a·bae·na
anab·a·sine
anab·a·sis
pl anab·a·ses
an·a·bat·ic
ana·bi·o·sis
pl ana·bi·o·ses
ana·bi·ot·ic
an·a·bo·lic
anab·o·lin
anab·o·lism
anab·o·lite
an·acid·i·ty
pl an·acid·i·ties
anac·la·sis
pl anac·la·ses
ana·clit·ic
ana·cul·ture
an·acu·sis
anae·mia
var of anemia
anae·mic
var of anemic
an·aer·obe
an·aer·o·bic
an·aer·o·bi·cal·ly
an·aero·bi·o·sis
pl an·aero·bi·o·ses
an·aes·the·sia
var of anesthesia
an·aes·thet·ic
var of anesthetic
an·aes·the·tist
var of anesthetist
an·aes·the·ti·za·tion
var of anesthetization
an·aes·the·tize
var of anesthetize
ana·gen·e·sis
pl ana·gen·e·ses
ana·gen·et·ic
anal
an·a·lep·tic
an·al·ge·sia
an·al·ge·sic
an·al·get·ic
anal·i·ty
pl anal·i·ties
an·a·log
also an·a·logue
anal·o·gous
anal·y·sand

anal·y·sis
pl anal·y·ses

an·a·lyst
an·a·lyt·ic
or an·a·lyt·i·cal

an·a·lyze
an·a·lyzed
an·a·lyz·ing
an·a·lyz·er
an·am·ne·sis
pl an·am·ne·ses

an·am·nes·tic
an·am·ni·on·ic
an·am·ni·ot·ic
ana·mor·pho·sis
pl ana·mor·pho·ses

ana·phase
an·aph·ro·di·sia
an·aph·ro·dis·i·ac
ana·phy·lac·tic
ana·phy·lac·tin
ana·phy·lac·to·gen
ana·phy·lac·to·gen·ic
ana·phy·lac·toid
ana·phyl·a·tox·in
ana·phy·lax·is
pl ana·phy·lax·es

an·a·pla·sia
ana·plas·ma
pl ana·plas·ma·ta
or ana·plas·mas

an·a·plas·mo·sis
pl an·a·plas·mo·ses

an·a·plas·tic
ana·pro·tas·pis
pl ana·pro·tas·pes

an·a·rith·mia
an·ar·thria
ana·sar·ca
ana·sar·cous
ana·state
an·astig·mat·ic
anas·to·mose
anas·to·mosed
anas·to·mos·ing
anas·to·mo·sis
pl anas·to·mo·ses

anas·to·mot·ic
an·as·tral
an·a·tom·ic
or an·a·tom·i·cal

an·a·tom·i·co·path·o·log·ic
anat·o·mist
anat·o·mize
anat·o·mized
anat·o·miz·ing
anat·o·my
pl anat·o·mies

ana·tox·in
an·au·dia
an·chor·age
an·chy·lose
var of ankylose

an·chy·lo·sis
var of ankylosis

an·chy·lot·ic
var of ankylotic

an·cil·lary
pl an·cil·lar·ies

an·cip·i·tal
an·cip·i·tous
an·co·nal
an·co·ne·al
an·co·ne·us
pl an·co·nei

an·co·noid
an·cy·lose
var of ankylose

an·cy·lo·sis
var of ankylosis

An·cy·los·to·ma
an·cy·lo·sto·mi·a·sis
pl an·cy·lo·sto·mi·a·ses

an·cy·lot·ic
var of ankylotic

an·cy·roid
var of ankyroid

An·di·ra
an·dro·cyte
an·dro·gam·one
an·dro·gen
an·dro·gen·e·sis
pl an·dro·gen·e·ses

an·dro·gen·ic
an·drog·e·nous
an·dro·gyne
an·drog·y·nism
an·drog·y·nous
an·drog·y·ny
pl an·drog·y·nies

an·droid
an·drom·e·da
an·drom·edo·tox·in

an·dro·mi·met·ic
an·dro·pho·bia
an·dro·stane
an·dro·stene·di·one
an·dros·te·rone
an·elec·tro·ton·ic
an·elec·trot·o·nus
ane·mia
also anae·mia
ane·mic
also anae·mic
an·e·mom·e·ter
an·en·ce·phal·ic
an·en·ceph·a·lous
an·en·ceph·a·lus
pl an·en·ceph·a·li
an·en·ceph·a·ly
also an·en·ce·pha·lia
pl an·en·ceph·a·lies
also an·en·ce·pha·lias
an·en·ter·ous
an·er·gic
an·er·gy
pl an·er·gies
an·er·oid
an·er·y·throp·sia
an·es·the·sia
also an·aes·the·sia
an·es·the·si·ol·o·gist
an·es·the·si·ol·o·gy
pl an·es·the·si·ol·o·gies
an·es·thet·ic
also an·aes·thet·ic

an·es·the·tist
also an·aes·the·tist
an·es·the·ti·za·tion
also an·aes·the·ti·za·tion
an·es·the·tize
also an·aes·the·tize
an·es·the·tized
also an·aes·the·tized
an·es·the·tiz·ing
also an·aes·the·tiz·ing
an·es·tric
an·es·trous
also an·oes·trous
an·es·trum
also an·oes·trum
pl an·es·tra *also* an·oes·tra
an·es·trus
also an·oes·trus
pl an·es·tri *also* an·oes·tri
an·e·thole
an·e·to·der·ma
an·eu·ploid
an·eu·ploi·dy
pl an·eu·ploi·dies
aneu·ri·lem·mic
an·eu·rin
also an·eu·rine
an·eu·rysm
also an·eu·rism
an·eu·rys·mal
also an·eu·ris·mal
an·frac·tu·os·i·ty
pl an·frac·tu·os·i·ties

an·gel·i·ca
an·gi·ec·to·my
pl an·gi·ec·to·mies
an·gi·i·tis
pl an·gi·it·i·des
an·gi·na
an·gi·nal
an·gi·na pec·to·ris
an·gi·noid
an·gi·nose
an·gi·nous
an·gio·blast
an·gio·blas·to·ma
pl an·gio·blas·to·mas *or* an·gio·blas·to·ma·ta
an·gio·car·di·og·ra·phy
pl an·gio·car·di·og·ra·phies
an·gio·cho·li·tis
an·gio·cyst
an·gio·ede·ma
pl an·gio·ede·mas *or* an·gio·ede·ma·ta
an·gio·fi·bro·ma
pl an·gio·fi·bro·mas *also* an·gio·fi·bro·ma·ta
an·gio·gen·e·sis
pl an·gio·gen·e·ses
an·gio·gen·ic
an·gio·gram
an·gi·og·ra·phy
pl an·gi·og·ra·phies
an·gi·oid
an·gi·ol·o·gy
pl an·gi·ol·o·gies

an·gi·o·ma
pl an·gi·o·mas
or an·gi·o·ma·ta

an·gi·o·ma·to·sis
pl an·gi·o·ma·to·ses

an·gi·o·ma·tous
an·gio·neu·rot·ic
an·gi·op·a·thy
pl an·gi·op·a·thies

an·gio·sar·co·ma
pl an·gio·sar·co·mas
or an·gio·sar·co·ma·ta

an·gio·scle·ro·sis
pl an·gio·scle·ro·ses

an·gio·sco·to·ma
pl an·gio·sco·to·mas
or an·gio·sco·to·ma·ta

an·gio·sco·tom·e·try
pl an·gio·sco·tom·e·tries

an·gio·spasm
an·gio·spas·tic
an·gi·os·to·my
pl an·gi·os·to·mies

an·gio·ten·sin
an·gio·ten·sin·ase
an·gio·ton·ic
an·gio·to·nin
an·gos·tu·ra
ang·strom
an·gu·la·tion
an·gu·lus
pl an·gu·li

an·ha·lo·ni·um
an·he·do·nia
an·hi·dro·sis
or an·hy·dro·sis
also an·idro·sis
pl an·hi·dro·ses
or an·hy·dro·ses
also an·idro·ses

an·hi·drot·ic
or an·hy·drot·ic
also an·idrot·ic

an·his·tic
an·his·tous
an·hy·drase
an·hy·dra·tion
an·hy·dre·mia
also an·hy·drae·mia

an·hy·dride
an·hy·drous
an·ic·ter·ic
anile
an·i·lide
an·i·line
ani·lin·gus
or ani·linc·tus

an·i·lin·ism
anil·i·ty
pl anil·i·ties

an·i·ma
an·i·mal
an·i·mal·cule
an·i·mal·i·ty
pl an·i·mal·i·ties

an·i·ma·tion
an·i·mism
an·i·mus
an·ion
an·ion·ic
an·ion·i·cal·ly
an·ion·ot·ro·py
pl an·ion·ot·ro·pies
an·irid·ia
an·is·ate
an·ise
an·is·ei·ko·nia
anis·ic
an·iso·co·ria
an·iso·cy·to·sis
pl an·iso·cy·to·ses

an·isog·a·mous
also an·iso·gam·ic

an·isog·a·my
pl an·isog·a·mies

an·isog·na·thous
an·is·ole
an·iso·me·tro·pia
an·iso·me·trop·ic
an·iso·spore
an·iso·trop·ic
an·isot·ro·pous
an·kle
an·kle·bone
an·ky·lo·glos·sia
an·ky·lose
also an·chy·lose
or an·cy·lose

an·ky·lo·sis
also an·chy·lo·sis
or an·cy·lo·sis
pl an·ky·lo·ses
also an·chy·lo·ses
or an·cy·lo·ses

An·ky·los·to·ma
an·ky·lo·sto·mi·a·sis
pl an·ky·lo·sto·mi·a·ses

an·ky·lot·ic
also an·chy·lot·ic
or an·cy·lot·ic

an•ky•roid
also an•cy•roid

an•la•ge
pl an•la•gen
also an•la•ges

an•neal

an•nec•tent
also an•nec•tant

an•nexa

an•not•to

an•nu•lar

an•nu•lus
pl an•nu•li
also an•nu•lus•es

an•od•al

an•ode

an•od•ic

an•o•don•tia

an•o•dyne

an•o•dyn•ia

an•o•e•sia

an•oes•trous
var of anestrous

an•oes•trum
var of anestrum

an•oes•trus
var of anestrus

an•o•et•ic

anoia

anom•a•ly
pl anom•a•lies

an•o•mer

ano•mia

an•o•mie
or an•o•my
pl an•o•mies

an•o•nych•ia

anon•y•ma
pl anon•y•mae
or anon•y•mas

ano•op•sia
or an•op•sia

Anoph•e•les

anoph•e•line

anoph•e•lism

an•oph•thal•mia

an•oph•thal•mos

an•oph•thal•mus

An•o•pla

ano•plas•ty
pl ano•plas•ties

An•op•lo•ceph•a•la

an•or•chism

ano•rec•tal

an•o•rec•tic
also an•o•ret•ic

an•orex•ia

an•orexi•ant

an•orex•i•gen•ic

an•or•gan•ic

an•or•tho•pia

ano•scope

an•os•mat•ic

an•os•mia

an•os•mic

an•os•phre•sia
pl an•os•phra•sia

an•ovu•lant

an•ovu•la•tion

an•ovu•la•to•ry

an•ox•emia
also an•ox•aemia

an•ox•emic
also an•ox•aemic

an•ox•ia

an•ox•ic

an•sa
pl an•sae

an•sate
or an•sat•ed

an•ser•ine

an•si•form

ant•ac•id

an•tag•o•nism

an•tag•o•nist

an•tag•o•nis•tic

an•te•brach•i•al

an•te•bra•chi•um

an•te•car•di•um
var of anticardium

an•te•cor•nu
pl an•te•cor•nua

an•te•cu•bi•tal

an•te•flex•ion

an•te•mor•tem

an•te•na•tal

an•te•par•tum

an•te•po•si•tion

an•te•ri•or

an•tero•grade

an•tero•lat•er•al

an•tero•pos•te•ri•or

an•te•ver•sion

an•te•vert

ant•he•lix
var of antihelix

an•thel•min•tic
also an•thel•min•thic

an·tho·cy·an·in
also an·tho·cy·an

an·tho·xan·thin
an·thra·cene
an·thrac·nose
an·thra·coid
an·thra·co·sil·i·co·sis
pl an·thra·co·sil·i·co·ses

an·thra·co·sis
pl an·thra·co·ses

an·thra·cot·ic
an·thra·gal·lol
an·thra·lin
an·thra·ni·late
an·thra·nil·ic
an·thra·qui·none
an·thrax
pl an·thra·ces

an·throne
an·thro·po·gen·e·sis
pl an·thro·po·gen·e·ses

an·thro·po·ge·net·ic
an·thro·po·gen·ic
an·thro·pog·e·ny
pl an·thro·pog·e·nies

an·thro·pog·o·ny
pl an·thro·pog·o·nies

an·thro·pog·ra·phy
pl an·thro·pog·ra·phies

an·thro·poid
An·thro·poi·dea

an·thro·pol·o·gy
pl an·thro·pol·o·gies

an·thro·pom·e·ter
an·thro·po·met·ric
an·thro·pom·e·try
pl an·thro·pom·e·tries

an·thro·po·mor·phism
an·thro·pop·a·thy
pl an·thro·pop·a·thies

an·thro·poph·a·gy
pl an·thro·poph·a·gies

an·thro·po·phil·ic
an·thro·pos·o·phy
pl an·thro·pos·o·phies

an·ti·abor·tion
an·ti·abor·tion·ist
an·ti·ac·id
an·ti·al·ler·gic
also an·ti·al·ler·gen·ic

an·ti·am·y·lase
an·ti·ana·phy·lax·is
pl an·ti·ana·phy·lax·es

an·ti·ane·mic
an·ti·anx·i·ety
an·ti·ar·rhyth·mic
an·ti·ar·thrit·ic
an·ti·aux·in
an·ti·bac·te·ri·al
an·ti·bi·ont

an·ti·bi·o·sis
pl an·ti·bi·o·ses

an·ti·bi·ot·ic
an·ti·body
pl an·ti·bod·ies

an·ti·bra·chi·um
pl an·ti·bra·chia

an·ti·can·cer
also an·ti·can·cer·ous

an·ti·car·di·um
or an·te·car·di·um
pl an·ti·car·dia
or an·te·car·dia

an·ti·car·i·ous
an·ti·cath·ode
an·ti·cho·lin·er·gic
an·ti·cho·lin·es·ter·ase
an·ti·cli·nal
an·tic·ne·mi·on
an·ti·co·ag·u·lant
an·ti·co·ag·u·late
an·ti·co·ag·u·lat·ed
an·ti·co·ag·u·lat·ing
an·ti·co·ag·u·la·tion
an·ti·co·ag·u·la·tive
an·ti·co·ag·u·lin
an·ti·co·don
an·ti·com·ple·ment
an·ti·com·ple·men·ta·ry

an·ti·con·vul·sant
an·ti·con·vul·sive
an·ti·cus
an·ti·de·pres·sant
an·ti·de·pres·sive
an·ti·di·a·bet·ic
an·ti·di·ar·rhe·al
an·ti·di·u·ret·ic
an·ti·dot·al
an·ti·dot·al·ly
an·ti·dote
an·ti·drom·ic
an·ti·emet·ic
an·ti·en·zyme
an·ti·fe·brile
an·ti·fer·til·i·ty
an·ti·fi·bri·nol·y·sin
an·ti·flu·o·ri·da·tion·ist
an·ti·fun·gal
an·ti·gen
an·ti·gen·ic
an·ti·ge·ni·ci·ty
pl an·ti·ge·nic·i·ties

an·ti·glob·u·lin
an·ti·he·lix
or ant·he·lix
pl an·ti·he·li·ces *or* an·ti·he·lix·es *or* ant·he·li·ces *or* ant·he·lix·es

an·ti·he·mo·phil·ic
an·ti·his·ta·mine
an·ti·hor·mone
an·ti·hu·man
an·ti·hy·per·ten·sive
an·ti-in·flam·ma·to·ry
an·ti·leu·ke·mic
an·ti·lo·bi·um
pl an·ti·lo·bia

an·ti·lu·et·ic
an·ti·lym·pho·cyte
or an·ti·lym·pho·cyt·ic

an·ti·ly·sin
an·ti·ly·sis
pl an·ti·ly·ses

an·ti·lyt·ic
an·ti·ma·lar·i·al
an·ti·mere
an·ti·me·tab·o·lite
an·ti·mi·cro·bi·al
an·ti·mi·cro·bic
an·ti·mi·tot·ic
an·ti·mo·ni·al
an·ti·mon·ic
an·ti·mo·nide
an·ti·mo·ny
pl an·ti·mo·nies

an·ti·mo·nyl
an·ti·mu·ta·gen·ic
an·ti·my·cin
an·ti·my·cot·ic
an·ti·neo·plas·tic
an·ti·neu·rit·ic
an·tin·i·al
an·tin·i·on
an·tin·o·my
pl an·tin·o·mies

an·ti·ox·i·dant
an·ti·par·a·sit·ic
an·tip·a·thy
pl an·tip·a·thies

an·ti·pe·ri·od·ic
an·ti·peri·stal·sis
pl an·ti·peri·stal·ses

an·ti·peri·stal·tic
an·ti·per·spi·rant
an·ti·phlo·gis·tic
an·ti·plas·tic
an·ti·pneu·mo·coc·cic
an·tip·o·dal
an·ti·pode
pl an·ti·po·des

an·ti·pol·lu·tion
an·ti·pol·lu·tion·ist
an·ti·pros·tate
an·ti·pro·throm·bin
an·ti·pru·rit·ic
an·ti·psy·chot·ic
an·ti·py·re·sis
pl an·ti·py·re·ses

an·ti·py·ret·ic
an·ti·py·rine
an·ti·ra·chit·ic
an·ti·re·flec·tion
an·ti·rheu·mat·ic
an·ti·scor·bu·tic
an·ti·sep·sis
pl an·ti·sep·ses

an·ti·sep·tic

an·ti·sep·ti·cize
an·ti·sep·ti·cized
an·ti·sep·ti·ciz·ing
an·ti·ser·um
pl an·ti·ser·ums
or an·ti·sera
an·ti·sid·er·ic
an·ti·so·cial
an·ti·spas·mod·ic
an·ti·strep·tol·y·sin
an·ti·syph·i·lit·ic
an·ti·the·nar
an·ti·throm·bin
an·ti·thy·roid
an·ti·tox·ic
an·ti·tox·in
an·ti·trag·i·cus
pl an·ti·trag·i·ci
an·ti·tra·gus
pl an·ti·tra·gi
an·ti·trope
an·ti·trop·ic
an·ti·tryp·sin
an·ti·tryp·tic
an·ti·tu·ber·cu·lous
also an·ti·tu·ber·cu·lar
an·ti·tu·mor
also an·ti·tu·mor·al
an·ti·tus·sive
an·ti·ven·in
an·ti·vi·ral
an·ti·vi·ta·min
an·ti·vivi·sec·tion·ist
an·ti·xe·roph·thal·mic
an·tral
an·trorse
an·trorse·ly
an·tros·to·my
pl an·tros·to·mies
an·trot·o·my
pl an·trot·o·mies
an·trum
pl an·tra
an·ure·sis
pl an·ure·ses
an·uret·ic
an·uria
anus
pl anus·es
or ani
anx·i·ety
pl anx·i·eties
aor·ta
pl aor·tas
or aor·tae
aor·tal
aor·tic
aor·ti·tis
aor·tog·ra·phy
pl aor·tog·ra·phies
ap·a·thet·ic
ap·a·thy
pl ap·a·thies
ap·a·tite
a mineral (*see* appetite)
ape·ri·ent
ape·ri·od·ic
aper·i·tive
ap·er·tom·e·ter
ap·er·ture
apex
pl apex·es
or api·ces
apha·gia
apha·kia
also apha·cia
apha·kic
apha·sia
apha·si·ac
apha·sic
Aphas·mid·ia
aph·e·li·ot·ro·pism
aphe·mia
aphe·mic
apho·nia
aphon·ic
aphra·sia
aph·ro·di·sia
aph·ro·dis·i·ac
aph·tha
pl aph·thae
aph·thoid
aph·tho·sis
pl aph·tho·ses
aph·thous
ap·i·cal
api·ci·tis
pl api·ci·tes
api·co·ec·to·my
pl api·co·ec·to·mies
api·co·lo·ca·tor
api·col·y·sis
pl api·col·y·ses

api·gen·in
Api·um
apla·cen·tal
aplan·a·tism
apla·sia
aplas·tic
ap·nea
or ap·noea
ap·ne·ic
or ap·noe·ic
ap·neu·sis
pl ap·neu·ses
ap·neus·tic
apo·chro·mat·ic
apoc·o·pe
apo·crine
apoc·y·nin
Apoc·y·num
ap·o·dal
apo·dia
apo·en·zyme
apo·fer·ri·tin
apo·lar
apo·mict
apo·mic·tic
apo·mic·ti·cal·ly
apo·mix·is
pl apo·mix·es
apo·mor·phine
apo·neu·ro·sis
pl apo·neu·ro·ses
apo·neu·rot·ic
apoph·y·se·al
also apoph·y·si·al
or aphoph·y·sary
apoph·y·sis
pl apoph·y·ses
apoph·y·si·tis
ap·o·plec·tic
ap·o·plec·ti·form
ap·o·plexy
pl ap·o·plex·ies
apo·ria
pl apo·rias
or apo·ri·ae
apos·ta·sis
ap·o·stax·is
pl ap·o·stax·es
ap·os·teme
apoth·e·car·ies' mea·sure
apoth·e·car·ies' weight
apoth·e·cary
pl apoth·e·car·ies
ap·o·them
ap·o·zem
apoz·e·ma
apo·zy·mase
ap·pa·ra·tus
pl ap·pa·ra·tus·es
or ap·pa·ra·tus
ap·pear·ance
ap·pend·age
ap·pen·dec·to·my
pl ap·pen·dec·to·mies
ap·pen·di·ceal
or ap·pen·di·cal
or ap·pen·di·cial
ap·pen·di·cec·to·my
pl ap·pen·di·cec·to·mies
ap·pen·di·ci·tis
ap·pen·di·cos·to·my
pl ap·pen·di·cos·to·mies
ap·pen·dic·u·lar
ap·pen·dix
pl ap·pen·dix·es
or ap·pen·di·ces
ap·per·ceive
ap·per·ceived
ap·per·ceiv·ing
ap·per·cep·tion
ap·per·cep·tive
ap·per·son·a·tion
ap·pe·stat
ap·pe·tite
an instinctive desire (*see* apatite)
ap·pe·ti·tion
ap·pe·ti·tive
ap·pla·nate
ap·pla·na·tion
ap·pli·ance
ap·pli·ca·tor
ap·pli·qué
ap·po·si·tion
aprac·tic
aprax·ia
aprax·ic
apri·cot
apros·ex·ia
apty·a·lia
apty·a·lism
ap·y·rase
apy·ret·ic

apy•rex•ia
also apy•rexy
pl apy•rex•ias
also apy•rex•ies

apy•rex•i•al
aq•ua
aquat•ic
aq•ue•duct
aq•ue•duct of Syl•vi•us
aque•ous
aquos•i•ty
pl aquos•i•ties

ar•a•ban
ar•a•bic
arab•i•nose
ara•bi•no•side
arab•i•tol
ar•a•chid•ic
also arach•ic

ar•a•chi•don•ic
ar•a•chis
Arach•ni•da
arach•nid•ism
ar•ach•ni•tis
arach•no•dac•ty•ly
pl arach•no•dac•ty•lies

arach•noid
ar•ach•noi•dal
Arach•noi•dea
arach•noid•ism
arach•noid•i•tis
arach•no•ly•sin
ar•ach•no•pia
ara•lia
ar•al•kyl
ara•ro•ba
ar•bo•res•cent
ar•bo•ri•za•tion
ar•bo•rize
ar•bo•rized
ar•bo•riz•ing
ar•bor•vi•tae
ar•bo•vi•rus
ar•bu•tin
ar•bu•tus
ar•cade
ar•chaeo•cyte
also ar•cheo•cyte

ar•cha•ic
ar•che•go•ni•al
ar•che•go•ni•ate
ar•che•go•ni•um
pl ar•che•go•nia

arch•en•ter•on
pl arch•en•tera

ar•che•spore
or ar•che•spo•ri•um
pl ar•che•spores
or ar•che•spo•ria

ar•che•type
ar•che•us
also ar•chae•us
pl ar•chei
also ar•chaei

ar•chi•a•ter
ar•chil
also or•chil

ar•chi•pal•li•um
ar•chi•plasm
ar•chi•tec•ton•ics
ar•chi•tec•ture
arch of Cor•ti
ar•cho•plasm
ar•ci•form
arc•to•staph•y•los
ar•cu•al
ar•cu•ate
ar•cu•a•tion
ar•cus
ar•dor
ar•dor uri•nae
ar•ea opa•ca
ar•ea pel•lu•ci•da
ar•ea pla•cen•ta•lis
ar•ea vas•cu•lo•sa
are•ca
are•co•line
are•flex•ia
ar•e•na•ceous
are•o•la
pl are•o•lae
or are•o•las

are•o•lar
ar•e•om•e•ter
Ar•gas
Ar•gas•i•dae
ar•gen•taf•fin
or ar•gen•taf•fine

ar•gen•taf•fi•no•ma
ar•gen•tic
ar•gen•tine
ar•gen•to•phil
or ar•gen•to•phile
or ar•gen•to•phil•ic

ar•gen•tous
ar•gen•tum
ar•gi•nase
ar•gi•nine

ar·gon
Ar·gyll-Rob·ert·son pu·pil
ar·gyr·ia
ar·gyr·ic
ar·gyr·o·phil
or ar·gyr·o·phile
or ar·gyr·o·phil·ic
ar·gy·ro·sis
pl ar·gy·ro·ses
ari·bo·fla·vin·o·sis
pl ari·bo·fla·vin·o·ses
ar·ma·men·tar·i·um
pl ar·ma·men·tar·ia
or ar·ma·men·tar·iums
ar·mar·i·um
pl ar·mar·ia
or ar·mar·i·ums
arm·pit
ar·ni·ca
ar·o·mat·ic
aro·ma·tize
aro·ma·tized
aro·ma·tiz·ing
ar·o·yl
ar·rec·tor
pl ar·rec·to·res
or ar·rec·tors
ar·rest
ar·rhe·no·blas·to·ma
pl ar·rhe·no·blas·to·mas
also ar·rhe·no·blas·to·ma·ta
ar·rhyth·mia
also ar·ryth·mia
ar·rhyth·mic
or ar·rhyth·mi·cal
ar·row·root
ar·se·nate
ar·se·nic
ar·sen·i·cal
ar·sen·i·cal·ism
ar·se·nide
ar·se·ni·ous
ar·se·nite
ar·se·ni·um
ar·sen·iu·ret·ted
or ar·sen·iu·ret·ed
ar·se·no·ther·a·py
pl ar·se·no·ther·a·pies
ar·se·nous
ar·sen·ox·ide
ar·sine
ar·son·ic
ar·so·ni·um
ars·phen·a·mine
ar·te·fac, ar·te·fact
vars of artifact
ar·te·mis·ia
ar·te·re·nol
ar·te·ria
ar·te·ri·al
ar·te·ri·al·i·za·tion
ar·te·ri·al·ize
ar·te·ri·al·ized
ar·te·ri·al·iz·ing
ar·te·rio·cap·il·lary
ar·te·rio·gram
ar·te·ri·og·ra·phy
pl ar·te·ri·og·ra·phies
ar·te·ri·o·lar
ar·te·ri·ole
ar·te·ri·o·lo·scle·ro·sis
pl ar·te·ri·o·lo·scle·ro·ses
ar·te·rio·ma·la·cia
ar·te·rio·ne·cro·sis
pl ar·te·rio·ne·cro·ses
ar·te·rio·plas·ty
pl ar·te·rio·plas·ties
ar·te·ri·or·rha·phy
pl ar·te·ri·or·rha·phies
ar·te·rio·rrhex·is
pl ar·te·rio·rrhex·es
ar·te·rio·scle·ro·sis
pl ar·te·rio·scle·ro·ses
ar·te·rio·scle·rot·ic
ar·te·rio·spasm
ar·te·rio·ste·no·sis
pl ar·te·rio·ste·no·ses
ar·te·rio·tome
ar·te·ri·ot·o·my
pl ar·te·ri·ot·o·mies
ar·te·rio·ve·nous
ar·te·ri·tis
ar·tery
pl ar·ter·ies
ar·thral
ar·thral·gia

ar·threc·to·my
pl ar·threc·to·mies

ar·thrit·ic

ar·thri·tis
pl ar·thrit·i·des

ar·thri·tis de·for·mans

ar·thro·cele

ar·thro·cen·te·sis
pl ar·thro·cen·te·ses

ar·throd·e·sis
pl ar·throd·e·ses

ar·thro·dia

ar·thro·di·al

ar·throg·e·nous

ar·thro·gram

ar·throg·ra·phy
pl ar·throg·ra·phies

ar·thro·kat·a·dy·sis
pl ar·thro·kat·a·dy·ses

ar·thro·lith

ar·throl·o·gy
pl ar·throl·o·gies

ar·throl·y·sis
pl ar·throl·y·ses

ar·throp·a·thy
pl ar·throp·a·thies

ar·thro·plas·ty
pl ar·thro·plas·ties

ar·thro·pod

Ar·throp·o·da

ar·throp·o·dous

ar·thro·sis
pl ar·thro·ses

ar·thro·spore

ar·thro·spor·ic
or ar·thro·spo·rous

ar·thros·to·my
pl ar·thros·to·mies

ar·throt·o·my
pl ar·throt·o·mies

Ar·thus phe·nom·e·non

ar·ti·ad

ar·ti·cle

ar·tic·u·lar

ar·tic·u·late
ar·tic·u·lat·ed
ar·tic·u·lat·ing

ar·tic·u·la·tio
pl ar·tic·u·la·ti·on·es

ar·tic·u·la·tion

ar·tic·u·la·tor

ar·tic·u·la·to·ry

ar·tic·u·lus
pl ar·tic·u·li

ar·ti·fact
or ar·te·fact
also ar·te·fac

ar·ti·fac·ti·tious

ar·ti·fi·cial

Ar·ti·o·dac·ty·la

ary·epi·glot·tic

ar·yl

ar·y·te·no·epi·glot·tid·e·an

ar·y·te·noid

ar·y·te·noi·dec·to·my
pl ar·y·te·noi·dec·to·mies

asa·fet·i·da
or asa·foet·i·da
or as·sa·fet·i·da
or as·sa·foet·i·da

as·a·rum

as·bes·to·sis
pl as·bes·to·ses

as·ca·ri·a·sis
pl as·ca·ri·a·ses

as·car·i·cide

as·ca·rid

As·ca·rid·ia

as·car·i·di·a·sis
pl as·car·i·di·a·ses

as·ca·ris
pl as·car·i·des

As·ca·rops

as·cer·tain·ment

Asch·heim-Zon·dek test

Aschoff body
or Aschoff nod·ule

as·ci·tes
pl as·ci·tes

as·cit·ic

as·cle·pi·ad

as·cle·pi·as

as·co·carp

as·co·car·pous

as·co·go·ni·um
pl as·co·go·nia

as·co·my·cete

As·co·my·ce·tes

as·co·my·ce·tous

ascor·bate

ascor·bic

as·co·spore

as·co·spor·ic
or as·co·spor·ous

as·cus
pl as·ci

ase·mia
asep·sis
pl asep·ses

asep·tic
asex·u·al
asex·u·al·i·za·tion
aso·cial
as·pa·rag·i·nase
as·par·a·gine
as·pa·rag·i·nyl
as·par·a·gus
as·par·tase
as·par·tate
as·par·tic
as·par·to·ki·nase
as·par·to·yl
also as·par·tyl

as·pect
As·per·gil·la·les
as·per·gil·lin
as·per·gil·lo·sis
pl as·per·gil·lo·ses

as·per·gil·lus
pl as·per·gil·li

asper·ma·tism
asper·mia
as·per·sion
aspher·ic
as·phyx·ia
as·phyx·i·al
as·phyx·i·ant
as·phyx·i·ate
as·phyx·i·at·ed
as·phyx·i·at·ing
as·phyx·i·a·tion
as·pid·i·nol
as·pid·i·um
pl as·pid·ia

as·pi·do·sper·ma
as·pi·do·sper·mine
as·pi·rate
as·pi·rat·ed
as·pi·rat·ing
as·pi·ra·tion
as·pi·ra·tor
as·pi·rin
As·ple·ni·um
aspo·ro·gen·ic
aspo·rog·e·nous
aspo·rous
aspo·ru·late
as·sa·fet·i·da, as·sa·foet·i·da
vars of asafetida

as·say
as·sim·i·la·ble
as·sim·i·late
as·sim·i·lat·ed
as·sim·i·lat·ing
as·sim·i·la·tion
as·sim·i·la·tive
as·so·ci·a·tion
as·so·cia·tive
as·so·nance
asta·sia
asta·sia-aba·sia
astat·ic
as·ta·tine
as·ter
aster·e·og·no·sis
pl aster·e·og·no·ses

as·te·ri·on
pl as·te·ria

aster·nal
as·tero·coc·cus
pl as·tero·coc·ci

as·ter·oid
as·the·nia
as·then·ic
as·the·no·co·ria
as·the·no·pia
as·the·nop·ic
asth·ma
asth·mat·ic
asth·mo·gen·ic
as·tig·mat·ic
astig·mat·ism
astig·ma·tom·e·ter
astig·mia
astig·mom·e·ter
astig·mom·e·try
pl astig·mom·e·tries

astig·mo·scope
asto·ma·tous
asto·mia
asto·mous
as·trag·a·lar
as·trag·a·lec·to·my
pl as·trag·a·lec·to·mies

as·trag·a·lus
pl as·trag·a·li
or as·trag·a·lus·es

as·tral
as·tric·tion
as·tringe
  as·tringed
  as·tring·ing
as·trin·gent
as·tro·bi·o·log·i·cal
as·tro·bi·ol·o·gy
  pl as·tro·bi·ol·o·gies
as·tro·blast
as·tro·blas·to·ma
  pl as·tro·blas·to·mas
  or as·tro·blas·to·ma·ta
as·tro·cyte
as·tro·cy·to·ma
  pl as·tro·cy·to·mas
  or as·tro·cy·to·ma·ta
as·troid
as·tro·sphere
asyl·la·bia
asy·lum
asym·bo·lia
asym·met·ri·cal
asym·me·try
  pl asym·me·tries
asymp·to·mat·ic
asyn·ap·sis
  pl asyn·ap·ses
asyn·clit·ism
asyn·de·sis
  pl asyn·de·ses
asyn·er·gia
asyn·er·gic
asyn·er·gy
  pl asyn·er·gies
asys·tem·at·ic
asys·to·le
asys·tol·ic
atac·tic
at·a·rac·tic
  or at·a·rax·ic
at·a·rax·ia
at·a·vic
at·a·vism
at·a·vis·tic
atax·apha·sia
  or ataxi·apha·sia
atax·ia
  also ataxy
  pl atax·ias
  also atax·ies
atax·ia·gram
atax·ia·graph
atax·ic
at·el·ec·ta·sis
  pl at·el·ec·ta·ses
at·el·ec·tat·ic
at·el·i·o·sis
  pl at·el·i·o·ses
at·el·i·ot·ic
athe·lia
ather·man·cy
  pl ather·man·cies
ather·ma·nous
ather·mic
ath·ero·gen·e·sis
  pl ath·ero·gen·e·ses
ath·ero·gen·ic
ath·er·o·ma
  pl ath·er·o·mas
  also ath·er·o·ma·ta
ath·er·o·ma·to·sis
  pl ath·er·o·ma·to·ses
ath·er·o·ma·tous
ath·ero·scle·ro·sis
  pl ath·ero·scle·ro·ses
ath·e·te·sis
  pl ath·e·te·ses
ath·e·toid
ath·e·to·sic
ath·e·to·sis
  pl ath·e·to·ses
ath·e·tot·ic
ath·lete's foot
athrep·sia
athrep·tic
ath·ro·cyte
ath·ro·cy·to·sis
  pl ath·ro·cy·to·ses
athy·re·o·sis
  or athy·ro·sis
at·lan·tad
at·lan·to·ax·i·al
at·lan·to-oc·cip·i·tal
at·las
at·loid
at·mol·y·sis
  pl at·mol·y·ses
at·mom·e·ter
at·mo·sphere
ato·cia
at·om
atom·ic
at·o·mic·i·ty
  pl at·o·mic·i·ties
at·om·ism
at·om·is·tic
at·om·i·za·tion

at·om·ize
at·om·ized
at·om·iz·ing
at·om·iz·er
ato·nia
aton·ic
ato·nic·i·ty
pl ato·nic·i·ties
at·o·ny
pl at·o·nies
ato·pen
atop·ic
atop·og·no·sis
pl atop·og·no·ses
at·o·py
pl at·o·pies
atox·ic
ATPase
atre·mia
atre·sia
atre·sic
atret·ic
atri·al
atrich·ia
at·rich·o·sis
pl at·rich·o·ses
at·ri·chous
atrio·sep·to·pexy
pl atrio·sep·to·pex·ies
atrio·ven·tric·u·lar
atri·um
pl atria
At·ro·pa
atro·phia
at·ro·pho·der·ma

at·ro·phy
noun
pl at·ro·phies
at·ro·phy
verb
at·ro·phied
at·ro·phy·ing
at·ro·pine
at·ro·pin·iza·tion
at·ro·pin·ize
at·ro·pin·ized
at·ro·pin·iz·ing
at·ro·scine
at·tach·ment
at·tar
at·ten·u·ate
at·ten·u·at·ed
at·ten·u·at·ing
at·ten·u·a·tion
at·ti·co·an·trot·o·my
pl at·ti·co·an·trot·o·mies
at·ti·co·mas·toid
at·ti·cot·o·my
pl at·ti·cot·o·mies
at·ti·tude
at·ti·tu·di·nal
at·trac·tion
at·tri·tion
atyp·ia
a·typ·i·cal
atyp·ism
au·dile
au·dio·gen·ic
au·dio·gram
au·di·ol·o·gist

au·di·ol·o·gy
pl au·di·ol·o·gies
au·di·om·e·ter
au·di·om·e·trist
au·di·om·e·try
pl au·di·om·e·tries
au·dio·vis·u·al
au·di·tion
au·di·tive
au·di·to·ry
Auer·bach's plex·us
au·la
pl au·las
or au·lae
au·ra
pl au·ras
or au·rae
au·ral
of the ear or hearing (*see* oral)
au·ral·ly
au·ric
au·ri·cle
au·ric·u·la
pl au·ric·u·las
also au·ric·u·lae
au·ric·u·lar
au·ric·u·lare
pl au·ric·u·lar·ia
au·ric·u·la·ris
pl au·ric·u·la·res
au·ric·u·late
au·ric·u·lo·tem·po·ral
au·ric·u·lo·ven·tric·u·lar
au·ri·form

au·rin
au·ro·thio·glu·
cose
au·rum
aus·cul·tate
aus·cul·tat·ed
aus·cul·tat·ing
aus·cul·ta·tion
aus·cul·ta·to·ry
aus·ten·it·ic
au·ta·coid
au·te·cious
au·tism
au·tis·tic
au·to·ag·glu·ti·
na·tion
au·to·ag·glu·tin·
nin
au·to·an·ti·body
pl au·to·an·ti·bod·ies
au·to·ca·tal·y·sis
pl au·to·ca·tal·y·ses
au·to·cat·a·lyt·ic
au·toch·tho·nous
au·to·clav·able
au·to·clave
au·to·cy·tol·y·sis
pl au·to·cy·tol·y·ses
au·to·di·ges·tion
au·toe·cious
au·to·erot·ic
au·to·erot·i·cism
au·to·erot·ism
au·tog·a·mous
au·tog·a·my
pl au·tog·a·mies

au·to·gen·e·sis
pl au·to·gen·e·ses
au·to·ge·net·ic
au·to·gen·ic
au·tog·e·nous
au·tog·no·sis
pl au·tog·no·ses
au·to·graft
au·to·he·mol·y·sis
pl au·to·he·mol·y·ses
au·to·he·mo·ther·
a·py
pl au·to·he·mo·ther·
a·pies
au·to·im·mune
au·to·im·mu·ni·ty
pl au·to·im·mu·ni·
ties
au·to·im·mu·ni·
za·tion
au·to·im·mu·nize
au·to·im·mu·
nized
au·to·im·mu·
niz·ing
au·to·in·fec·tion
au·to·in·oc·u·la·
ble
au·to·in·oc·u·la·
tion
au·to·in·tox·i·ca·
tion
au·to·ki·ne·sis
pl au·to·ki·ne·ses
au·to·ki·net·ic
au·tol·o·gous
au·tol·y·sate

au·tol·y·sin
au·tol·y·sis
pl au·tol·y·ses
au·to·lyt·ic
au·to·lyze
au·to·lyzed
au·to·lyz·ing
au·to·ma·nip·u·
la·tion
au·to·ma·nip·u·
la·tive
au·tom·a·tism
au·to·mato·graph
au·to·mix·is
pl au·to·mix·es
au·tom·ne·sia
au·to·my·so·pho·
bia
au·to·nom·ic
au·ton·o·mous
au·ton·o·my
pl au·ton·o·mies
au·to-ox·i·da·tion
au·to·pha·gia
au·toph·a·gic
au·toph·a·gy
pl au·toph·a·gies
au·to·pho·bia
au·to·plas·tic
au·to·ploid
au·to·ploidy
pl au·to·ploi·dies
au·to·poly·ploid
au·to·poly·ploidy
pl au·to·poly·ploi·
dies

au·top·sy
pl au·top·sies

au·to·ra·dio·gram
au·to·ra·di·og·ra·phy
pl au·to·ra·di·og·ra·phies

au·to·reg·u·la·tion
au·to·reg·u·la·tive
au·to·reg·u·la·to·ry
au·to·scope
au·to·sen·si·ti·za·tion
au·to·se·rum
au·to·sex·ing
au·to·site
au·to·so·mal
au·to·so·mal·ly
au·to·some
au·to·sug·gest·ibil·i·ty
pl au·to·sug·gest·ibil·i·ties

au·to·sug·ges·tion
au·to·tel·ic
au·to·tet·ra·ploi·dy
pl au·to·tet·ra·ploi·dies

au·to·ther·a·py
pl au·to·ther·a·pies

au·tot·o·mize
au·tot·o·mized
au·tot·o·miz·ing
au·tot·o·my
pl au·tot·o·mies

au·to·tox·emia
au·to·tox·in
au·to·trans·plant
au·to·trans·plan·ta·tion
au·to·troph
au·to·tro·phic
au·tox·i·da·tion
aux·an·ogram
aux·ano·graph·ic
aux·a·nog·ra·phy
pl aux·a·nog·ra·phies

aux·e·sis
pl aux·e·ses

aux·et·ic
aux·in
auxo·chrome
auxo·cyte
auxo·drome
auxo·ton·ic
auxo·troph
auxo·tro·phic
aux·ot·ro·phy
pl aux·ot·ro·phies

aval·vu·lar
avas·cu·lar
Av·ena
ave·nin
or ave·nine

aver·sion
aver·sive
aver·sive·ly
avi·an
avi·an·ize
avi·an·ized
avi·an·iz·ing

av·i·din
avir·u·lent
avi·ta·min·osis
pl avi·ta·min·oses

Avo·ga·dro num·ber
or Avo·ga·dro con·stant

avoid·ance
avoid·ant
av·oir·du·pois
avulse
avulsed
avuls·ing
avul·sion
axen·ic
ax·i·al
ax·il
ax·ile
ax·il·la
pl ax·il·lae
or ax·il·las

ax·il·lar
ax·il·lary
pl ax·il·lar·ies

ax·is
pl ax·es

ax·ite
axo·den·drite
ax·om·e·ter
ax·on
ax·o·nal
ax·one
axo·neme
axo·nom·e·ter
axo·plasm
axo·style

Ayer•za'a dis•ease
aza•ser•ine
aza•thi•o•prine
az•e•la•ic
azeo•trope
azide
azo•ic
azo•lit•min
azo•pro•tein
azo•sper•mia
azo•sul•fa•mide
azote
azo•te•mia
az•oth
azo•to•bacter
az•o•tom•e•ter
azo•tu•ria
azure
azy•gos
azy•gous

B

bab•bitt met•al
Bab•cock test
ba•be•sia
bab•e•si•a•sis
pl ba•be•si•a•ses
Ba•be•si•i•dae
ba•be•si•o•sis
pl ba•be•si•o•ses
Ba•bin•ski re•flex
or Ba•bin•ski sign
also Ba•bin•ski's re•flex
or Ba•bin•ski's sign
bac•cate
Bac•il•la•ce•ae
ba•cil•lar
bac•il•lary
bac•il•le•mia
bac•il•li•form
bac•il•lo•sis
pl bac•il•lo•ses
bac•il•lu•ria
ba•cil•lus
pl ba•cil•li
bac•i•tra•cin
back•ache
back•bone
back•cross
bac•te•re•mia
or bac•te•ri•e•mia
also bac•te•ri•ae•mia
bac•te•ria
pl of bacterium
bac•te•ri•al
bac•te•ri•cid•al
also bac•te•rio•cid•al
bac•te•ri•cid•al•ly
bac•te•ri•cide
bac•te•ri•cid•in
or bac•te•ri•o•cid•in
bac•ter•id
bac•ter•in
bac•te•rio•chlo•ro•phyll
bac•te•rio•cin
bac•te•rio•gen•ic
bac•te•ri•og•e•nous
bac•te•ri•o•log•ic
or bac•te•rio•log•i•cal
bac•te•ri•ol•o•gist
bac•te•ri•ol•o•gy
pl bac•te•ri•ol•o•gies
bac•te•rio•ly•sin
bac•te•ri•ol•y•sis
pl bac•te•ri•ol•y•ses
bac•te•rio•lyt•ic
bac•te•rio•phage
bac•te•ri•o•sis
pl bac•te•ri•o•ses
bac•te•rio•sta•sis
pl bac•te•rio•sta•ses
bac•te•rio•stat
bac•te•rio•stat•ic
bac•te•rio•tox•in
bac•te•rio•trop•ic
bac•te•ri•ot•ro•pin
bac•te•ri•um
sing of bacteria
bac•te•ri•uria
bac•te•ri•za•tion
bac•te•rize
bac•te•rized
bac•te•riz•ing
bac•te•roid
also bac•te•ri•oid
bac•te•roi•dal
also bac•te•ri•oi•dal
bac•te•roi•des
bac•u•lum
pl bac•u•lums
or bac•u•la
bag•as•so•sis
pl bag•as•so•ses
Bain•bridge re•flex
bak•ers' yeast
ba•lan•ic

Bal·a·ni·tes
bal·a·ni·tis
bal·a·no·pos·thi·tis
bal·an·tid·i·al
or bal·an·tid·ic
bal·an·ti·di·a·sis
also bal·an·tid·i·o·sis
pl bal·an·ti·di·a·ses
also bal·an·tid·i·o·ses
bal·an·tid·i·um
pl bal·an·tid·ia
bald·ness
ball-and-sock·et
ball·ing iron
or ball·ing gun
bal·ling scale
bal·lism
bal·lis·mus
bal·lis·to·car·dio·gram
bal·lis·to·car·dio·graph
bal·lis·to·car·di·og·ra·phy
pl bal·lis·to·car·di·og·ra·phies
bal·lot·ta·ble
bal·lotte·ment
bal·ne·a·tion
bal·ne·ol·o·gy
pl bal·ne·ol·o·gies
bal·neo·ther·a·peu·tics
bal·neo·ther·a·py
pl bal·neo·ther·a·pies
bal·sam
bal·sam·ic
ba·nal
ban·dage
bandy-leg
ban·dy-legged
bane
bang
var of bhang
Bang's dis·ease
ban·ting
ban·ting·ism
Ban·ti's dis·ease
or Ban·ti's syn·drome
bar·ag·no·sis
pl bar·ag·no·ses
Bá·rá·ny chair
barb·al·o·in
bar·ber·ry
pl bar·ber·ries
bar·ber's itch
bar·bi·tal
bar·bi·tone
bar·bi·tu·rate
bar·bi·tu·ric
bar·bi·tu·rism
bar·bo·ne
bare·foot
bar·es·the·sia
bar·ia·tri·cian
bar·iat·rics
bar·ic
ba·ri·lla
bar·i·um
bar·og·no·sis
pl bar·og·no·ses
baro·graph
baro·graph·ic
baro·met·ro·graph
baro·phil·ic
baro·re·cep·tor
also baro·cep·tor
baro·scope
Ba·ros·ma
baro·stat
baro·tax·is
pl baro·tax·es
baro·ti·tis
baro·trau·ma
pl baro·trau·ma·ta
or baro·trau·mas
bar·ren
bar·tho·lin·itis
pl bar·tho·lin·ites
Bar·tho·lin's gland
Bar·ton·el·la
Bar·ton·el·la·ce·ae
bar·ton·el·lo·sis
pl bar·ton·el·lo·ses
bar·ye
bary·la·lia
ba·ry·ta
ba·sad
bas·al
ba·sa·lis
pl ba·sa·les
Ba·se·dow's dis·ease
base·ment
base·plate
ba·sic·i·ty
pl ba·sic·i·ties

ba·si·cra·ni·al
ba·sid·i·al
Ba·sid·io·my·ce·tes
ba·sid·io·my·ce·tous
ba·sid·io·spore
ba·sid·i·um
pl ba·sid·ia
ba·si·fa·cial
ba·si·hy·al
ba·si·hy·oid
bas·i·lar
ba·si·oc·cip·i·tal
ba·si·on
ba·sip·e·tal
ba·si·sphe·noid
ba·si·sphe·noi·dal
ba·si·tem·po·ral
ba·si·ver·te·bral
ba·so·cyte
ba·so·phil
ba·so·phile
ba·so·phil·ia
ba·so·phil·ic
ba·soph·i·lous
bas·so·rin
bath
bath·mo·trop·ic
ba·tracho·tox·in
bat·tle fa·tigue
bat·yl
Bau·mé scale
bay·ber·ry
pl bay·ber·ries
B cell
B com·plex
BCG vac·cine
bdel·li·um
bdel·lo·vi·brio
pl bdel·lo·vi·bri·os
beak·er
bear·ber·ry
pl bear·ber·ries
be·bee·rine
Bech·te·rew's nu·cle·us
Bec·que·rel ray
bed·bug
bed·lam
bed·pan
bed·side
bed·so·nia
pl bed·so·ni·ae
bed·sore
bed-wet·ting
Beer's law
bees·wax
be·hav·ior
be·hav·ior·al
be·hav·ior·ism
be·hav·ior·ist
be·hen·ic
bej·el
bel
belch
bel·em·noid
bel·la·don·na
Bel·li·ni's duct
also Bel·li·ni's tu·bule
bel·lows
bel·ly
pl bel·lies
bel·ly·ache
bel·ly but·ton
be·me·gride
Bence-Jones pro·tein
Ben·der Ge·stalt test
bends
Ben·e·dict's test
be·nign
ben·ne
also bene
ben·ton·ite
benz·al·de·hyde
ben·zal·ko·ni·um
benz·an·thra·cene
ben·zene
ben·zes·trol
ben·zi·dine
benz·imid·azole
ben·zine
also ben·zin
ben·zo·ate
ben·zo·caine
ben·zo·ic
ben·zo·in
ben·zol
ben·zo·py·rene
or benz·py·rene
ben·zo·qui·none
ben·zo·sul·fi·mide
ben·zo·yl
benz·pyr·in·i·um
ben·zyl
ben·zyl·ic

ben•zyl•i•dene
ben•zyl•pen•i•cil•lin
ber•ba•mine
ber•ber•ine
ber•ber•is
ber•dache
ber•ga•mot
ber•gap•ten
or ber•gap•tene

beri•beri
berke•li•um
Ber•lin blue
ber•serk
Ber•tin's col•umn
be•ryl•li•o•sis
also ber•yl•lo•sis
pl be•ryl•li•o•ses
also ber•yl•lo•ses

be•ryl•li•um
bes•ti•al•i•ty
pl bes•ti•al•i•ties

be•ta
be•ta-ad•ren•er•gic
be•ta•cism
be•ta glob•u•lin
be•ta•ine
be•ta-ox•i•da•tion
be•ta-re•cep•tor
be•ta•tron
be•tel
Bet•u•la
bet•u•lin
bet•u•lin•ol
be•tween•brain
Betz cell
be•zoar
bhang
also bang
bi•ar•tic•u•lar
bi•au•ric•u•lar
bib•lio•clast
bib•lio•klept
bib•lio•klep•to•ma•nia
bib•lio•ma•nia
bib•lio•ther•a•peu•tic
bib•lio•ther•a•pist
bib•lio•ther•a•py
pl bib•lio•ther•a•pies

bib•u•lous
bi•cam•er•al
bi•cap•su•lar
bi•car•bon•ate
bi•cau•dal
bi•cau•date
bi•cel•lu•lar
bi•ceps
bi•chlo•ride
bi•chro•mate
bi•cil•i•ate
bi•cip•i•tal
bi•con•cave
bi•con•vex
bi•cor•nate
bi•cor•nu•ate
bi•cor•nu•ous
bi•cus•pid
Bid•der's gan•gli•on
Bid•der's or•gan
bi•det
Bie•brich scar•let
Bier•mer's ane•mia
or Bier•mer's dis•ease

bi•fid
bi•fla•gel•late
bi•fo•cal
bi•fo•rate
bi•fur•cate
bi•fur•cat•ed
bi•fur•ca•tion
bi•gem•i•nal
bi•gem•i•ny
pl bi•gem•i•nies

big•head
big toe
bi•lat•er•al
bi•lat•er•al•ism
bi•lay•er
bile
bil•har•zia
bil•har•zi•a•sis
or bil•har•zi•o•sis
pl bil•har•zi•a•ses
or bil•har•zi•o•ses

bil•i•ary
bil•i•cy•a•nin
bil•i•fi•ca•tion
bil•i•fus•cin
bil•i•hu•min
bil•i•neu•rine
bil•ious
bil•i•ru•bin
bil•i•ru•bi•ne•mia
or bil•i•ru•bi•nae•mia

bil•i•ru•bi•nuria

bil·i·uria
bil·i·ver·din
bi·lo·bate
bi·lob·u·lar
bi·loc·u·lar
bi·loc·u·late
bi·loph·o·dont
bi·man·u·al
bi·mas·toid
bi·mod·al
bi·mo·lec·u·lar
bi·na·ry
pl bi·na·ries

bin·au·ral
Bi·net age
Bi·net-Si·mon test
bin·io·dide
bin·oc·u·lar
bi·no·mi·al
bin·ovu·lar
bin·ox·ide
bi·nu·cle·ar
bi·nu·cle·ate
bi·nu·cle·o·late
bio·acous·tics
bio·ac·tiv·i·ty
pl bio·ac·tiv·i·ties

bio·as·say
bio·as·tro·nau·ti·cal
bio·as·tro·nau·tics
bio·au·to·graph
bio·au·to·graph·ic
bio·au·tog·ra·phy
pl bio·au·tog·ra·phies

bio·cat·a·lyst
bio·ce·no·sis
or bio·coe·no·sis
pl bio·ce·no·ses
or bio·coe·no·ses

bio·chem·i·cal
bio·chem·is·try
pl bio·chem·is·tries

bio·che·mor·phol·ogy
pl bio·che·mor·phol·o·gies

bio·cid·al
bio·cide
bio·clean
bio·cli·ma·tol·o·gy
pl bio·cli·ma·tol·o·gies

bio·col·loid
bio·cy·tin
bio·de·grad·abil·i·ty
pl bio·de·grad·abil·i·ties

bio·de·grad·able
bio·deg·ra·da·tion
bio·de·grade
bio·de·grad·ed
bio·de·grad·ing
bio·dy·nam·ic
bio·dy·nam·ics
bio·ecol·o·gy
pl bio·ecol·o·gies

bio·elec·tric
or bio·elec·tri·cal
bio·elec·tric·i·ty
pl bio·elec·tric·i·ties

bio·elec·tro·gen·e·sis
pl bio·elec·tro·gen·e·ses

bio·elec·tron·ics
bio·en·er·get·ics
bio·en·gi·neer·ing
bio·en·vi·ron·men·tal
bio·feed·back
bio·fla·vo·noid
bio·gen·e·sis
pl bio·gen·e·ses

bio·ge·ne·tic
bio·gen·ic
bio·geo·chem·is·try
pl bio·geo·chem·is·tries
bio·haz·ard
bio·in·stru·men·ta·tion
bio·ki·net·ics
bi·o·log·ic
or bi·o·log·i·cal
bi·ol·o·gist
bi·ol·o·gy
pl bi·ol·o·gies
bio·lu·mi·nes·cence
bi·ol·y·sis
pl bi·ol·y·ses
bio·lyt·ic
bio·ma·te·ri·al
bio·math·e·mat·ics

bio•me•chan•ics
bio•med•i•cal
bio•med•i•cine
bi•om•e•ter
bio•me•tri•cian
bio•met•rics
bio•mi•cro•scope
bio•mi•cros•co•py
pl bio•mi•cros•co•pies
bi•on•ics
bi•o•nom•ics
bi•on•o•my
pl bi•on•o•mies
bio•or•gan•ic
bi•oph•a•gous
bi•oph•a•gy
pl bi•oph•a•gies
bi•o•phore
bio•pho•tom•e•ter
bio•phys•ics
bio•phys•i•og•ra•phy
pl bio•phys•i•og•ra•phies
bi•o•plasm
bi•o•plas•mic
bio•poly•mer
bi•op•sy
pl bi•op•sies
bio•psy•chol•o•gy
pl bio•psy•chol•o•gies
bi•or•bit•al
bio•re•search
bio•rhythm
bio•rhyth•mic
bio•rhyth•mic•i•ty
pl bio•rhyth•mic•i•ties

bi•os
pl bi•oi
or bi•os•es
bio•sat•el•lite
bio•sci•ence
bio•sci•en•tist
bio•sen•sor
bio•sphere
bio•sta•tis•tics
bio•syn•the•sis
pl bio•syn•the•ses
bio•tech•no•log•i•cal
bio•tech•nol•o•gy
pl bio•tech•nol•o•gies
bio•tel•e•met•ric
bio•te•lem•e•try
pl bio•te•lem•e•tries
bi•ot•ic
bi•o•tin
bio•trans•for•ma•tion
bio•tron
bio•type
bi•ovu•lar
bi•pa•ren•tal
bi•pa•ri•etal
bip•a•rous
bi•ped
bi•ped•al
bi•pen•ni•form
bi•phe•nyl
bi•po•lar
bi•po•ten•ti•al•i•ty
pl bi•po•ten•ti•al•i•ties
bi•ra•mous
also bi•ra•mose

bi•re•frac•tive
bi•re•frin•gent
bi•ro•ta•tion
birth con•trol
birth•mark
birth pang
bis•cuit
bi•sex•u•al
bis•fer•i•ous
bish•op
bis•hy•droxy•cou•ma•rin
bis•muth
bis•muth•yl
bis•tou•ry
pl bis•tou•ries
bi•stra•tal
bi•sul•fate
bi•sul•fide
bi•sul•fite
bi•tar•trate
bi•tem•po•ral
bite•wing
Bi•tot's spots
bi•tro•chan•ter•ic
bi•u•ret
bi•va•lence
bi•va•len•cy
pl bi•va•len•cies
bi•va•lent
bi•ven•ter
bi•ven•tral
bix•in
bi•zy•go•mat•ic
black-and-blue
black eye
black•head

black·leg
black lung
black·out
black vom·it
black·wa·ter
blad·der
blain
Bla·lock-Taus·sig op·er·a·tion
blast
blas·te·ma
pl blas·te·mas
or blas·te·ma·ta
blas·tem·ic
blas·tic
blas·tin
blas·to·coel
or blas·to·coele
blas·to·coe·lic
blas·to·cyst
blas·to·cyte
blas·to·derm
blas·to·der·mic
blas·to·disc
also blas·to·disk
blas·to·gen·e·sis
pl blas·to·gen·e·ses
blas·to·gen·ic
blas·to·ma
pl blas·to·mas
or blas·to·ma·ta
blas·to·mere
Blas·to·my·ces
blas·to·my·cete
Blas·to·my·ce·tes
blas·to·my·ce·tic
blas·to·my·co·sis
pl blas·to·my·co·ses

blas·to·neu·ro·pore
blas·toph·tho·ria
also blas·toph·tho·ry
pl blas·toph·tho·rias
or blas·toph·tho·ries
blas·toph·thor·ic
blas·to·por·al
or blas·to·por·ic
blas·to·pore
blas·to·sphere
blas·to·spher·ic
blas·to·spore
blas·tot·o·my
pl blas·tot·o·mies
blas·tu·la
pl blas·tu·las
or blas·tu·lae
blas·tu·lar
blas·tu·la·tion
Blat·ta
Blaud's pill
blear-eyed
bleary
blear·i·er
blear·i·est
bleb
bleed
bled
bleed·ing
bleed·er
blem·ish
blen·noid
blen·nor·rhea
also blen·nor·rhoea
blen·nor·rhe·al
also blen·nor·rhoe·al

bleph·a·ral
bleph·a·rism
bleph·a·ri·tis
pl bleph·a·rit·i·des
bleph·a·ro·con·junc·ti·vi·tis
bleph·a·ro·plast
bleph·a·ro·plas·tic
bleph·a·ro·spasm
bleph·a·ro·stat
blind gut
blind·ness
blind spot
blis·ter
block·ade
block·er
blood bank
blood cell
blood count
blood fluke
blood group
blood heat
blood·less
blood·let·ting
blood·line
blood·mo·bile
blood plate·let
blood poi·son·ing
blood pres·sure
blood·root
blood se·rum
blood·shot
blood·stream
blood·suck·er
blood sug·ar
blood test

blood-type
blood ves·sel
blood·worm
blotch
blow·fly
pl blow·flies

blow·pipe
blue baby
blue mold
blue·tongue
B lym·pho·cyte
Bo·dan·sky unit
bodi·ly
Bo·do
body louse
body wall
Boeck's sar·coid
or Boeck's dis·ease

Bohr the·o·ry
bol·dine
Bol·ling·er body
bo·lom·e·ter
bo·lus
bone·let
bone·set·ter
Bo·oph·i·lus
boost·er
bo·rac·ic
bo·rate
bo·rat·ed
bo·rax
bor·bo·ryg·mic
also bor·bo·ryg·mat·ic

bor·bo·ryg·mus
pl bor·bo·ryg·mi

bor·bo·ryg·my
pl bor·bo·ryg·mies

Bor·det-Gen·gou ba·cil·lus
Bor·det-Gen·gou test
bo·ric
bor·nane
bor·ne·ol
bo·ron
Bor·rel body
Bor·rel·ia
boss
bos·se·lat·ed
bot
bo·tan·i·cal
botch
bot·fly
pl bot·flies

Both·rio·ceph·a·lus
both·ri·um
pl both·ria
or both·ri·ums

bot·ry·oid
bot·ryo·my·co·sis
pl bot·ryo·my·co·ses

bot·ryo·my·cot·ic
bot·tle
bot·u·lin
bot·u·li·nal
bot·u·li·num
also bot·u·li·nus

bot·u·lism
bou·gie
bou·gi·nage
or bou·gie·nage

bouil·lon
Bou·in's flu·id
or Bou·in's so·lu·tion

bou·lim·ia
var of bulimia

bou·quet
bou·ton
bou·ton·niere
bou·ton ter·mi·nal
pl bou·tons ter·mi·naux

Bo·vic·o·la
bo·vine
bow·el
Bow·en's dis·ease
bow·leg
bow·legged
Bow·man's cap·sule
Bow·man's glands
Bow·man's mem·brane
Boyle's law
brace·let
bra·chi·al
bra·chi·al·gia
bra·chi·ate
bra·chi·at·ed
bra·chi·at·ing
bra·chi·a·tion
bra·chi·um
pl bra·chia

brachy·ce·phal·ic
brachy·ceph·a·lism

brachy·ceph·a·ly
pl brachy·ceph·a·lies
brachy·dac·ty·lous
brachy·dac·ty·ly
also brachy·dac·tyl·ia
pl brachy·dac·ty·lies
also brachy·dac·tyl·ias
brachy·dont
also brachy·o·dont
brachy·fa·cial
brachy·uran·ic
Brad·ford frame
brad·sot
brady·car·dia
slow heart action (*see* tachycardia)
brady·crot·ic
bra·dy·ki·nin
brad·yp·nea
braille
brain·case
brain·pan
brain·sick
brain stem
brain·wash
bran·chia
pl bran·chi·ae
bran·chi·al
bran·chi·og·e·nous
bran·chio·mere
bran·chi·om·er·ism
brash
braxy
pl brax·ies

bra·yera
braze
brazed
braz·ing
break
broke
bro·ken
break·ing
break·bone fe·ver
break·down
break·through
breast
breast·bone
breath
breathe
breathed
breath·ing
breech
breed
bred
breed·ing
breed·er
breg·ma
pl breg·ma·ta
breg·mat·ic
brei
pl breis
bridge·work
Bright's dis·ease
Brill's dis·ease
brim·stone
Bri·nell hard·ness
Bri·nell num·ber
bris·ket
bris·tle

Brit·ish an·ti-lew·is·ite
broad-spec·trum
Bro·ca's apha·sia
Bro·ca's ar·ea
Bro·ca scale
Bro·ca's con·vo·lu·tion
or Bro·ca's gy·rus
Bro·ca's point
Brod·mann ar·ea
or Brod·mann's ar·ea
broke
past of break
bro·ken
bro·mate
bro·me·lin
bro·mic
bro·mide
bro·mi·dro·sis
also brom·hi·dro·sis
pl bro·mi·dro·ses
also brom·hi·dro·ses
bro·mine
bro·min·ism
bro·mism
bro·mo
pl bro·mos
bro·mo·ac·e·tone
also brom·ac·e·tone
bro·mo·ben·zyl
bro·mo·cre·sol
also brom·cre·sol
bro·mo·form
bro·mo·phe·nol
or brom·phe·nol
bro·mo·ura·cil

bron•chi•al
bron•chi•al•ly
bron•chi•ec•ta•sia
bron•chi•ec•ta•sis
pl bron•chi•ec•ta•ses
bron•chio•gen•ic
bron•chi•ole
bron•chi•ol•itis
bron•chi•o•lus
pl bron•chi•o•li
bron•chit•ic
bron•chi•tis
pl bron•chit•i•des
bron•chi•um
pl bron•chia
bron•cho•cele
bron•cho•con•strict•tor
bron•cho•di•la•tor
bron•cho•ede•ma
pl bron•cho•ede•mas
also bron•cho•ede•ma•ta
bron•cho•gen•ic
bron•cho•gram
bron•cho•graph•ic
bron•chog•ra•phy
pl bron•chog•ra•phies
bron•cho•pneu•mo•nia
bron•cho•pul•mo•na•ry
bron•chor•rhea
bron•cho•scope
bron•chos•co•py
pl bron•chos•co•pies
bron•cho•spasm
bron•cho•spi•rom•e•try
pl bron•cho•spi•rom•e•tries
bron•cho•ste•no•sis
pl bron•cho•ste•no•ses
bron•chot•o•my
pl bron•chot•o•mies
bron•chus
pl bron•chi
bron•coph•o•ny
pl bron•coph•o•nies
bron•to•pho•bia
broth
pl broths
brown fat
bru•cel•la
pl bru•cel•lae
or bru•cel•las
Bru•cel•la•ce•ae
bru•cel•ler•gen
or bru•cel•ler•gin
bru•cel•lin
bru•cel•lo•sis
pl bru•cel•lo•ses
bruc•ine
bruise
bruised
bruis•ing
bruit
Brun•ner's gland
Brunn's mem•brane
brush bor•der
brush•ite
brux•ism
bruxo•ma•nia
bry•o•nia
bu•bo
pl bu•boes
bu•bon•al•gia
bu•bon•ic
bu•bon•o•cele
buc•ca
buc•cal
buc•ci•na•tor
buc•co•ax•i•al
buc•co•cer•vi•cal
buc•co•clu•sal
buc•co•dis•tal
buc•co•gin•gi•val
buc•cu•la
pl buc•cu•lae
Büch•ner fun•nel
bu•chu
buck•bean
buck•thorn
buck•tooth
pl buck•teeth
buck-toothed
Buer•ger's dis•ease
bu•fa•gin
buff•er
buffy coat
bu•fo•gen•in
Bu•fon•i•dae
bu•fo•tal•in
bu•fo•ten•ine
bu•fo•tox•in
bug•gery
pl bug•ger•ies

bul·bar
bul·bo·cap·nine
bul·bo·cav·er·no·sus
pl bul·bo·cav·er·no·si
bul·bo·ure·thral
bul·bous
bul·bus
pl bul·bi
bu·lim·ia
also bou·lim·ia
bul·la
pl bul·lae
bul·late
or bul·lat·ed
bull neck
bull·necked
bull·nose
bull·ock
bul·lous
also bul·lose
bun·ion
bu·no·dont
Bu·nos·to·mum
Bun·sen burn·er
buph·thal·mia
buph·thal·mos
bur
or burr
bur·dock
bu·rette
or bu·ret
Bur·kitt's lym·pho·ma
or Bur·kitt lym·pho·ma
Burr·kitt's tu·mor
or Bur·kitt tu·mor
bur·sa
pl bur·sas
or bur·sae
bur·sal
bur·sec·to·my
pl bur·sec·to·mies
bur·si·tis
bur·su·la
pl bur·su·lae
bu·sul·fan
bu·ta·caine
bu·tane
bu·ta·no·ic
bu·ta·nol
bu·to·py·ro·nox·yl
but·ter
but·ter·fat
but·ter·fly
pl but·ter·flies
but·ter·milk
but·ter·nut
but·tock
but·ton·hole
bu·tyl
bu·tyl·amine
bu·tyl·ate
bu·tyr·a·ceous
bu·tyr·ate
bu·tyr·ic
bu·tyr·om·e·ter
bu·tyr·ous
bu·tyr·yl
by·pass
bys·si·no·sis
pl bys·si·no·ses

C

caa·pi
Cab·ot's ring
or Cab·ot ring
ca·chec·tic
ca·chet
ca·chex·ia
also ca·chexy
pl ca·chex·ias
also ca·chex·ies
cach·in·nate
cach·in·nat·ed
cach·in·nat·ing
cach·in·na·tion
caco·de·mo·nia
or caco·de·mo·no·ma·nia
cac·o·dyl
cac·o·dyl·ate
cac·o·dyl·ic
cac·o·ë·thes
caco·gen·e·sis
pl caco·gen·e·ses
caco·gen·ic
caco·gen·ics
ca·cu·mi·nal
ca·dav·er
ca·dav·er·ic
ca·dav·er·ine
ca·dav·er·ous
ca·dav·er·ous·ly
cad·mi·um
ca·du·ceus
pl ca·du·cei
cae·cal
var of cecal

cae•cum
var of cecum

cae•no•gen•e•sis
var of cenogenesis

cae•no•ge•net•ic
var of cenogenetic

cae•sar•e•an,
cae•sar•ian
vars of cesarean

cae•si•um
var of cesium

caf•fe•ic
caf•feine
caf•fein•ic
caf•fe•ol
also caf•fe•one

ca•hin•ca
or ca•in•ca

cais•son dis•ease
caj•e•put
or caj•a•put
or caj•u•put

caj•e•put•ol
or caj•u•put•ol

cal•a•mine
cal•a•mus
pl cal•a•mi

cal•ca•ne•al
also cal•ca•ne•an

cal•ca•neo•cu•boid
cal•ca•ne•um
pl cal•ca•nea

cal•ca•ne•us
pl cal•ca•nei

cal•car
pl cal•car•ia

cal•car avis
pl cal•car•ia avi•um

cal•car•e•ous
also cal•car•i•ous

cal•car•e•ous•ly
cal•car•e•ous•ness
cal•ca•rine
cal•ces
pl of calx

cal•cic
cal•ci•co•sis
pl cal•ci•co•ses

cal•cif•er•ol
cal•cif•er•ous
cal•cif•ic
cal•ci•fi•ca•tion
cal•ci•fy
cal•ci•fied
cal•ci•fy•ing
cal•cim•e•ter
cal•ci•na•tion
cal•cine
cal•cined
cal•cin•ing
cal•ci•no•sis
pl cal•ci•no•ses

cal•ci•pe•nia
cal•ci•phy•lac•tic
cal•ci•phy•lac•ti•cal•ly
cal•ci•phy•lax•is
pl cal•ci•phy•lax•es

cal•cite
cal•ci•to•nin
cal•ci•um
cal•co•sphe•rite
or cal•co•sphae•rite

cal•cu•lo•sis
pl cal•cu•lo•ses

cal•cu•lous
cal•cu•lus
pl cal•cu•li
also cal•cu•lus•es

cal•e•fa•cient
ca•len•du•la
ca•len•du•lin
cal•en•ture
cal•i•ber
or cal•i•bre

cal•i•brate
cal•i•brat•ed
cal•i•brat•ing
cal•i•bra•tion
cal•i•bra•tor
or cal•i•brat•er

cal•i•ce•al
or cal•y•ce•al

cal•i•per
or cal•li•per

cal•i•saya bark
cal•is•then•ics
ca•lix
pl ca•li•ces

Cal•liph•o•ra
cal•liph•o•rid
Cal•li•phor•i•dae
cal•liph•o•rine
Cal•li•tro•ga
cal•lo•sal
cal•lose
cal•los•i•ty
pl cal•los•i•ties

cal•lo•sum
pl cal•lo•sa

cal·lous
cal·lus
or cal·lous
pl cal·lus·es
or cal·lous·es
also cal·li

calm·ative
cal·o·mel
cal·or
cal·o·res·cence
cal·o·res·cent
ca·lo·ric
cal·o·rie
also cal·o·ry
pl cal·o·ries

ca·lo·ri·fa·cient
cal·o·rif·ic
ca·lo·ri·gen·ic
cal·o·rim·e·ter
cal·o·ri·met·ric
or cal·o·ri·met·ri·cal

cal·o·ri·met·ri·cal·ly
cal·o·rim·e·try
pl cal·o·rim·e·tries

ca·lum·ba
or co·lom·bo

cal·var·ia
pl cal·var·ias

cal·var·i·al
cal·var·i·um
pl cal·var·ia

cal·vi·ti·es
pl cal·vi·ti·es

calx
pl calx·es
or cal·ces

cal·y·ce·al
var of caliceal

ca·ly·cine
also ca·lyc·i·nal

ca·ly·cle
ca·lyc·u·late
ca·lyc·u·lus
pl ca·lyc·u·li

Ca·lym·ma·to·bac·te·ri·um
ca·lyx
pl ca·lyx·es
or ca·ly·ces

cam·bo·gia
cam·era lu·ci·da
pl cam·era lu·ci·das

cam·era ob·scu·ra
pl cam·era ob·scu·ras

cam·i·sole
cam·o·mile
var of chamomile

cam·phane
cam·phene
cam·phor
cam·pho·ra·ceous
cam·phor·ate
cam·phor·at·ed
cam·phor·at·ing
cam·phor·ic
cam·pim·e·ter
camp·to·cor·mia
can·a·dine
can·a·lic·u·lar
can·a·lic·u·la·tion
also can·a·lic·u·li·za·tion

can·a·lic·u·lus
pl can·a·lic·u·li

can·a·line
ca·na·lis
pl ca·na·les

ca·na·li·za·tion
can·a·lize
can·a·lized
can·a·liz·ing
can·a·val·in
can·a·van·ine
can·cel·late
or can·cel·lat·ed

can·cel·lous
can·cel·lus
pl can·cel·li

can·cer
can·cer·ate
can·cer·iza·tion
can·cer·o·ci·dal
can·cer·o·gen·ic
or can·cer·i·gen·ic

can·cer·ol·o·gist
can·cer·ol·o·gy
pl can·cer·ol·o·gies

can·cer·o·lyt·ic
can·cer·ous
can·cer·ous·ly
can·cer·pho·bia
or can·cer·o·pho·bia

can·croid
can·crum oris
pl can·cra oris

can·de·la
can·di·ci·din
can·di·da

can·di·di·a·sis
pl can·di·di·a·ses

ca·nic·o·la fe·ver
Can·i·dae
ca·nine
ca·ni·ni·form
Ca·nis
ca·ni·ti·es
pl ca·ni·ti·es

can·ker
can·kered
can·ker·ing
can·ker·ous
can·na·bi·di·ol
ca·na·bin
can·na·bi·nol
can·na·bis
can·na·bism
can·non bone
can·nu·la
also can·u·la
pl can·nu·las
or can·nu·lae
also can·u·las
or can·u·lae

can·nu·late
can·nu·lat·ed
can·nu·lat·ing
can·nu·la·tion
can·thal
can·thar·i·dal
can·thar·i·date
can·thar·i·dat·ed
can·thar·i·dat·ing
can·tha·rid·i·an
or can·tha·rid·e·an
can·thar·i·din
can·thar·i·dism
can·thar·i·dize
can·thar·i·dized
can·thar·i·diz·ing
can·tha·ris
pl can·thar·i·des

can·thus
pl can·thi

caou·tchouc
ca·pac·i·tance
ca·pac·i·tate
ca·pac·i·tat·ed
ca·pac·i·tat·ing
ca·pac·i·ta·tion
ca·pac·i·tive
also ca·pac·i·ta·tive

ca·pac·i·tor
ca·pac·i·ty
pl ca·pac·i·ties

cap·e·line
cap·il·lar·ec·ta·sia
cap·il·lar·ia
ca·pil·la·ri·a·sis
also cap·il·lar·i·o·sis
pl ca·pil·la·ri·a·ses
also cap·il·lar·i·o·ses

cap·il·lar·id
cap·il·lar·i·ty
pl cap·il·lar·i·ties

cap·il·lar·o·scope
cap·il·la·ros·co·py
also cap·il·lar·i·os·co·py
pl cap·il·la·ros·co·pies
also cap·il·lar·i·os·co·pies

cap·il·lary
pl cap·il·lar·ies

ca·pil·li·cul·ture
ca·pil·lus
pl ca·pil·li

ca·pi·ta
pl of caput

cap·i·tate
cap·i·tel·lum
pl cap·i·tel·la

ca·pit·u·lar
ca·pit·u·lum
pl ca·pit·u·la

ca·pon·iza·tion
ca·pon·ize
ca·pon·ized
ca·pon·iz·ing
cap·rate
cap·ric
cap·rin
cap·ro·ate
ca·pro·ic
cap·ro·in
cap·ro·yl
cap·ry·late
ca·pryl·ic
cap·sa·icin
cap·si·cum
cap·sid
cap·sid·al
cap·so·mere

cap•su•la
pl cap•su•lae

cap•su•lar

cap•su•late
or cap•su•lat•ed

cap•su•la•tion

cap•sule
cap•suled
cap•sul•ing

ca•put
pl ca•pi•ta

ca•put mor•tu•um
pl ca•pi•ta mor•tua

ca•put suc•ce•da•ne•um
pl ca•pi•ta suc•ce•da•nea

car•a•geen
var of carrageen

car•at

ca•ra•te

car•ba•chol

car•ba•mate

car•bam•ic

carb•amide

carb•ami•no

car•ba•myl
or car•bam•o•yl

car•bar•sone

car•ba•ryl

car•ba•zide

car•ba•zole

carb•azot•ic

car•ben•i•cil•lin

carb•he•mo•glo•bin
or car•bo•he•mo•glo•bin

car•bide

car•bi•nol

car•bo

car•bo•ben•zoxy
or car•bo•ben•zy•loxy

car•bo•cy•clic

car•bo•hy•drase

car•bo•hy•drate

car•bo•hy•drat•uria

car•bo•late
car•bo•lat•ed
car•bo•lat•ing

car•bol•fuch•sin

car•bol•ic

car•bo•line

car•bo•lize
car•bo•lized
car•bo•liz•ing

car•bol•xy•lene

car•bo•my•cin

car•bon•ate
car•bon•at•ed
car•bon•at•ing

car•bon•ic

car•bon•iza•tion

car•bon•ize
car•bon•ized
car•bon•iz•ing

car•bon•yl

car•boxy•he•mo•glo•bin

car•box•yl

car•box•yl•ase

car•box•yl•ate
car•box•yl•at•ed
car•box•yl•at•ing

car•box•yl•ation

car•box•yl•ic

car•boxy•meth•yl

car•boxy•pep•ti•dase

car•bro•mal

car•bun•cle
inflammation with pus
(*see* caruncle, furuncle)

car•bun•cu•lar

car•bun•cu•lo•sis
pl car•bun•cu•lo•ses

car•bu•ret
car•bu•ret•ed
also car•bu•ret•ted
car•bu•ret•ing
also car•bu•ret•ting

car•ce•ag

car•cin•o•gen

car•ci•no•gen•e•sis
pl car•ci•no•gen•e•ses

car•ci•no•gen•ic

car•ci•noid

car•ci•no•lyt•ic

car•ci•no•ma
pl car•ci•no•mas
or car•ci•no•ma•ta

car•ci•no•ma•toid

car•ci•no•ma•to•sis
pl car•ci•no•ma•to•ses

car•ci•no•ma•tous

car·ci·no·sar·co·ma
pl car·ci·no·sar·co·mas
or car·ci·no·sar·co·ma·ta

car·ci·no·sis
pl car·ci·no·ses

car·da·mom
also car·da·mum
or car·da·mon

car·dia
pl car·di·ae
or car·di·as

car·di·ac

car·di·al·gia

car·di·ec·to·my
pl car·di·ec·to·mies

car·dio·ac·cel·er·a·tion

car·dio·dy·nam·ic

car·dio·dy·nam·ics

car·dio·gram

car·dio·graph

car·di·og·ra·pher

car·dio·graph·ic

car·di·og·ra·phy
pl car·di·og·ra·phies

car·dio·he·pat·ic

car·di·oid

car·dio·in·hib·i·to·ry

car·dio·ki·net·ic

car·dio·lip·in

car·di·ol·o·gist

car·di·ol·o·gy
pl car·di·ol·o·gies

car·di·ol·y·sis
pl car·di·ol·y·ses

car·dio·meg·a·ly
pl car·dio·meg·a·lies

car·di·om·e·ter

car·dio·met·ric

car·di·om·e·try
pl car·di·om·e·tries

car·dio·my·op·a·thy
pl car·dio·my·op·a·thies

car·dio·path

car·di·op·a·thy
pl car·di·op·a·thies

car·dio·peri·car·dio·pexy
pl car·dio·peri·car·dio·pex·ies

car·dio·peri·car·di·tis

car·dio·pho·bia

car·dio·plas·ty
pl car·dio·plas·ties

car·dio·ple·gia

car·dio·pneu·mat·ic

car·dio·pul·mo·nary

car·dio·re·nal

car·dio·re·spi·ra·to·ry

car·di·or·rha·phy
pl car·di·or·rha·phies

car·dio·scope

car·dio·spasm

car·dio·spas·tic

car·dio·ta·chom·e·ter

car·dio·ther·a·py
pl car·dio·ther·a·pies

car·di·ot·o·my
pl car·di·ot·o·mies

car·dio·ton·ic

car·dio·tox·ic

car·dio·vas·cu·lar

car·di·tis

Car·i·ca

car·ies
pl car·ies

ca·ri·na
pl ca·ri·nas
or ca·ri·nae

car·i·nate
also car·i·nat·ed

car·io·gen·ic

car·i·ous

ca·ri·so·pro·dol

carm·al·um

car·mi·na·tive

car·mine

car·min·ic

car·nas·si·al

car·ni·fi·ca·tion

car·ni·tive

Car·niv·o·ra

car·ni·vore

car·niv·o·rous

car·no·sine

car·ob

car·o·tene
also car·o·tin

car·o·ten·emia
or car·o·ten·aemia
also car·o·tin·emia

ca·rot·enoid
also ca·rot·i·noid

ca·rot·ic
ca·rot·i·co·tym·pan·ic
ca·rot·id
car·oto·dyn·ia
car·pa·ine
car·pal
car·pa·le
car·pec·to·my
pl car·pec·to·mies

car·phol·o·gy
also car·pho·lo·gia
pl car·phol·o·gies
also car·pho·lo·gi·as

car·pi·tis
car·po·meta·car·pal
car·po·ped·al
car·pus
pl car·pi
wrist (*see* corpus)

car·ra·geen
or car·ra·gheen
also car·a·geen

car·ra·geen·an
or car·ra·geen·in
also car·ra·gheen·in

car·ri·er
Car·ri·on's dis·ease
car·ron oil
car·sick
car·sick·ness
Car·te·sian
Car·tha·mus
car·ti·lage
car·ti·lag·i·noid
car·ti·lag·i·nous
also car·ti·la·gin·e·ous

Ca·rum
car·un·cle
small fleshy eminence
(*see* carbuncle, furuncle)

ca·run·cu·la
pl ca·run·cu·lae

car·va·crol
carv·er
cas·cara
cas·cara amar·ga
cas·cara sa·gra·da
cas·ca·ril·la
ca·se·ate
ca·se·at·ed
ca·se·at·ing
ca·se·a·tion
case·book
ca·sein
ca·sein·ate
ca·sein·o·gen
ca·se·ous
casque
cas·sette
cas·sia
Cas·ta·nea
Cas·tel·la·ni's paint
Cas·tile soap
cast·ing
cas·tor
cas·trate
cas·trat·ed
cas·trat·ing
cas·tra·tion
ca·su·al·ty
pl ca·su·al·ties

ca·su·is·tics
cata·bi·o·sis
pl cata·bi·o·ses

cata·bi·ot·ic
cat·a·bol·ic
ca·tab·o·lism
also ka·tab·o·lism

ca·tab·o·lite
ca·tab·o·lize
ca·tab·o·lized
ca·tab·o·liz·ing
cata·chro·ma·sis
var of katachromasis

cata·di·op·tric
also cata·di·op·tri·cal

cata·gen·e·sis
pl cata·gen·e·ses

cata·ge·net·ic
cat·a·lase
cat·a·lat·ic
cat·a·lep·sy
pl cat·a·lep·sies

cat·a·lep·tic
cat·a·lep·ti·cal·ly
cat·a·lep·toid
cat·a·lo·gia
ca·tal·y·sis
pl ca·tal·y·ses

cat·a·lyst
cat·a·lyt·ic
cat·a·lyt·i·cal·ly

cat·a·lyze
cat·a·lyzed
cat·a·lyz·ing
cat·a·lyz·er
cat·a·me·nia
cat·a·me·ni·al
cat·a·mite
cat·am·ne·sis
pl cat·am·ne·ses
cat·am·nes·tic
cata·pha·sia
cat·a·pho·re·sis
pl cat·a·pho·re·ses
cat·a·pho·ret·ic
cat·a·pho·ret·i·cally
cat·a·phor·ic
cat·a·pla·sia
cat·a·plasm
cat·a·plas·tic
cat·a·plec·tic
cat·a·plexy
pl cat·a·plex·ies
cat·a·ract
cat·a·rac·tal
cat·a·ract·ous
ca·tar·ia
ca·tarrh
ca·tarrh·al
ca·tarrh·al·ly
Cat·ar·rhi·na
cat·ar·rhine
also cat·a·rhine
cat·ar·rhin·i·an
ca·tas·ta·sis
pl ca·tas·ta·ses
cata·state
cata·stat·ic
cata·ther·mom·e·ter
var of katathermometer
cata·to·nia
also cata·to·ny
pl cata·to·nias
also cata·to·nies
cata·ton·ic
cat·e·chin
cat·e·chol
cat·e·chol·amine
cat·e·chu
cat·elec·tro·ton·ic
cat·elec·trot·o·nus
cat·e·nate
cat·e·nat·ed
cat·e·nat·ing
cat·e·noid
ca·ten·u·late
cat·gut
Catha
ca·thar·sis
also ka·thar·sis
pl ca·thar·ses
also ka·thar·ses
ca·thar·tic
also ka·thar·tic
ca·thect
ca·thec·tic
ca·thep·sin
cath·e·ter
cath·e·ter·iza·tion
cath·e·ter·ize
cath·e·ter·ized
cath·e·ter·iz·ing
ca·thex·is
pl ca·thex·es
cath·ode
cath·od·ic
cath·od·i·cal·ly
ca·thol·i·con
cat·ion
cat·ion·ic
cat·ion·i·cal·ly
cat·nip
also cat·nep
ca·top·tric
also ca·top·tri·cal
ca·top·tri·cal·ly
cat·ta·lo
pl cat·ta·loes
or cat·ta·los
cat·tery
pl cat·ter·ies
cau·da
pl cau·dae
cau·dad
cau·da equi·na
pl cau·dae equi·nae
cau·da he·li·cis
pl cau·dae he·li·cis
cau·dal
cau·dal·ly
cau·date
also cau·dat·ed
cau·da·tion
cau·da·to·len·tic·u·lar
caul
cau·li·flou·er
cau·sal·gia
cau·sal·gic

caus·tic
cau·ter
cau·ter·ant
cau·ter·i·za·tion
cau·ter·ize
cau·ter·ized
cau·ter·iz·ing
cau·tery
pl cau·ter·ies

ca·va
pl ca·vae

ca·va
var of kava

ca·val
cav·al·ry bone
cava·scope
cav·ern
cav·er·no·ma
pl cav·er·no·mas
or cav·er·no·ma·ta

cav·er·nos·to·my
pl cav·er·nos·to·mies

cav·ern·ous
Ca·via
Ca·vi·i·dae
cav·i·tary
cav·i·tate
cav·i·tat·ed
cav·i·tat·ing
cav·i·ta·tion
cav·i·ty
pl cav·i·ties

ca·vum
pl ca·va

ca·vy
pl ca·vies

ceb·a·dil·la
var of sabadilla

ce·cal
or cae·cal

ce·cec·to·my
pl ce·cec·to·mies

ce·ci·tis
ce·co·pexy
pl ce·co·pex·ies

ce·co·pli·ca·tion
ce·cop·to·sis
pl ce·cop·to·ses

ce·cor·rha·phy
pl ce·cor·rha·phies

ce·co·sig·moid·os·to·my
pl ce·co·sig·moid·os·to·mies

ce·cos·to·my
pl ce·cos·to·mies

ce·cot·o·my
pl ce·cot·o·mies

ce·cum
or cae·cum
pl ce·ca
or cae·ca

ce·dar·wood
ce·la·tion
cel·en·ter·on
var of coelenteron

cel·ery
pl cel·er·ies

ce·li·ac
or coe·li·ac

ce·lio·col·pot·o·my
pl ce·lio·col·pot·o·mies

ce·lio·en·ter·ot·o·my
pl ce·lio·en·ter·ot·o·mies

ce·li·os·co·py
pl ce·li·os·co·pies

ce·li·ot·o·my
pl ce·li·ot·o·mies

cel·la
pl cel·lae

cel·lif·u·gal
or cel·lu·lif·u·gal

cel·lip·e·tal
or cel·lu·lip·e·tal

cel·lo·bi·ose
cell of Clau·di·us
cell of Cor·ti
cel·loi·din
cel·lose
cel·lu·la
pl cel·lu·lae

cel·lu·lar
cel·lu·lar·i·ty
pl cel·lu·lar·i·ties

cel·lu·lase
cel·lule
cel·lu·lin
cel·lu·li·tis
cel·lu·lo·lyt·ic
cel·lu·los·an
cel·lu·lose
cel·lu·los·ic
ce·lom
var of coelom

ce·lom·ic
var of coelomic

Cel·si·us

ce·ment
ce·men·ta·tion
ce·ment·i·cle
ce·ment·i·fi·ca·tion
ce·ment·ite
ce·ment·o·blast
ce·men·to·ma
pl ce·men·to·mas
or ce·men·to·ma·ta
ce·men·tum
pl ce·men·ta
ce·nes·the·sia
also coe·nes·the·sia
ce·no·gen·e·sis
or coe·no·gen·e·sis
also cae·no·gen·e·sis
pl ce·no·gen·e·ses
or coe·no·gen·e·ses
or cae·no·gen·e·ses
ce·no·ge·net·ic
or coe·no·ge·net·ic
also cae·no·ge·net·ic
cen·o·site
cen·sor
cen·sor·ship
cen·ter
cen·te·sis
pl cen·te·ses
cen·ti·bar
cen·ti·grade
cen·ti·gram
cen·ti·li·ter
cen·ti·me·ter
cen·ti·nor·mal
cen·ti·pede
cen·ti·poise
cen·ti·stoke
cen·trad
cen·tral
cen·tric
cen·trif·u·gal
cen·trif·u·gal·i·za·tion
cen·trif·u·gal·ize
cen·trif·u·gal·ized
cen·trif·u·gal·iz·ing
cen·trif·u·ga·tion
cen·tri·fuge
cen·tri·fuged
cen·tri·fug·ing
cen·tri·ole
cen·trip·e·tal
cen·tro·lec·i·thal
cen·tro·mere
cen·tro·mer·ic
cen·tro·plasm
cen·tro·some
cen·tro·so·mic
cen·tro·sphere
cen·trum
pl cen·trums
or cen·tra
Cen·tru·roi·des
ce·pha·eline
Cepha·elis
ceph·a·lad
ceph·a·lal·gia
ceph·al·he·ma·to·ma
pl ceph·al·he·ma·to·mas
or ceph·al·he·ma·to·ma·ta
ceph·al·hy·dro·cele
ce·phal·ic
ceph·a·lin
also keph·a·lin
ceph·a·li·za·tion
ceph·a·lo·cau·dal
ceph·a·lo·cele
ceph·a·lo·cen·te·sis
pl ceph·a·lo·cen·te·ses
ceph·a·lo·gy·ric
ceph·a·lo·he·ma·to·cele
ceph·a·lo·me·nia
ceph·a·lom·e·ter
ceph·a·lo·met·ric
ceph·a·lom·e·try
pl ceph·a·lom·e·tries
ceph·a·lop·a·thy
pl ceph·a·lop·a·thies
ceph·a·lo·pel·vic
ceph·a·lo·pha·ryn·ge·us
ceph·a·lor·i·dine
ceph·a·lo·spo·rin
Ceph·a·lo·spo·ri·um
ceph·a·lo·thin
ceph·a·lo·tho·rac·ic
ceph·a·lot·o·my
pl ceph·a·lot·o·mies
ceph·a·lo·tribe
ceph·a·lo·trip·sy
pl ceph·a·lo·trip·sies

ce•ra
ce•ra•ceous
Cer•a•sus
ce•rate
cer•a•tin
var of keratin

cer•a•ti•tis
var of keratitis

cer•a•to•con•junc•
ti•vi•tis
var of keratocon-
junctivitis

Cer•a•to•phyl•lus
cer•a•tose
var of keratose

cer•car•ia
pl cer•car•iae

cer•clage
Cer•com•o•nas
Cer•co•pi•the•cus
cer•cus
pl cer•ci

cere
cered
cer•ing
ce•rea flex•i•bil•i•
tas
ce•re•al
cer•e•bel•lar
cer•e•bel•lo•ru•
bral
cer•e•bel•lo•ru•
bro•spi•nal
cer•e•bel•lo•spi•
nal
cer•e•bel•lum
pl cer•e•bel•lums
or cer•e•bel•la

ce•re•bral
ce•re•bral-pal•
sied
cer•e•brate
cer•e•brat•ed
cer•e•brat•ing
cer•e•bra•tion
ce•re•bri•form
cer•e•brif•u•gal
cer•e•brip•e•tal
cer•e•broid
ce•re•bro•med•ul•
lary
cer•e•bron•ic
ce•re•bro•scle•ro•
sis
pl ce•re•bro•scle•ro•
ses

cer•e•brose
ce•re•bro•side
ce•re•bro•spi•nal
ce•re•bro•to•nia
ce•re•bro•vas•cu•
lar
ce•re•brum
pl ce•re•brums
or ce•re•bra

cere•cloth
cere•ment
Ce•ren•kov ra•di•
a•tion
or Che•ren•kov ra•di•
a•tion

cer•e•sin
also cer•e•sine

Ce•re•us
ce•ria
ce•ri•um
ce•roid
ce•ro•tic
cer•ti•fi•a•ble
cer•ti•fi•ca•tion
cer•ti•fy
cer•ti•fied
cer•ti•fy•ing
ce•ru•lo•plas•min
ce•ru•men
ce•ru•mi•no•sis
pl ce•ru•mi•no•ses

ce•ru•mi•nous
also ce•ru•mi•nal

ce•ruse
cer•vi•cal
cer•vi•cec•to•my
pl cer•vi•cec•to•mies

cer•vi•ci•tis
cer•vi•co•buc•cal
cer•vi•co•dyn•ia
cer•vi•co•fa•cial
cer•vi•co•la•bi•al
cer•vi•co•lin•gual
cer•vi•co•ves•i•cal
cer•vix
pl cer•vi•ces
or cer•vix•es

cer•vix ute•ri
ce•ryl
ce•sar•e•an
also ce•sar•i•an
or cae•sar•e•an
or cae•sar•i•an

ce•si•um
also cae•si•um

Ces•to•da
ces•to•dan
ces•tode
ces•to•di•a•sis
pl ces•to•di•a•ses

ces•toid
Ces•toi•dea
ces•toi•de•an
ce•ta•ce•um
Ce•trar•ia
ce•tyl
ce•tyl•pyr•i•din•i•um
cev•a•dil•la
cev•a•dine
ce•vi•tam•ic acid
ceys•sa•tite
Cha•ber•tia
chae•ta
pl chae•tae

chae•tal
Cha•gas' dis•ease
cha•go•ma
pl cha•go•mas
or cha•go•ma•ta

cha•la•za
pl cha•la•zae
or cha•la•zas

cha•la•zi•on
pl cha•la•zia

chal•cone
also chal•kone

chal•co•sis
chal•i•co•sis
pl chal•i•co•ses

chalk•stone
chal•lenge
chal•lenged
chal•leng•ing
chal•one
cha•lyb•e•ate
Cham•ber•land fil•ter
cham•o•mile
or cam•o•mile

chan•cre
chan•cri•form
chan•croid
chan•croi•dal
chan•crous
chan•nel
chan•neled
or chan•nelled
chan•nel•ing
or chan•nel•ling

char•ac•ter•iza•tion
char•ac•ter•olog•i•cal
also char•ac•ter•o•log•ic

char•ac•ter•olog•i•cal•ly
char•ac•ter•ol•o•gist
char•ac•ter•ol•o•gy
pl char•ac•ter•ol•o•gies

cha•ras
char•bon
char•coal

Char•cot joint
char•la•tan
char•la•tan•ism
Charles's law
char•ley horse
char•ta
pl char•tae

chart•ing
char•tu•la
pl char•tu•lae

Chas•tek pa•ral•y•sis
chaul•moo•gra
also chaul•mu•gra
or chaul•mau•gra

check•bite
check•er•ber•ry
pl check•er•ber•ries

check•up
cheek
cheek•bone
chei•lec•to•my
pl chei•lec•to•mies

cheil•ec•tro•pi•on
also chil•ec•tro•pi•on

chei•li•tis
or chi•li•tis

chei•lo•plas•ty
pl chei•lo•plas•ties

chei•los•chi•sis
pl chei•los•chi•ses

chei•lo•sis
pl chei•lo•ses

chei•rog•no•my
or chi•rog•no•my
pl chei•rog•no•mies
or chi•rog•no•mies

chei·rol·o·gy
or chi·rol·o·gy
pl chei·rol·o·gies
or chi·rol·o·gies

chei·ro·meg·a·ly
or chi·ro·meg·a·ly
pl chei·ro·meg·a·lies
or chi·ro·meg·a·lies

chei·ro·plas·ty
or chi·ro·plas·ty
pl chei·ro·plas·ties
or chi·ro·plas·ty

chei·ro·pom·pho·lyx
chei·ro·spasm
or chi·ro·spasm

che·late
che·la·tion
che·la·tor
che·lic·era
pl che·lic·er·ae

Chel·i·do·ni·um
che·li·ped
che·loid
var of keloid

Che·lo·nia
che·lo·ni·an
chem·i·cal
chem·i·cal·ly
che·mi·lu·mi·nes·cence
che·mise
chem·ist
chem·is·try
pl chem·is·tries

che·mo·au·to·troph
che·mo·au·to·tro·phic
che·mo·au·to·tro·phi·cal·ly
chemo·au·tot·ro·phy
pl chemo·au·tot·ro·phies

che·mo·dec·to·ma
pl che·mo·dec·to·mas
or che·mo·dec·to·ma·ta

che·mo·dif·fer·en·ti·a·tion
che·mo·ki·ne·sis
pl che·mo·ki·ne·ses

che·mo·ki·net·ic
che·mo·pro·phy·lac·tic
che·mo·pro·phy·lax·is
pl che·mo·pro·phy·lax·es

che·mo·re·cep·tion
che·mo·re·cep·tive
che·mo·re·cep·tiv·i·ty
pl che·mo·re·cep·tiv·i·ties

che·mo·re·cep·tor
che·mo·re·flex
che·mo·re·sis·tance
che·mo·sen·si·tive
che·mo·sen·si·tiv·i·ty
pl che·mo·sen·si·tiv·i·ties

che·mo·sen·so·ry
che·mo·sis
pl che·mo·ses

chem·os·mo·sis
pl chem·os·mo·ses

chem·os·mot·ic
che·mo·ster·il·ant
che·mo·ster·il·iza·tion
che·mo·ster·il·ize
che·mo·ster·il·ized
che·mo·ster·il·iz·ing
che·mo·sur·gi·cal
che·mo·sur·gery
pl che·mo·sur·ger·ies

che·mo·syn·the·sis
pl che·mo·syn·the·ses

che·mo·syn·thet·ic
che·mo·tac·tic
che·mo·tac·ti·cal·ly
che·mo·tax·is
also che·mo·taxy
pl che·mo·tax·es
also che·mo·tax·ies

che·mo·ther·a·peu·tic
or che·mo·ther·a·peu·ti·cal

che·mo·ther·a·peu·ti·cal·ly
che·mo·ther·a·peu·tics
che·mo·ther·a·pist
che·mo·ther·a·py
pl che·mo·ther·a·pies
che·mot·ic
che·mo·trop·ic
che·mot·ro·pism
che·no·de·oxy·cho·lic
Che·no·po·di·um
Che·ren·kov ra·di·a·tion
var of Cerenkov radiation
chev·on
Cheyne-Stokes res·pi·ra·tion
or Cheyne-Stokes breath·ing
chi·asm
chi·as·ma
pl chi·as·ma·ta
or chi·as·mas
chi·as·mat·ic
chick·en pox
chig·ger
chig·oe
chil·blain
child·bear·ing
child·bed
child·birth
child·hood
chil·ec·tro·pi·on
var of cheilectropion
chi·li·tis
var of cheilitis
Chi·lo·mas·tix
Chi·lop·o·da
chi·lop·o·dan
chi·lop·o·dous
chi·me·ra
or chi·mae·ra
chi·me·rism
chim·pan·zee
chi·myl
chin·a·crin, chin·a·crine
vars of quinacrine
chin·bone
chinch
chin·cho·na, chin·co·na
vars of cinchona
chine
chi·ni·o·fon
chin·o·line
var of quinoline
chi·on·ablep·sia
chip·blow·er
chi·rog·no·my
var of cheirognomy
chi·rol·o·gy
var of cheirology
chi·ro·meg·a·ly
var of cheiromegaly
chi·ro·plas·ty
var of cheiroplasty
chi·ro·po·di·al
chi·rop·o·dist
chi·rop·o·dy
pl chi·rop·o·dies
chi·ro·prac·tic
chi·ro·prac·tor
chi·ro·prax·is
pl chi·ro·prax·es
chi·ro·spasm
var of cheirospasm
Chla·myd·ia
Chla·myd·i·a·ce·ae
chlam·ydo·mo·nas
chla·myd·o·spore
chla·myd·o·spor·ic
chlo·as·ma
pl chlo·as·ma·ta
chlor·ac·ne
chlo·ral
chlo·ra·lose
chlo·ram·bu·cil
chlo·ram·ine
chlor·am·phen·i·col
chlor·ane·mia
or chlor·anae·mia
chlor·ane·mic
chlor·bu·tol
chlor·cy·cli·zine
chlor·dane
or chlor·dan
chlor·di·az·epox·ide
chlor·e·mia
or chlor·ae·mia
chlor·hy·dria
chlo·rine
chlor·mer·o·drin

chlo·ro·az·o·din
chlo·ro·bu·ta·nol
also chlor·bu·ta·nol
chlo·ro·gua·nide
or chlor·gua·nide
chlo·ro·leu·ke·mia
or chlo·ro·leu·kae·mia
chlo·ro·ma
pl chlo·ro·mas
or chlo·ro·ma·ta
chlo·rom·a·tous
chlo·ro·meth·ane
chlo·ro·phane
chlo·ro·phe·nol
also chlor·phe·nol
chlo·ro·phen·o·thane
chlo·ro·pia
chlo·ro·pic·rin
also chlor·pic·rin
Chlo·rop·i·dae
chlo·ro·pro·caine
chlo·rop·sia
chlo·ro·quine
chlo·ro·sis
pl chlo·ro·ses
chlo·ro·then
chlo·rot·ic
chlo·rot·i·cal·ly
chlo·ro·thy·mol
chlo·rous
chlor·prom·a·zine
chlor·prop·amide
chlor·tet·ra·cy·cline
cho·a·na
pl cho·a·nae
cho·a·nate
Cho·a·no·tae·nia
cho·lae·mia
var of cholemia
cho·la·gog·ic
cho·la·gogue
chol·an·gi·ec·ta·sis
pl chol·an·gi·ec·ta·ses
chol·an·gio·gas·tros·to·my
pl chol·an·gio·gas·tros·to·mies
chol·an·gio·gram
chol·an·gio·graph·ic
chol·an·gi·og·ra·phy
pl chol·an·gi·og·ra·phies
chol·an·gi·ole
chol·an·gio·lit·ic
chol·an·gio·li·tis
pl chol·an·gio·lit·i·des
chol·an·gi·o·ma
pl chol·an·gi·o·mas
also chol·an·gi·o·ma·ta
chol·an·gi·os·to·my
pl chol·an·gi·os·to·mies
chol·an·gi·ot·o·my
pl chol·an·gi·ot·o·mies
chol·an·gi·tis
pl chol·an·git·i·des
chol·an·threne
cho·le·cal·cif·er·ol
cho·le·cyst
also cho·le·cys·tis
cho·le·cyst·a·gogue
cho·le·cys·tec·ta·sia
cho·le·cys·tec·to·my
pl cho·le·cys·tec·to·mies
cho·le·cys·tic
cho·le·cys·ti·tis
pl cho·le·cys·tit·i·des
cho·le·cys·to·du·o·de·nos·to·my
pl cho·le·cys·to·du·o·de·nos·to·mies
cho·le·cys·to·gas·tros·to·my
pl cho·le·cys·to·gas·tros·to·mies
cho·le·cys·to·gram
cho·le·cys·to·graph·ic
cho·le·cys·tog·ra·phy
pl cho·le·cys·tog·ra·phies
cho·le·cys·to·ki·nin
cho·le·cys·to·pexy
pl cho·le·cys·to·pex·ies

cho·le·cys·tos·to·my
pl cho·le·cys·tos·to·mies

cho·le·cys·tot·o·my
pl cho·le·cys·tot·o·mies

cho·le·doch
or cho·le·doch·al

cho·led·o·chi·tis

cho·led·o·cho·li·thi·a·sis
pl cho·led·o·cho·li·thi·a·ses

cho·led·o·cho·li·thot·o·my
pl cho·led·o·cho·li·thot·o·mies

cho·led·o·chos·to·my
pl cho·led·o·chos·to·mies

cho·led·o·chus
pl cho·led·o·chi

cho·le·glo·bin

cho·le·ic

cho·le·lith

cho·le·li·thi·a·sis
pl cho·le·li·thi·a·ses

cho·lem·e·sis

cho·le·mia
or cho·lae·mia

cho·lem·ic

cho·le·poi·e·sis
pl cho·le·poi·e·ses

cho·le·poi·et·ic

chol·era

chol·er·a·ic

chol·era in·fan·tum

chol·era mor·bus

cho·le·re·sis
pl cho·le·re·ses

cho·le·ret·ic

cho·ler·ic

cho·ler·i·form

chol·er·oid

chol·er·rha·gia

cho·les·te·a·to·ma
pl cho·les·te·a·to·mas
or cho·les·te·a·to·ma·ta

cho·les·ter·ic

cho·les·ter·ol

cho·les·ter·ol·emia
also cho·les·ter·ol·ae·mia
or cho·les·ter·emia
or cho·les·ter·ae·mia

cho·les·ter·o·sis
pl cho·les·ter·o·ses

cho·line

cho·lin·er·gic

cho·lin·es·ter·ase

cho·li·no·lyt·ic

cho·li·no·mi·met·ic

chol·uria

chon·dral

chon·drec·to·my
pl chon·drec·to·mies

chon·dri·fi·ca·tion

chon·dri·fy
chon·dri·fied
chon·dri·fy·ing

chon·drin

chon·dri·tis

chon·dro·blast

chon·dro·blas·tic

chon·dro·clast

chon·dro·cos·tal

chon·dro·cra·ni·um
pl chon·dro·cra·ni·ums
or chon·dro·cra·nia

chon·dro·cyte

chon·dro·dys·pla·sia

chon·dro·dys·tro·phic

chon·dro·dys·tro·phy
or chon·dro·dys·tro·phia
pl chon·dro·dys·tro·phies
or chon·dro·dys·tro·phi·as

chon·dro·gen·e·sis
pl chon·dro·gen·e·ses

chon·dro·ge·net·ic

chon·dro·gen·ic
or chon·drog·e·nous

chon·dro·glos·sus
pl chon·dro·glos·si

chon·droid

chon·droi·tin

chon·drol·o·gy
pl chron·drol·o·gies

chon·dro·ma
pl chon·dro·mas
also chon·dro·ma·ta

chon·dro·ma·la·cia
chon·drom·a·tous
chon·dro·mu·coid
chon·dro·os·teo·dys·tro·phy
pl chon·dro·os·teo·dys·tro·phies

chon·drop·a·thy
pl chon·drop·a·thies

chon·dro·pha·ryn·ge·us
pl chon·dro·pha·ryn·gei

chon·dro·phyte
chon·dro·plast
chon·dro·plas·ty
pl chon·dro·plas·ties

chon·dro·sar·co·ma
pl chon·dro·sar·co·mas
also chon·dro·sar·co·ma·ta

chon·dro·sis
pl chon·dro·ses

chon·dro·skel·e·ton
chon·dro·ster·nal
chon·dro·tome
chon·drot·o·my
pl chon·drot·o·mies

chon·dro·xi·phoid
chon·drus
pl chon·dri

Cho·part's joint

chor·da
pl chor·dae

chord·al
chor·da·me·so·derm
or chor·do·me·so·derm

chor·da·me·so·der·mal
or chor·do·me·so·der·mal

chor·da ten·di·nea
pl chor·dae ten·di·ne·ae

chor·dee
chor·di·tis
chor·do·ma
pl chor·do·mas
or chor·do·ma·ta

chor·dot·o·my
pl chor·dot·o·mies

cho·rea
cho·re·al
cho·re·at·ic
cho·re·ic
cho·re·i·form
cho·reo·ath·e·toid
or cho·reo·ath·e·tot·ic

cho·reo·ath·e·to·sis
pl cho·reo·ath·e·to·ses

cho·re·oid
cho·rio·al·lan·to·ic
also cho·rio·al·lan·to·id

cho·rio·al·lan·to·is
pl cho·rio·al·lan·to·i·des

cho·rio·car·ci·no·ma
pl cho·rio·car·ci·no·mas
or cho·rio·car·ci·no·ma·ta

cho·rio·cele
cho·rio·ep·i·the·li·o·ma
pl cho·rio·ep·i·the·li·o·mas
or cho·rio·ep·i·the·li·o·ma·ta

cho·rio·ep·i·the·li·o·ma·tous
cho·ri·oid
var of choroid

cho·ri·o·ma
pl cho·ri·o·mas
also cho·ri·o·ma·ta

cho·rio·men·in·gi·tis
pl cho·rio·men·in·git·i·des

cho·ri·on
cho·ri·on·ep·i·the·li·o·ma
pl cho·ri·on·ep·i·the·li·o·mas
or cho·ri·on·ep·i·the·li·o·ma·ta

cho·ri·on·ic
Cho·ri·op·tes
cho·ri·op·tic

cho·rio·ret·i·ni·tis
also cho·roido·ret·i·ni·tis
pl cho·rio·ret·i·nit·i·des
also cho·roido·ret·i·nit·i·des

cho·roid
also cho·ri·oid

cho·roi·dal
cho·roi·di·tis
or cho·ri·oi·di·tis

cho·roi·do·cy·cli·tis
cho·roi·do·iri·tis
Christ·mas dis·ease
chro·maf·fin
also chro·maf·fine

chro·maf·fi·no·ma
pl chro·maf·fi·no·mas
or chro·maf·fi·no·ma·ta

chro·ma·phil
chro·mat·ic
chro·mat·i·cal·ly
chro·ma·tism
chro·ma·tog·e·nous
chro·mato·gram
chro·mato·graph
chro·mato·graph·ic
chro·mato·graph·i·cal·ly
chro·ma·tog·ra·phy
pl chro·ma·tog·ra·phies

chro·ma·tol·y·sis
pl chro·ma·tol·y·ses

chro·mato·lyt·ic
chro·ma·tom·e·ter
chro·ma·top·a·thy
pl chro·ma·top·a·thies

chro·mat·o·phil
or chro·mat·o·phile

chro·mato·phil·ia
also chro·moph·i·ly
pl chro·mato·phil·ias
also chro·moph·i·lies

chro·mato·phore
chro·mato·phor·ic
or chro·ma·toph·o·rous

chro·ma·top·sia
chrom·es·the·sia
chro·mi·dro·sis
or chrom·hi·dro·sis
pl chro·mi·dro·ses
or chrom·hi·dro·ses

chro·mi·um
chro·mo·bac·te·ri·um
pl chro·mo·bac·te·ria

chro·mo·blast
chro·mo·blas·to·my·co·sis
pl chro·mo·blas·to·my·co·ses

chro·mo·cyte
chro·mo·gen
chro·mo·gen·e·sis
pl chro·mo·gen·e·ses

chro·mo·gen·ic
chro·mo·phil
or chro·mo·phile

chro·mo·phil·ic
chro·moph·i·ly
var of chromatophilia

chro·mo·phobe
chro·mo·pho·bic
chro·mo·pro·tein
chro·mo·scope
chro·mo·scop·ic
chro·mos·co·py
pl chro·mos·co·pies

chro·mo·som·al
chro·mo·som·al·ly
chro·mo·some
chro·mo·so·mic
chro·mo·ther·a·py
pl chro·mo·ther·a·pies

chro·mo·trich·i·al
chro·nax·ie
or chro·naxy
also chro·nax·ia
pl chro·nax·ies
also chro·nax·ias

chro·nax·im·e·ter
chro·nax·i·met·ric
chro·nax·im·e·try
pl chro·nax·im·e·tries

chron·ic

chro·nic·i·ty
pl chro·nic·i·ties
chro·no·trop·ic
chro·not·ro·pism
chrys·a·ro·bin
Chrys·o·mya
Chrys·o·my·ia
Chrys·ops
chryso·ther·a·py
pl chryso·ther·a·pies
chyl·an·gi·o·ma
pl chyl·an·gi·o·mas
or chyl·an·gi·o·ma·ta
chyle
chy·le·mia
chy·li·fac·tion
chy·li·fac·tive
chy·lif·er·ous
chy·li·fi·ca·tion
chy·li·form
chy·lo·cele
chy·lo·cyst
chy·lo·mi·cron
chy·lo·poi·e·sis
pl chy·lo·poi·e·ses
chy·lo·poi·et·ic
or chy·lo·po·et·ic
chy·lor·rhea
chy·lo·sis
pl chy·lo·ses
chy·lo·tho·rax
pl chy·lo·tho·rax·es
or chy·lo·tho·ra·ces
chy·lous
chy·lu·ria
chyme
chy·mi·fi·ca·tion
chy·mo·tryp·sin
chy·mo·tryp·sin·o·gen
chy·mous
cic·a·tri·cial
cic·a·trix
pl cic·a·tri·ces
also cic·a·trix·es
cic·a·tri·zant
cic·a·tri·za·tion
cic·a·trize
cic·a·trized
cic·a·triz·ing
cic·u·tox·in
cil·i·ary
Cil·i·a·ta
cil·i·ate
or cil·i·at·ed
Cil·i·oph·o·ra
cil·i·oph·o·ran
cil·io·scle·ral
cil·i·um
pl cil·ia
cil·lo·sis
ci·mex
pl cim·i·ces
cin·cho·na
also chin·cho·na
or chin·co·na
cin·chon·i·dine
cin·cho·nine
cin·cho·nism
cin·cho·nize
cin·cho·nized
cin·cho·niz·ing
cin·cho·phen
cine·an·gio·car·dio·graph·ic
cine·an·gio·car·di·og·ra·phy
pl cine·an·gio·car·di·og·ra·phies
cine·an·gio·graph·ic
cine·an·gi·og·ra·phy
pl cine·an·gi·og·ra·phies
cine·flu·o·ro·graph·ic
cine·flu·o·rog·ra·phy
pl cine·flu·o·rog·ra·phies
ci·ne·mat·ics
var of kinematics
cin·e·mat·o·graph
also kin·e·mat·o·graph
cin·e·mat·o·graph·ic
cin·e·mat·o·graph·i·cal·ly
cin·e·ma·tog·ra·phy
pl cin·e·ma·tog·ra·phies
cin·e·ole
also cin·e·ol
cin·e·plas·tic
cin·e·plas·ty
also kin·e·plas·ty
pl cin·e·plas·ties
also kin·e·plas·ties
cine·ra·di·og·ra·phy
pl cine·ra·di·og·ra·phies

ci•ne•rea
ci•ne•re•al
cin•er•in
cine•roent•gen•og•ra•phy
pl cine•roent•gen•og•ra•phies
ci•ne•sis
var of kinesis
ci•neto•plast
var of kinetoplast
cin•gu•lec•to•my
pl cin•gu•lec•to•mies
cin•gu•lum
pl cin•gu•la
ci•on
var of scion
cir•ca•di•an
circ•an•nu•al
cir•ci•nate
cir•cle of Wil•lis
cir•cu•late
cir•cu•lat•ed
cir•cu•lat•ing
cir•cu•la•tion
cir•cu•la•to•ry
cir•cu•lus
pl cir•cu•li
cir•cum•anal
cir•cum•ar•tic•u•lar
cir•cum•cise
cir•cum•cised
cir•cum•cis•ing
cir•cum•ci•sion
cir•cum•cor•ne•al
cir•cum•duc•tion
cir•cum•flex
cir•cum•in•su•lar
cir•cum•len•tal
cir•cum•oral
cir•cum•val•late
cir•cum•vas•cu•lar
cir•rho•sis
pl cir•rho•ses
cir•rhot•ic
cir•rus
pl cir•ri
cir•sec•to•my
pl cir•sec•to•mies
cir•soid
cis•tern
cis•ter•na
pl cis•ter•nae
cis•ter•na chy•li
pl cis•ter•nae chy•li
cis•ter•nal
cis•ter•na mag•na
pl cis•ter•nae mag•nae
ci•tri•nin
cit•ro•nel•la
ci•trul•line
Clad•o•spo•ri•um
clair•voy•ance
also clair•voy•an•cy
pl clair•voy•anc•es
also clair•voy•an•cies
clar•i•fi•a•ble
cla•rif•i•cant
clar•i•fi•ca•tion
clar•i•fi•er
clar•i•fy
clar•i•fied
clar•i•fy•ing
Clarke's col•umn
or Clarke's nu•cle•us
clas•mato•cyte
clas•mato•cyt•ic
clas•ma•to•sis
pl clas•ma•to•ses
clas•si•fi•ca•tion
clas•si•fy
clas•si•fied
clas•si•fy•ing
clas•tic
clath•rate
clath•ra•tion
clau•di•ca•tion
claus•tro•phobe
claus•tro•pho•bia
claus•tro•pho•bic
or claus•tro•pho•bi•ac
claus•trum
pl claus•tra
cla•va
pl cla•vae
clav•a•cin
cla•val
cla•vate
also cla•vat•ed
cla•vate•ly
cla•va•tion
clav•i•cle
cla•vic•u•la
pl cla•vic•u•lae
cla•vic•u•lar

cla•vus
pl cla•vi

Clay•ton gas
clei•do•cos•tal
clei•do•cra•ni•al
cle•oid
clep•to•ma•nia
var of kleptomania

clep•to•ma•ni•ac
var of kleptomaniac

cli•mac•te•ri•al
cli•mac•ter•ic
cli•mac•te•ri•um
pl cli•mac•te•ria

cli•ma•to•ther•a•py
pl cli•ma•to•ther•a•pies

clin•ic
clin•i•cal
clin•i•cal•ly
cli•ni•cian
clin•i•co•patho•log•ic
also clin•i•co•patho•log•i•cal

cli•noid
cli•nom•e•ter
cli•no•met•ric
also cli•no•met•ri•cal

cli•nom•e•try
pl cli•nom•e•tries

clit•i•on
pl clit•ia

cli•to•ral
or cli•tor•ic

cli•to•rid•e•an
cli•to•ri•dec•to•my
pl cli•to•ri•dec•to•mies

cli•to•ri•di•tis
cli•to•ris
cli•to•ri•tis
cli•vus
pl cli•vi

clo•a•ca
pl clo•a•cae

clo•a•cal
clo•a•ci•tis
clo•fi•brate
clo•mi•phene
clon•ic
clo•nic•i•ty
pl clo•nic•i•ties

clo•nism
clo•nor•chi•a•sis
also clo•nor•chi•o•sis
pl clo•nor•chi•a•ses
also clo•nor•chi•o•ses

Clo•nor•chis
clo•nus
clos•trid•i•al
or clos•trid•i•an

clos•trid•i•um
pl clos•trid•ia

clot
clot•ted
clot•ting
clox•a•cil•lin
club•foot
pl club•feet

club•foot•ed
club•hand
clu•ne•al
clu•pe•ine
also clu•pe•in

clut•ter•ing
cly•sis
pl cly•ses

clys•ma
pl clys•ma•ta

clys•ter
cne•mi•al
cne•mis
pl cnem•i•des

cni•do•blast
co•ac•er•vate
co•ac•er•vat•ed
co•ac•er•vat•ing
co•ac•er•va•tion
co•ag•u•la•bil•i•ty
pl co•ag•u•la•bil•i•ties

co•ag•u•la•ble
co•ag•u•lant
co•ag•u•lase
co•ag•u•late
co•ag•u•lat•ed
co•ag•u•lat•ing
co•ag•u•la•tion
co•ag•u•la•tive
co•ag•u•lin
co•ag•u•lom•e•ter
co•ag•u•lum
pl co•ag•u•la

co•apt
co•ap•ta•tion
co•arct
co•arc•tate
co•arc•ta•tion
coat

co·bal·a·min
also co·bal·a·mine

co·ca
co·caine
co·cain·ism
co·cain·i·za·tion
co·cain·ize
co·cain·ized
co·cain·iz·ing
co·car·box·yl·ase
coc·cal
coc·ci
pl of coccus

Coc·cid·ia
coc·cid·i·al
coc·cid·i·an
coc·cid·i·oi·dal
Coc·cid·i·oi·des
coc·cid·i·oi·din
coc·cid·i·oi·do·my·co·sis
also coc·cid·io·my·co·sis
pl coc·cid·i·oi·do·my·co·ses
also coc·cid·io·my·co·ses

coc·cid·io·sis
pl coc·cid·io·ses

coc·cid·io·stat
coc·cid·i·um
pl coc·cid·ia

coc·co·ba·cil·la·ry
coc·co·ba·cil·lus
pl coc·co·ba·cil·li

coc·co·gen·ic
or coc·ci·gen·ic

coc·coid
or coc·coi·dal

coc·cus
pl coc·ci

coc·cy·al·gia
coc·cy·dyn·ia
coc·cy·geal
coc·cy·gec·to·my
pl coc·cy·gec·to·mies

coc·cyg·e·us
pl coc·cyg·ei

coc·cy·go·dyn·ia
coc·cyx
pl coc·cy·ges
also coc·cyx·es

co·chi·neal
co·chlea
pl co·chle·as
or co·chle·ae

co·chle·ar
co·chle·are
co·chle·ar·i·form
co·chleo·ves·tib·u·lar
Co·chlio·my·ia
co·chro·mato·graph
co·chro·ma·tog·ra·phy
pl co·chro·ma·tog·ra·phies

co·con·scious
co·con·scious·ness
co·de·hy·drog·enase
co·deine
co·dex
pl co·di·ces

cod-liv·er oil

Coel·en·ter·a·ta
coel·en·ter·ate
coel·en·ter·on
or cel·en·ter·on
pl coel·en·tera
or cel·en·tera

coe·li·ac
var of celiac

coe·lom
also coe·lome
or ce·lom
pl coe·loms
or coe·lo·ma·ta
also coe·lomes
or ce·loms

coe·lom·ic
or ce·lom·ic

coe·nes·the·sia
var of cenesthesia

coe·no·gen·e·sis
var of cenogenesis

coe·no·ge·net·ic
var of cenogenetic

coe·nu·ri·a·sis
pl coe·nu·ri·a·ses

coe·nu·ro·sis
pl coe·nu·ro·ses

coe·nu·rus
pl coe·nu·ri

co·en·zy·mat·ic
co·en·zy·mat·i·cal·ly
co·en·zyme
co·fac·tor
cog·ni·tion
cog·ni·tive
Cohn·heim's ar·ea
co·ho·ba

co·ital
co·ition
co·ito·pho·bia
co·itus
co·itus in·ter·rup·tus
also co·itus re·ser·va·tus
pl co·itus in·ter·rup·ti
also co·itus re·ser·va·ti

co·la nut
var of kola nut

co·la·mine
col·chi·cine
col·chi·cum
col·ec·to·my
pl col·ec·to·mies

co·li
co·li·bac·il·le·mia
co·li·bac·il·luria
co·lic
adjective
relating to the colon

col·ic
noun
paroxysmal abdominal pain

co·li·cin
also co·li·cine

col·i·ci·no·ge·nic
col·i·ci·no·ge·nic·i·ty
pl col·i·ci·no·ge·nic·i·ties

col·i·ci·nog·e·ny
pl col·i·ci·nog·e·nies

col·icky
co·li·form
co·li·phage
co·lis·tin
co·li·tis
col·la·gen
col·la·ge·nase
col·la·gen·ic
col·la·gen·o·lyt·ic
col·la·ge·no·sis
pl col·la·ge·no·ses

col·lag·e·nous
col·lapse
col·lapsed
col·laps·ing
col·lar·bone
col·lat·er·al
Col·les's frac·ture
col·li·mate
col·li·mat·ed
col·li·mat·ing
col·li·ma·tion
col·li·ma·tor
col·li·qua·tion
col·liq·ua·tive
col·lo·di·on
also col·lo·di·um

col·loid
col·loi·dal
col·loi·dal·ly
col·lum
pl col·la

col·lu·nar·i·um
pl col·lu·nar·ia

col·lu·to·ri·um
pl col·lu·to·ria

col·lyr·i·um
pl col·lyr·ia
or col·lyr·i·ums

col·o·bo·ma
pl col·o·bo·ma·ta

col·o·bo·ma·tous
co·lo·co·lic
co·lo·co·los·to·my
pl co·lo·co·los·to·mies

col·o·cynth
co·lom·bo
var of calumba

co·lon
co·lon·ic
co·lo·pexy
pl co·lo·pex·ies

co·lo·proc·tos·to·my
pl co·lo·proc·tos·to·mies

col·or-blind
col·or·im·e·ter
col·or·im·e·try
pl col·or·im·e·tries

co·lo·sig·moid·os·to·my
pl co·lo·sig·moid·os·to·mies

co·los·to·my
pl co·los·to·mies

co·los·tral
also co·los·tric
or co·los·trous

co·los·trum
co·lot·o·my
pl co·lot·o·mies

col·pal·gia

col·pa·tre·sia
col·pec·ta·sia
col·pec·to·my
pl col·pec·to·mies
col·pi·tis
col·po·cele
col·po·clei·sis
pl col·po·clei·ses
col·po·per·i·neo·plas·ty
pl col·po·per·i·neo·plas·ties
col·po·pexy
pl col·po·pex·ies
col·po·plas·ty
pl col·po·plas·ties
col·por·rha·phy
pl col·por·rha·phies
col·po·scope
col·pos·co·py
pl col·pos·co·pies
col·po·stat
col·pot·o·my
pl col·pot·o·mies
col·u·mel·la
pl col·u·mel·lae
col·u·mel·la au·ris
col·u·mel·lar
col·u·mel·late
co·lum·na
pl co·lum·nae
co·lum·nar
col·umn of Ber·tin
co·ma
co·ma·tose
com·e·do
pl com·e·do·nes
com·e·do·car·ci·no·ma
pl com·e·do·car·ci·no·mas
or com·e·do·car·ci·no·ma·ta
co·mes
pl com·i·tes
com·mi·nute
com·mi·nut·ed
com·mi·nut·ing
com·mi·nu·tion
com·mis·su·ra
pl com·mis·su·rae
com·mis·sur·al
com·mis·sure
com·mis·sur·ot·o·my
pl com·mis·sur·ot·o·mies
com·mo·tio
com·mu·ni·ca·bil·i·ty
pl com·mu·ni·ca·bil·i·ties
com·mu·ni·ca·ble
com·pac·ta
com·par·o·scope
also com·par·a·scope
com·pat·i·bil·i·ty
pl com·pat·i·bil·i·ties
com·pat·i·ble
com·pen·sate
com·pen·sat·ed
com·pen·sat·ing
com·pen·sa·tion
com·pen·sa·to·ry
com·pe·tence
com·pe·ten·cy
pl com·pe·ten·cies
com·pe·tent
com·pet·i·tive
com·ple·ment
com·ple·men·ta·ry
com·plex·ion
com·plex·ion·al
com·plex·ioned
com·plex·us
pl com·plex·us
com·pli·ance
or com·pli·an·cy
pl com·pli·an·ces
or com·pli·an·cies
com·pli·cate
com·pli·cat·ed
com·pli·cat·ing
com·pli·ca·tion
com·pos men·tis
com·press
com·pres·sion
com·pres·sor
com·pul·sion
com·pul·sive
con·al·bu·min
co·nar·i·um
pl co·nar·ia
co·na·tion
co·na·tion·al
co·na·tive
con·can·a·val·in
con·cave

con·cav·i·ty
pl con·cav·i·ties

con·ca·vo-con·cave
con·ca·vo-con·vex
con·ceive
con·ceived
con·ceiv·ing
con·cen·trate
con·cen·trat·ed
con·cen·trat·ing
con·cen·tra·tion
con·cep·tion
con·cep·tive
con·cep·tus
pl con·cep·tus·es
also con·cep·ti

con·cha
pl con·chae

con·chi·tis
con·choi·dal
con·choi·dal·ly
con·cho·tome
con·cre·ment
con·cres·cence
con·cres·cent
con·cre·tion
con·cuss
con·cus·sion
jarring brain injury (*see* contusion, convulsion)

con·cus·sive
con·cus·sive·ly
con·di·tion
con·di·tion·al
con·di·tion·al·ly
con·di·tioned
con·di·tion·ing
con·dom
con·duc·tion
con·duc·tiv·i·ty
pl con·duc·tiv·i·ties

con·duc·tor
con·du·ran·go
pl con·du·ran·gos

con·dy·lar
con·dy·lar·thro·sis
pl con·dy·lar·thro·ses

con·dyle
con·dy·lec·to·my
pl con·dy·lec·to·mies

con·dyl·i·on
con·dy·loid
con·dy·lo·ma
pl con·dy·lo·mas
or con·dy·lo·ma·ta

con·dy·lo·ma·tous
con·dy·lot·o·my
pl con·dy·lot·o·mies

con·fab·u·la·tion
con·fec·tio
pl con·fec·ti·o·nes

con·fec·tion
con·fer·tus
con·fig·u·ra·tion
con·fig·u·ra·tion·al
con·fig·u·ra·tion·al·ly
con·fig·u·ra·tive
con·fine·ment
con·flict
con·for·ma·tion·al
con·for·ma·tion·al·ly
con·fu·sion
con·fu·sion·al
con·geal
con·ge·la·tion
con·gen·i·tal
con·gen·i·tal·ly
con·gest
con·ges·tion
con·ges·tive
con·glo·bate
con·glo·ba·tion
con·glom·er·ate
con·glom·er·at·ed
con·glom·er·at·ing
con·glom·er·a·tion
con·glu·ti·nant
con·glu·ti·nate
con·glu·ti·nat·ed
con·glu·ti·nat·ing
con·glu·ti·na·tion
con·glu·ti·nin
con·hy·drine
co·ni
pl of conus

co·nid·i·al
co·nid·io·phore
co·nid·i·oph·o·rous

co·nid·io·spore
co·nid·i·um
pl co·nid·ia

co·ni·ine
co·ni·ol·o·gy
var of koniology

co·ni·om·e·ter
var of konimeter

co·ni·um
con·iza·tion
con·ju·gal
con·ju·gal·i·ty
pl con·ju·gal·i·ties

con·ju·gal·ly
con·ju·gant
con·ju·ga·ta
pl con·ju·ga·tae

con·ju·gate
con·ju·gat·ed
con·ju·gat·ing
con·ju·ga·tion
con·junc·ti·va
pl con·junc·ti·vas
or con·junc·ti·vae

con·junc·ti·val
con·junc·ti·vi·tis
con·nec·tive
con·nec·tor
also con·nect·er

co·noid
or co·noi·dal

con·qui·nine
con·san·guin·e·ous
con·san·guin·e·ous·ly
con·san·guin·i·ty
pl con·san·guin·i·ties

con·scious
con·scious·ly
con·scious·ness
con·sen·su·al
con·sen·su·al·ly
con·serve
con·sol·i·date
con·sol·i·dat·ed
con·sol·i·dat·ing
con·sol·i·da·tion
con·so·lute
con·sti·pate
con·sti·pat·ed
con·sti·pat·ing
con·sti·pa·tion
con·sti·tu·tion
con·sti·tu·tion·al
con·strict
con·stric·tion
con·stric·tor
con·sult
con·sul·tant
con·sul·ta·tion
con·sum·ma·to·ry
con·sump·tion
con·sump·tive
con·sump·tive·ly
con·ta·gion
con·ta·gious
con·ta·gious·ly
con·ta·gious·ness
con·ta·gium
pl con·ta·gia
con·tam·i·nant
con·tam·i·nate
con·tam·i·nat·ed
con·tam·i·nat·ing
con·tam·i·na·tion
con·ti·gu·ity
pl con·ti·gu·ities

con·tig·u·ous
con·tig·u·ous·ly
con·tig·u·ous·ness
con·ti·nence
con·ti·nent
con·tra·cep·tion
con·tra·cep·tive
con·tract
con·trac·tile
con·trac·til·i·ty
or con·tract·ibil·i·ty
pl con·trac·til·i·ties
or con·tract·ibil·i·ties

con·trac·tion
con·trac·tor
con·trac·ture
con·tra·in·di·cate
con·tra·in·di·cat·ed
con·tra·in·di·cat·ing
con·tra·in·di·ca·tion
con·tra·in·dic·a·tive
con·tra·lat·er·al
con·tra·stim·u·lant

con·tre·coup
con·trec·ta·tion
con·tuse
con·tused
con·tus·ing
con·tu·sion
bruise (*see* concussion, convulsion)

co·nus
pl co·ni

Co·nus
co·nus ar·te·ri·o·sus
pl co·ni ar·te·ri·o·si

con·va·lesce
con·va·lesced
con·va·lesc·ing
con·va·les·cence
con·va·les·cent
con·vec·tion
con·vec·tive
con·ver·gence
con·ver·gent
con·ver·sion
con·vex
con·vex·i·ty
pl con·vex·i·ties

con·vexo-con·cave
con·vexo-con·vex
con·vo·lute
con·vo·lut·ed
con·vo·lut·ing
con·vo·lute·ly
con·vo·lu·tion
con·vol·vu·lin
con·vol·vu·lus
pl con·vol·vu·lus·es *or* con·vol·vu·li

con·vul·sant
con·vulse
con·vulsed
con·vuls·ing
con·vul·sion
involuntary muscular contraction (*see* concussion, contusion)

con·vul·sive
con·vul·sive·ly
Coo·ley's ane·mia
also Coo·ley's dis·ease

Coo·lidge tube
Coo·pe·ria
coo·per·id
Coo·per's lig·a·ment
co·or·di·na·tion
co·os·si·fi·ca·tion
co·os·si·fy
co·os·si·fied
co·os·si·fy·ing
coo·tie
co·pai·ba
Co·pep·o·da
co·pol·y·mer
co·pol·y·mer·ic
co·po·ly·mer·iza·tion
co·po·ly·mer·ize
co·po·ly·mer·ized
co·po·ly·mer·iz·ing
cop·per
cop·per·as
cop·per·head
cop·rem·e·sis
pl cop·rem·e·ses

cop·ro·lag·nia
cop·ro·lag·nist
cop·ro·la·lia
cop·ro·lith
co·prol·o·gy
pl co·prol·o·gies

cop·ro·pha·gia
cop·ro·phag·ic
co·proph·a·gist
co·proph·a·gous
co·proph·a·gy
pl co·proph·a·gies

cop·ro·phil·ia
cop·ro·phil·i·ac
cop·ro·phil·ic
cop·ro·pho·bia
cop·ro·por·phy·rin
co·pros·ta·nol
co·pros·ter·ol
cop·u·la
pl cop·u·las *also* cop·u·lae

cop·u·late
cop·u·lat·ed
cop·u·lat·ing
cop·u·la·tion
cop·u·la·to·ry
co·quille

cor·a·cid·i·um
pl cor·a·cid·ia

cor·a·co·bra·chi·a·lis
pl cor·a·co·bra·chi·a·les

cor·a·co·hu·mer·al
cor·a·coid
cor·al·line
or cor·al·lin

cor·date
cor·date·ly
cor·dec·to·my
pl cor·dec·to·mies

cor·dial
cor·di·form
cor·di·tis
cor·do·pexy
pl cor·do·pex·ies

cor·dot·o·my
pl cor·dot·o·mies

cor·ec·ta·sis
pl cor·ec·ta·ses

cor·ec·to·pia
core·di·al·y·sis
pl core·di·al·y·ses

co·rel·y·sis
pl co·rel·y·ses

cor·e·om·e·ter
co·re·pres·sor
cor·e·ste·no·ma
co·ri·um
pl co·ria

cor·nea
cor·ne·al
cor·ne·itis
cor·neo·bleph·a·ron
cor·ne·ous
cor·ne·um
pl cor·nea

cor·nic·u·late
cor·nic·u·lum
cor·ni·fi·ca·tion
cor·ni·fy
cor·ni·fied
cor·ni·fy·ing
cor·nu
pl cor·nua

cor·nu·al
co·ro·na
cor·o·nal
cor·o·nale
co·ro·na ra·di·a·ta
pl co·ro·nae ra·di·a·tae

cor·o·nary
pl cor·o·nar·ies

cor·o·ner
cor·o·net
co·ro·ni·on
pl co·ro·nia

cor·o·ni·tis
cor·o·noid
cor·po·re·al
cor·po·re·al·ly
corps·man
pl corps·men

cor·pu·lence
or cor·pu·len·cy
pl cor·pu·lences
or cor·pu·len·cies

cor·pu·lent
cor pul·mo·na·le
pl cor·dia pul·mo·na·lia

cor·pus
pl cor·po·ra
body (*see* carpus)

cor·pus al·bi·cans
pl cor·po·ra al·bi·can·tia

cor·pus cal·lo·sum
pl cor·po·ra cal·lo·sa

cor·pus ca·ver·no·sum
pl cor·po·ra ca·ver·no·sa

cor·pus·cle
cor·pus·cle of Has·sall
or cor·pus·cle of Has·sal

cor·pus·cle of Herbst
cor·pus·cle of Krau·se
cor·pus·cle of Va·ter
cor·pus·cu·lar
cor·pus de·lic·ti
pl cor·po·ra de·lic·ti

cor·pus lu·te·um
pl cor·po·ra lu·tea

cor·pus stri·a·tum
pl cor·po·ra stri·a·ta

cor·re·spon·dence
cor·re·spond·ing
Cor·ri·gan pulse

cor•ri•gent
cor•rode
  cor•rod•ed
  cor•rod•ing
cor•ro•sion
cor•ro•sive
cor•ros•ive•ly
cor•ros•ive•ness
cor•ru•ga•tor
cor•tex
  pl cor•ti•ces
  or cor•tex•es
cor•tex•one
cor•ti•cal
cor•ti•cal•ly
cor•ti•cate
cor•ti•cif•u•gal
cor•ti•cip•e•tal
cor•ti•co•af•fer•
  ent
cor•ti•co•ef•fer•
  ent
cor•ti•coid
cor•ti•co•spi•nal
cor•ti•co•ste•roid
cor•ti•cos•te•rone
cor•ti•co•tha•lam•
  ic
cor•ti•co•tro•pin
  or cor•ti•co•tro•phin
cor•tin
Cor•ti's gan•gli•on
cor•ti•sol
cor•ti•sone
Cor•ti's or•gan
co•run•dum
cor•us•ca•tion
co•ryd•a•lis
Co•ry•ne•bac•te•
  ri•a•ce•ae
co•ry•ne•bac•te•ri•
  al
co•ry•ne•bac•te•ri•
  um
  pl co•ry•ne•bac•te•ria
co•ryne•form
co•ry•za
co•ry•zal
cos•met•ic
cos•me•ti•cian
cos•ta
  pl cos•tae
cos•tal
cos•tal•gia
cos•tate
cos•tec•to•my
  pl cos•tec•to•mies
cos•tive
cos•tive•ness
cos•to•cen•tral
cos•to•chon•dral
cos•to•cla•vic•u•
  lar
cos•to•cor•a•coid
cos•to•scap•u•lar
cos•to•tome
cos•to•trans•verse
cos•to•trans•ver•
  sec•to•my
  pl cos•to•trans•ver•
  sec•to•mies
cos•to•ver•te•bral
cos•to•xi•phoid
co•tar•nine
co•trans•duc•tion
cot•y•loid
cou•ma•phos
cou•ma•rin
  also cu•ma•rin
coun•sel
  coun•seled
  or coun•selled
  coun•sel•ing
  or coun•sel•ling
coun•sel•or
  or coun•sel•lor
coun•ter•con•di•
  tion•ing
coun•ter•cur•rent
coun•ter•ir•ri•tant
coun•ter•ir•ri•ta•
  tion
coun•ter•open•ing
coun•ter•pho•bic
coun•ter•pul•sa•
  tion
coun•ter•punc•
  ture
coun•ter•shock
coun•ter•stain
coun•ter•trac•tion
coun•ter•trans•
  fer•ence
course
court plaster
cou•vade
co•va•lent
cov•er glass
cov•er•slip
cow•age
  or cow•hage

Cow·dria
cow hock
cow-hocked
cow·per·i·tis
Cow·per's gland
cow·pox
coxa
pl cox·ae
cox·al·gia
also cox·al·gy
pl cox·al·gias
also cox·al·gies
Cox·i·el·la
cox·i·tis
pl cox·it·i·des
cox·o·fem·o·ral
Cox·sack·ie vi·rus
cra·ni·al
cra·ni·al·ly
Cra·ni·a·ta
cra·ni·ate
cra·ni·ec·to·my
pl cra·ni·ec·to·mies
cra·nio·cele
cra·nio·ce·re·bral
cra·nio·cla·sis
pl cra·nio·cla·ses
cra·nio·fa·cial
cra·nio·graph
cra·ni·ol·o·gy
pl cra·ni·ol·o·gies
cra·ni·om·e·ter
cra·nio·met·ric
cra·ni·om·e·try
pl cra·ni·om·e·tries
cra·ni·op·a·gus
pl cra·ni·op·a·gi
cra·ni·op·a·thy
pl cra·ni·op·a·thies
cra·nio·pha·ryn·geal
cra·nio·pha·ryn·gi·o·ma
pl cra·nio·pha·ryn·gi·o·mas
or cra·nio·pha·ryn·gi·o·ma·ta
cra·nio·phore
cra·nio·plas·ty
pl cra·nio·plas·ties
cra·nio·ra·chis·chi·sis
pl cra·nio·ra·chis·chi·ses
cra·nio·sa·cral
cra·ni·os·chi·sis
pl cra·ni·os·chi·ses
cra·ni·os·co·py
pl cra·ni·os·co·pies
cra·nio·spi·nal
cra·nio·ste·no·sis
pl cra·nio·ste·no·ses
cra·nio·syn·os·to·sis
pl cra·nio·syn·os·to·ses
or cra·nio·syn·os·to·sis·es
cra·nio·ta·bes
pl cra·nio·ta·bes
cra·nio·tome
cra·ni·ot·o·my
pl cra·ni·ot·o·mies
cra·ni·um
pl cra·ni·ums
or cra·nia
crap·u·lence
crap·u·lent
crap·u·lous
cra·sis
pl cra·ses
cra·ter
craw-craw
C-re·ac·tive
cre·atine
cre·at·i·nine
cre·atin·uria
crèche
cre·mains
cre·mas·ter
crem·as·te·ri·al
crem·as·ter·ic
cre·mate
cre·mat·ed
cre·mat·ing
cre·ma·tion
cre·ma·to·ri·um
pl cre·ma·to·ri·ums
or cre·ma·to·ria
cre·ma·to·ry
pl cre·ma·to·ries
crème
cre·na
pl cre·nae
cre·nate
or cre·nat·ed
cre·na·tion
cren·o·cyte
cre·oph·a·gy
pl cre·oph·a·gies
cre·o·sol
cre·o·sote
crep·i·tant

crep·i·ta·tion
crep·i·tus
pl crep·i·tus

cre·pus·cu·lar
cres·cent
cres·cen·tic
cres·co·graph
cre·sol
cre·ta
cre·tin
cre·tin·ism
cre·tin·oid
cre·tin·ous
crev·ice
cre·vic·u·lar
crib·ber
crib·bing
crib·rate
cri·bra·tion
crib·ri·form
cri·ce·tid
Cri·cet·i·dae
cric·e·tine
Cri·ce·tu·lus
Cri·ce·tus
cri·co·ar·y·te·noid
cri·coid
cri du chat syn·
drome
crim·i·nol·o·gy
pl crim·i·nol·o·gies

crino·gen·ic
crip·ple
crip·pled
crip·pling
cri·sis
pl cri·ses

cris·pa·tion
cris·ta
pl cris·tae

cris·ta acus·ti·ca
pl cris·tae acus·ti·
cae

crith
cri·thid·ia
cri·thid·i·form
crit·i·cal
crit·i·cal·ly
crock
cro·cus
pl cro·cus·es

Crohn's dis·ease
cross·abil·i·ty
pl cross·abil·i·ties

cross-eye
cross-eyed
cross-fir·ing
cross match·ing
cross re·ac·tion
cross-re·ac·tive
cross-re·ac·tiv·i·ty
pl cross-re·ac·tiv·i·
ties

cross·way
cro·ta·lid
Cro·tal·i·dae
cro·ta·lin
cro·ta·line
cro·ta·lism
Cro·ta·lus
cro·taph·i·on
crotch
cro·tin
cro·ton

cro·ton·ic
cro·to·nyl
croup
croup·ous
croupy
croup·i·er
croup·i·est
cru·ci·ble
crup·per
cru·ral
crus
pl cru·ra

crus·ta
pl crus·tae

Crus·ta·cea
crus·ta·cean
crust·al
crutch
crux
pl crux·es
also cru·ces

cry·anes·the·sia
cryo·bi·o·log·i·cal
cryo·bi·o·log·i·
cal·ly
cryo·bi·ol·o·gist
cryo·bi·ol·o·gy
pl cryo·bi·ol·o·gies

cryo·gen
cryo·gen·ic
cryo·gen·i·cal·ly
cryo·gen·ics
cry·og·e·ny
pl cry·og·e·nies

cryo·glob·u·lin
cryo·glob·u·li·ne·
mia

cryo·hy·drate
cry·om·e·ter
cry·on·ics
cryo·phil·ic
cryo·pre·cip·i·tate
cryo·pre·cip·i·ta·tion
cryo·probe
cryo·pro·tec·tive
cryo·scope
cryo·scop·ic
or cryo·scop·i·cal

cry·os·co·py
pl cry·os·co·pies

cryo·sur·geon
cryo·sur·gi·cal
cryo·stat
cryo·ther·a·py
or cry·mo·ther·a·py
pl cryo·ther·a·pies
or cry·mo·ther·a·pies

crypt
crypt·es·the·sia
or crypt·aes·the·sia

cryp·tic
cryp·ti·cal·ly
cryp·ti·tis
cryp·to·bi·o·sis
pl cryp·to·bi·o·ses

crypt·to·coc·co·sis
pl cryp·to·coc·co·ses

cryp·to·coc·cus
pl cryp·to·coc·ci

cryp·to·crys·tal·line
crypt of Lie·ber·kühn
crypt of Mor·ga·gni
cryp·to·gam
Cryp·to·gam·ia
cryp·to·gam·ic
or cryp·tog·a·mous

cryp·to·ge·net·ic
cryp·to·gen·ic
cryp·to·lith
cryp·to·men·or·rhea
cryp·tom·ne·sia
cryp·tom·ne·sic
cryp·to·pine
cryp·to·pyr·role
crypt·or·chid
also crypt·or·chis

crypt·or·chi·dism
also crypt·or·chism

cryp·to·xan·thin
cryp·to·zo·ite
cryp·to·zy·gous
crys·tal
crys·tal·lin
crys·tal·line
crys·tal·lite
crys·tal·li·za·tion
crys·tal·lo·gram
crys·tal·lo·graph·ic
or crys·tal·lo·graph·i·cal

crys·tal·log·ra·phy
pl crys·tal·lo·graph·ies

crys·tal·loid
crys·tal·loi·dal
crys·tal·lu·ria
Cteno·ce·phal·i·des
cu·beb
cu·bi·tal
cu·bi·tus
pl cu·bi·ti

cu·boid
cu·boi·dal
cu·cum·ber
cud·bear
cui·rass
cul-de-sac
pl culs-de-sac
also cul-de-sacs

cul·do·cen·te·sis
pl cul·do·cen·te·ses

cul·do·scop·ic
cul·dos·co·py
pl cul·dos·co·pies

Cu·lex
Cu·lic·i·dae
cu·li·cide
cul·men
pl cul·mens
or cul·mi·na

cul·ti·vate
cul·ti·vat·ed
cul·ti·vat·ing
cul·ti·va·tion
cul·ture
cul·tured
cul·tur·ing
cu·ma·rin
var of coumarin

cu·mu·la·tive

cu·mu·lus
pl cu·mu·li

cu·mu·lus ooph·o·rus

cu·ne·ate
also cu·ne·at·ed

cu·ne·i·form

cu·neo·cu·boid

cu·neo·na·vic·u·lar

cu·ne·us
pl cu·nei

cu·nic·u·lus
pl cu·nic·u·li

cun·ni·lin·gu·ism

cun·ni·lin·gus
or cun·ni·linc·tus

cun·nus
pl cun·ni

cu·po·la

cu·pre·ine

cu·pric

cu·pu·la
pl cu·pu·lae

cur·able

cu·ra·re
or cu·ra·ri

cu·ra·ri·form

cu·ra·rine

cu·ra·ri·za·tion

cu·ra·rize
cu·ra·rized
cu·ra·riz·ing

cu·ra·tive

cu·ra·tive·ly

cur·cu·ma

cu·rett·age

cu·rette
or cu·ret

cu·rette·ment
also cu·ret·ment

cu·rie

cu·rine

cu·ri·um

cur·va·ture

Cush·ing's dis·ease
or Cush·ing's syn·drome

cush·ion

cus·pate
also cus·pat·ed

cus·pid

cus·pi·date
or cus·pi·dat·ed

cus·to·di·al

cu·ta·ne·ous

cu·ta·ne·ous·ly

cut·down

Cu·te·re·bra

cu·te·re·brid

Cu·te·reb·ri·dae

cu·te·re·brine

cu·ti·cle

cu·tic·u·la
pl cu·tic·u·lae

cu·tic·u·lar·iza·tion

cu·tic·u·lar·ized

cu·tin

cu·tis
or cu·tis ve·ra
pl cu·tes
or cu·tis·es
or cu·tes ve·rae

cu·tis an·se·ri·na
pl cu·tes an·se·ri·nae

cu·vette

cy·an·a·mide
also cy·an·a·mid

cy·a·nate

cy·an·ic

cy·a·nide

cy·an·i·din

cy·a·no·ace·tic

cy·a·no·ac·ry·late

cy·a·no·co·bal·a·min

cy·ano·gen

cy·a·no·gen·e·sis
pl cy·a·no·gen·e·ses

cy·a·no·ge·net·ic
also cy·a·no·gen·ic

cy·a·no·hy·drin
also cy·an·hy·drin

cy·a·no·met·he·mo·glo·bin
or cy·an·met·he·mo·glo·bin

cy·an·o·phile
also cy·an·o·phil

cy·a·noph·i·lous
also cy·a·no·phil·ic

cy·a·no·phy·ce·ae

cy·a·nosed

cy·a·no·sis
pl cy·a·no·ses

cy·a·not·ic

cy·an·u·ric

cy·as·ma

cy·ber·cul·tur·al

cy·ber·cul·ture

cy•ber•nat•ed
cy•ber•na•tion
cy•ber•net•ic
also cy•ber•net•i•cal
cy•ber•net•i•cal•ly
cy•ber•ne•ti•cian
cy•ber•net•i•cist
cy•ber•net•ics
cy•borg
cy•ca•sin
cyc•la•mate
cy•cla•min
cyc•lar•thro•sis
pl cyc•lar•thro•ses
cy•clase
cy•claz•o•cine
cy•clic AMP
cy•cli•cot•o•my
pl cy•cli•cot•o•mies
cy•cli•tis
cy•cli•tol
cy•clo•di•al•y•sis
pl cy•clo•di•al•y•ses
cy•clo•dia•ther•my
pl cy•clo•dia•ther•mies
cy•clo•gram
cy•clo•hex•i•mide
cy•cloid
cy•clo•pho•ria
cy•clo•phos•pha•mide
Cy•clo•phyl•lid•ea
cy•clo•phyl•lid•e•an
cy•clo•pia
also cy•clo•py
pl cy•clo•pias
also cy•clo•pies
cy•clo•ple•gia
cy•clo•thyme
cy•clo•thy•mia
cy•clo•thy•mic
cy•clo•pro•pane
cy•clops
pl cy•clo•pes
cy•clo•ser•ine
cy•clo•sis
pl cy•clo•ses
Cy•clo•sto•ma•ta
cy•clos•to•mate
also cy•clo•sto•ma•tous
cy•clo•stome
Cy•clos•to•mi
cy•clo•thy•mia
cy•clo•thy•mic
cy•clot•o•my
pl cy•clot•o•mies
Cy•do•nia
cy•e•sis
pl cy•e•ses
cyl•in•droid
cyl•in•dro•ma
pl cyl•in•dro•mas
or cyl•in•dro•ma•ta
cyl•in•dru•ria
cy•ma•rin
cy•ma•rose
cym•ba
pl cym•bae
cym•bo•ce•phal•ic
or cym•bo•ceph•a•lous
cym•bo•ceph•a•ly
pl cym•bo•ceph•a•lies
cy•mo•graph
var of kymograph
cy•nan•thro•py
pl cy•nan•thro•pies
cyn•o•ceph•a•lus
pl cyn•o•ceph•a•li
cy•no•mol•gus
pl cy•no•mol•gi
Cy•prin•i•dae
cy•pro•hep•ta•dine
cy•prot•er•one
cyr•tom•e•ter
cyr•to•sis
pl cyr•to•ses
cyst
cyst•ad•e•no•car•ci•no•ma
pl cyst•ad•e•no•car•ci•no•mas
or cyst•ad•e•no•car•ci•no•ma•ta
cyst•ad•e•no•ma
pl cyst•ad•e•no•mas
or cyst•ad•e•no•ma•ta
cys•tal•gia
cys•ta•mine
cys•ta•thi•o•nine
cys•te•amine
cys•tec•ta•sia
cys•tec•to•my
pl cys•tec•to•mies
cys•te•ic
cys•te•ine
cys•tic

cys·ti·cer·co·sis
pl cys·ti·cer·co·ses

cys·ti·cer·cus
pl cys·ti·cer·ci

cys·tig·er·ous

cys·tine

cys·ti·no·sis
pl cys·ti·no·ses

cys·tin·uria

cys·ti·tis
pl cys·tit·i·des

cys·to·cele

cys·to·gram

cys·tog·ra·phy
pl cys·tog·ra·phies

cys·toid

cys·to·lith

cys·to·li·thi·a·sis
pl cys·to·li·thi·a·ses

cys·to·lith·ic

cys·to·ma
pl cys·to·mas
or cys·to·ma·ta

cys·tom·e·ter

cys·to·met·ro·gram

cys·to·pexy
pl cys·to·pex·ies

cys·to·plas·ty
pl cys·to·plas·ties

cys·to·py·eli·tis

cys·to·py·elog·ra·phy
pl cys·to·py·elog·ra·phies

cys·to·py·elo·ne·phri·tis
pl cys·to·py·elo·ne·phrit·i·des

cys·tor·rha·phy
pl cys·tor·rha·phies

cys·to·sar·co·ma
pl cys·to·sar·co·mas
or cys·to·sar·co·ma·ta

cys·to·scope

cys·to·scop·ic

cys·tos·co·pist

cys·tos·co·py
pl cys·tos·co·pies

cys·tos·to·my
pl cys·tos·to·mies

cys·to·tome

cys·tot·o·my
pl cys·tot·o·mies

cys·to·ure·ter·itis

cys·to·ure·thro·gram

cyst·ous

cy·ti·dine

cy·to·ar·chi·tec·ton·ic

cy·to·ar·chi·tec·ton·ics

cy·to·ar·chi·tec·tur·al

cy·to·ar·chi·tec·ture

cy·to·chem·i·cal

cy·to·chem·is·try
pl cy·to·chem·is·tries

cy·to·chrome

cy·toc·i·dal

cy·to·di·ag·no·sis
pl cy·to·di·ag·no·ses

cy·to·dif·fer·en·ti·a·tion

cy·to·ge·net·ic
also cy·to·ge·net·i·cal

cy·to·ge·net·i·cal·ly

cy·to·ge·net·i·cist

cy·to·ge·net·ics

cy·to·ki·ne·sis
pl cy·to·ki·ne·ses

cy·to·ki·net·ic

cy·to·ki·nin

cy·to·log·i·cal
or cy·to·log·ic

cy·to·log·i·cal·ly

cy·tol·o·gist

cy·tol·o·gy
pl cy·tol·o·gies

cy·to·lymph

cy·to·ly·sin

cy·tol·y·sis
pl cy·tol·y·ses

cy·to·lyt·ic

cy·to·me·gal·ic

cy·to·meg·a·lo·vi·rus

cy·to·mem·brane

cy·tom·e·ter

cy·to·mor·pho·log·i·cal

cy·to·mor·phol·o·gy
pl cy·to·mor·phol·o·gies

cy·ton

cy·to·path·ic
cy·to·patho·gen·ic
cy·to·patho·ge·nic·i·ty
pl cy·to·patho·ge·nic·i·ties
cy·to·pa·thol·o·gy
pl cy·to·pa·thol·o·gies
cy·to·pe·nia
cy·to·phag·ic
also cy·toph·a·gous
cy·toph·a·gy
pl cy·toph·a·gies
cy·to·phil
cy·to·phil·ic
cy·to·pho·tom·e·ter
cy·to·pho·to·met·ric
also cy·to·pho·to·met·ri·cal
cy·to·pho·to·met·ri·cal·ly
cy·to·pho·tom·e·try
pl cy·to·pho·tom·e·tries
cy·to·plasm
cy·to·plas·mic
cy·to·plas·mi·cal·ly
cy·to·pyge
cy·to·ryc·tes
also cy·tor·rhyc·tes
pl cy·to·ryc·tes
or cy·tor·rhyc·tes
cy·to·sine
cy·to·skel·e·ton
cy·to·sol
cy·to·some
cy·to·stat·ic
cy·to·stat·i·cal·ly
cy·to·tax·on·o·my
pl cy·to·tax·on·o·mies
cy·to·tech
cy·to·tech·nol·o·gist
cy·to·tech·nol·o·gy
pl cy·to·tech·nol·o·gies
cy·to·tox·ic
cy·to·tox·ic·i·ty
pl cy·to·tox·ic·i·ties
cy·to·tox·in
cy·to·tro·pho·blast
cy·to·tro·pic
cy·tot·ro·pism
cy·to·vi·rin

D

da·boia
dac·ry·ad·e·ni·tis
dac·ry·agogue
dac·ryo·ad·e·nal·gia
dac·ryo·ad·e·ni·tis
dac·ryo·blen·nor·rhea
dac·ryo·cyst
dac·ryo·cys·tec·to·my
pl dac·ryo·cys·tec·to·mies
dac·ryo·cys·ti·tis
dac·ryo·cys·to·blen·nor·rhea
dac·ryo·cys·to·cele
dac·ryo·cys·to·rhi·nos·to·my
pl dac·ryo·cys·to·rhi·nos·to·mies
dac·ryo·cys·to·tome
dac·ryo·cys·tot·o·my
pl dac·ryo·cys·tot·o·mies
dac·ryo·lith
dac·ryo·li·thi·a·sis
pl dac·ryo·li·thi·a·ses
dac·ry·oma
pl dac·ry·omas
or dac·ry·oma·ta
dac·ry·on
pl dac·rya
dac·ry·ops
dac·ry·or·rhea
dac·ryo·so·le·ni·tis
dac·ryo·ste·no·sis
pl dac·ryo·ste·no·ses
dac·ryo·syr·inx
pl dac·ryo·syr·in·ges
or dac·ryo·syr·inx·es
dac·tyl

dac·tyl·i·on
dac·ty·li·tis
dac·tyl·o·gram
dac·tyl·o·graph
dac·ty·log·ra·pher
dac·tyl·o·graph·ic
dac·ty·log·ra·phy
pl dac·ty·log·ra·phies
dac·ty·lol·o·gy
pl dac·ty·lol·o·gies
dac·tyl·o·scop·ic
dac·ty·los·co·pist
dac·ty·los·co·py
pl dac·ty·los·co·pies
dac·ty·lo·sym·phy·sis
pl dac·ty·lo·sym·phy·ses
dac·ty·lus
pl dac·ty·li
dah·lin
Dal·ton·ism
dan·druff
Da·nysz phe·nom·e·non
also Da·nysz ef·fect
dap·pen dish
also dap·pen glass
dap·sone
dark-field
D'Ar·son·val cur·rent
dar·tos
dar·trous
Das·y·proc·ta
das·y·proc·tid
das·y·proc·tine
Das·y·pus
da·tu·ra
da·tu·ric
dau·er·schlaf
dau·no·my·cin
de·acid·i·fi·ca·tion
de·acid·i·fy
de·acid·i·fied
de·acid·i·fy·ing
dead·ly night·shade
de·af·fer·en·ta·tion
deaf-mute
deaf-mut·ism
deaf·ness
de·al·co·hol·iza·tion
de·ar·te·ri·al·iza·tion
death
death rat·tle
de·bil·i·tant
de·bil·i·ty
pl de·bil·i·ties
de·bride
de·brid·ed
de·brid·ing
de·bride·ment
de·cal·ci·fi·ca·tion
de·cal·ci·fy
de·cal·ci·fied
de·cal·ci·fy·ing
de·cal·vant
deca·me·tho·ni·um
de·cap·i·tate
de·cap·i·tat·ed
de·cap·i·tat·ing
de·cap·i·ta·tion
de·cap·i·ta·tor
de·cap·su·late
de·cap·su·lat·ed
de·cap·su·lat·ing
de·cap·su·la·tion
de·car·bon·iza·tion
de·car·bon·ize
de·car·bon·ized
de·car·bon·iz·ing
de·car·box·yl·ase
de·car·box·yl·ate
de·car·box·yl·ation
de·cay
de·cer·e·brate
de·cer·e·brat·ed
de·cer·e·brat·ing
de·cer·e·bra·tion
de·chlo·ri·da·tion
de·chlo·ri·nate
de·chlo·ri·nat·ed
de·chlo·ri·nat·ing
de·chlo·ri·na·tion
de·chlo·ru·ra·tion
deci·bel
de·cid·ua
pl de·cid·u·ae

de·cid·u·al
de·cid·u·ate
de·cid·u·a·tion
de·cid·u·itis
de·cid·u·oma
pl de·cid·u·omas
or de·cid·u·oma·ta
de·cid·u·o·sis
pl de·cid·u·o·ses
or de·cid·u·o·sis·es
de·cid·u·ous
de·cip·a·ra
pl de·cip·a·ras
or de·cip·a·rae
dec·li·na·tion
de·clive
de·coct
de·coc·tion
de·coc·tum
pl de·coc·ta
de·col·late
de·col·lat·ed
de·col·lat·ing
de·col·la·tion
de·col·or·ation
de·col·or·iza·tion
de·com·pen·sate
de·com·pen·sat·ed
de·com·pen·sat·ing
de·com·pen·sa·tion
de·com·pose
de·com·posed
de·com·pos·ing
de·com·po·si·tion
de·com·press
de·com·pres·sion
de·com·pres·sive
de·con·di·tion
de·con·gest
de·con·ges·tant
de·con·ges·tion
de·con·ges·tive
de·con·tam·i·nate
de·con·tam·i·nat·ed
de·con·tam·i·nat·ing
de·con·tam·i·na·tion
de·cor·ti·cate
de·cor·ti·cat·ed
de·cor·ti·cat·ing
de·cor·ti·ca·tion
de·cu·ba·tion
de·cu·bi·tal
de·cu·bi·tus
pl de·cu·bi·ti
de·cur·rent
de·cus·sate
de·cus·sa·tion
de·den·ti·tion
de·dif·fer·en·ti·ate
de·dif·fer·en·ti·at·ed
de·dif·fer·en·ti·at·ing
de·dif·fer·en·ti·a·tion
deer·fly
de·fat
de·fat·ted
de·fat·ting
def·e·cate
def·e·cat·ed
def·e·cat·ing
def·e·ca·tion
de·fem·i·na·tion
def·er·ens
def·er·ent
de·fer·en·tec·to·my
pl def·er·en·tec·to·mies
def·er·en·tial
def·er·en·ti·tis
de·fer·ves·cence
de·fi·bril·late
de·fi·bril·lat·ed
de·fi·bril·lat·ing
de·fi·bril·la·tion
de·fi·bril·la·tive
de·fi·bril·la·tor
de·fi·bril·la·to·ry
de·fi·bri·nate
de·fi·bri·nat·ed
de·fi·bri·nat·ing
de·fi·bri·na·tion
de·fi·cien·cy
pl de·fi·cien·cies
de·fi·cient
de·flec·tion
de·flo·ra·tion
de·flo·res·cence
de·flu·vi·um
de·flux·ion

de•for•ma•tion
de•formed
de•for•mi•ty
pl de•for•mi•ties
de•gan•gli•on•ate
de•gen•er•a•cy
pl de•gen•er•a•cies
de•gen•er•ate
de•gen•er•at•ed
de•gen•er•at•ing
de•gen•er•a•tion
de•gen•er•a•tive
de•glov•ing
de•glu•ti•tion
de•gran•u•la•tion
de•gus•ta•tion
de•his•cence
de•hu•mid•i•fi•ca•tion
de•hu•mid•i•fi•er
de•hu•mid•i•fy
de•hu•mid•i•fied
de•hu•mid•i•fy•ing
de•hy•drant
de•hy•drase
de•hy•dra•tase
de•hy•drate
de•hy•drat•ed
de•hy•drat•ing
de•hy•dra•tion
de•hy•dro•ace•tic
also de•hy•dra•ce•tic
de•hy•dro•ascor•bic
de•hy•dro•chlo•ri•nase
de•hy•dro•chlo•ri•nate
de•hy•dro•chlo•ri•na•tion
de•hy•dro•cho•late
de•hy•dro•cho•les•ter•ol
de•hy•dro•cho•lic
de•hy•dro•cor•ti•co•ster•one
de•hy•dro•ge•nase
de•hy•dro•ge•na•tion
de•hy•dro•gen•ize
de•hy•dro•gen•ized
de•hy•dro•gen•iz•ing
de•hy•dro•iso•an•dros•ter•one
de•hyp•no•tize
de•hyp•no•tized
de•hyp•no•tiz•ing
Dei•ters' cell
Dei•ters' nu•cle•us
dé•jà vu
or dé•jà vue
de•jec•ta
de•jec•tion
de•lac•ta•tion
de•lead
del•e•te•ri•ous
de•lim•i•ta•tion
de•lin•quen•cy
pl de•lin•quen•cies
de•lin•quent
del•i•quesce
del•i•quesced
del•i•quesc•ing
del•i•ques•cence
del•i•ques•cent
de•lir•i•ant
de•liri•fa•cient
de•lir•i•ous
de•lir•i•um
pl de•lir•i•ums
also de•lir•ia
de•lir•i•um tre•mens
del•i•tes•cence
also del•i•tes•cen•cy
pl del•i•tes•cenc•es
also del•i•tes•cen•cies
de•liv•er
de•liv•ery
pl de•liv•er•ies
del•le
de•lo•mor•phous
or de•lo•mor•phic
de•louse
de•loused
de•lous•ing
del•phi•nine
del•toid
or del•toi•de•us
pl del•toids
or del•toi•dei
de•lu•sion
de•lu•sion•al
de•lu•sion•ary

de•mas•cu•lin•iza•tion
de•mas•cu•lin•ize
de•mas•cu•lin•ized
de•mas•cu•lin•iz•ing
dem•e•car•i•um
de•ment•ed
de•men•tia
de•men•tia par•a•lyt•i•ca
pl de•men•ti•ae par•a•lyt•i•cae

de•men•tia prae•cox
also de•men•tia pre•cox
pl de•men•ti•ae prae•co•ces
also de•men•ti•ae pre•co•ces

demi•lune
or demi•lune of Hei•den•hain
or demi•lune of Gia•nuz•zi

de•min•er•al•iza•tion
demi•pen•ni•form
de•mog•ra•phy
pl de•mog•ra•phies

de•mo•ni•ac
also de•mo•ni•a•cal

de•mor•phin•iza•tion
de•mul•cent
de•my•e•lin•ate
de•my•e•lin•at•ed
de•my•e•lin•at•ing
de•my•e•lin•ation
de•my•e•lin•iza•tion
de•nar•co•tize
de•nar•co•tized
de•nar•co•tiz•ing
de•na•tur•ant
de•na•tur•ation
de•na•ture
de•na•tured
de•na•tur•ing
den•dri•form
den•drite
den•drit•ic
den•droid
den•dron
pl den•drons
also den•dra

de•ner•vate
de•ner•vat•ed
de•ner•vat•ing
den•gue
den•i•da•tion
dens
pl den•tes

den•sim•e•ter
den•si•tom•e•ter
den•si•tom•e•try
pl den•si•tom•e•tries

den•tal
den•tal•gia
den•tate
or den•tat•ed

den•ta•tion
den•ti•cle
den•tic•u•late
or den•tic•u•lat•ed

den•ti•form
den•ti•frice
den•tig•er•ous
den•ti•la•bi•al
den•ti•lin•gual
den•tin
or den•tine

den•tin•al
den•tin•o•gen•e•sis
pl den•tin•o•gen•e•ses

den•ti•noid
den•ti•no•ma
pl den•ti•no•mas
also den•ti•no•ma•ta

den•tip•a•rous
den•tist
den•tist•ry
pl den•tist•ries

den•ti•tion
den•to•al•ve•o•lar
den•toid
den•tu•lous
den•ture
de•nu•cle•at•ed
de•nu•da•tion
de•ob•stru•ent
de•on•tol•o•gy
pl de•on•tol•o•gies

de•or•sum•duc•
tion
de•or•sum•ver•
gence
de•os•si•fi•ca•tion
de•ox•i•da•tion
also de•ox•i•di•za•
tion

de•ox•i•dize
de•ox•i•dized
de•ox•i•diz•ing
de•oxy•cho•late
de•oxy•cho•lic
de•oxy•cor•ti•co•
ste•rone
de•oxy•cor•tone
de•ox•y•gen•ate
de•ox•y•gen•at•
ed
de•ox•y•gen•at•
ing
de•ox•y•gen•ation
de•oxy•ri•bo•nu•
cle•ase
de•oxy•ri•bo•nu•
cle•ic
de•oxy•ri•bo•nu•
cleo•pro•tein
de•oxy•ri•bo•nu•
cle•o•tide
de•oxy•ri•bose
de•pan•cre•a•tize
de•pan•cre•a•
tized
de•pan•cre•a•
tiz•ing

de•per•son•al•iza•
tion
de•per•son•al•ize
de•per•son•al•
ized
de•per•son•al•
iz•ing
de•phos•phor•y•la•
tion
de•pig•men•ta•
tion
dep•i•late
dep•i•la•tion
de•pil•a•to•ry
pl de•pil•a•to•ries

de•plu•ma•tion
de•po•lar•iza•tion
de•po•lar•ize
de•po•lar•ized
de•po•lar•iz•ing
de•poly•mer•ase
de•pres•sant
de•pressed
de•press•ing
de•pres•sion
de•pres•sive
de•pres•sor
de•pri•va•tion
de•pu•li•za•tion
dep•u•rant
dep•u•rate
dep•u•rat•ed
dep•u•rat•ing
dep•u•ra•tion
de•re•al•iza•tion
de•re•ism

de•re•is•tic
der•en•ceph•a•lus
pl der•en•ceph•a•li

der•en•ceph•a•ly
pl der•en•ceph•a•lies

de•re•press
de•re•pres•sion
derm•abra•sion
Der•ma•cen•tor
der•mal
der•ma•my•ia•sis
Der•ma•nys•sus
der•ma•tal•gia
der•mat•ic
der•ma•ti•tis
pl der•ma•ti•ti•ses
or der•ma•tit•i•des

Der•ma•to•bia
der•ma•to•cel•lu•
li•tis
der•ma•to•cha•la•
sis
pl der•ma•to•cha•la•
ses
or der•ma•to•chal•
la•sis•es

der•ma•to•co•ni•o•
sis
pl der•ma•to•co•ni•o•
ses
or der•ma•to•co•ni•o•
sis•es

der•ma•to•cra•ni•
um
pl der•ma•to•cra•ni•
ums
or der•ma•to•cra•nia

der•ma•to•cyst

der•ma•to•fi•bro•ma
pl der•ma•to•fi•bro•mas
also der•ma•to•fi•bro•ma•ta

der•ma•to•fi•bro•sar•co•ma
pl der•ma•to•fi•bro•sar•co•mas
or der•ma•to•fi•bro•sar•co•ma•ta

der•ma•to•glyph•ics
der•ma•to•graph
der•ma•tog•ra•phy
pl der•ma•tog•ra•phies

der•ma•to•het•ero•plas•ty
pl der•ma•to•het•ero•plas•ties

der•ma•to•his•tol•o•gy
pl der•ma•to•his•tol•o•gies

der•ma•toid
der•ma•tol•o•gist
der•ma•tol•o•gy
pl der•ma•tol•o•gies

der•ma•tol•y•sis
pl der•ma•tol•y•ses

der•ma•tome
der•ma•to•meg•a•ly
pl der•ma•to•meg•a•lies

der•ma•to•mere

der•ma•to•mu•co•so•myo•si•tis
pl der•ma•to•mu•co•so•myo•si•tis•es
or der•ma•to•mu•co•so•myo•sit•i•des

der•ma•to•my•ces
pl der•ma•to•my•ce•tes

der•ma•to•my•co•sis
pl der•ma•to•my•co•ses

der•ma•to•my•o•ma
pl der•ma•to•my•o•mas
or der•ma•to•my•o•ma•ta

der•ma•to•my•o•si•tis
pl der•ma•to•my•o•si•tis•es
or der•ma•to•my•o•sit•i•des

der•ma•to•neu•ro•sis
pl der•ma•to•neu•ro•ses

der•ma•to•path•ia
also der•ma•top•a•thy
pl der•ma•to•path•ias
or der•ma•top•a•thies

der•ma•to•path•ic
der•ma•to•pa•thol•o•gy
pl der•ma•to•pa•thol•o•gies

der•ma•to•phi•lia•sis
pl der•ma•to•phi•lia•ses

der•ma•to•phyte
der•ma•to•phy•tid
der•ma•to•phy•to•sis
pl der•ma•to•phy•to•ses

der•ma•to•plas•ty
pl der•ma•to•plas•ties

der•ma•to•poly•neu•ri•tis
pl der•ma•to•poly•neu•ri•tis•es
or der•ma•to•poly•neu•rit•i•des

der•ma•tor•rha•gia
der•ma•to•scle•ro•sis
pl der•ma•to•scle•ro•ses

der•ma•tos•co•py
pl der•ma•tos•co•pies

der•ma•to•sis
pl der•ma•to•ses

der•ma•to•ther•a•py
pl der•ma•to•ther•a•pies

der•ma•to•thi•asia
der•ma•to•trop•ic
var of dermotropic

der•ma•to•zo•on
pl der•ma•to•zoa

der•ma•to•zo•on•o•sis
pl der•ma•to•zo•on•o•ses

der•mic
der•mis
der•mo•blast

der·mo·graph·ia
der·mog·ra·phism
der·mog·ra·phy
pl der·mog·ra·phies
der·moid
also der·moi·dal
der·moid·ec·to·my
pl der·moid·ec·to·mies
der·mo·li·po·ma
pl der·mo·li·po·mas *or* der·mo·li·po·ma·ta
der·mop·a·thy
pl der·mop·a·thies
der·mo·phle·bi·tis
der·mo·skel·e·ton
der·mo·ste·no·sis
pl der·mo·ste·no·ses
der·mo·sto·sis
pl der·mo·sto·ses
der·mo·syph·i·lop·a·thy
pl der·mo·syph·i·lop·a·thies
der·mo·trop·ic
also der·ma·to·trop·ic
der·o·did·y·mus
der·ren·ga·de·ra
des·ce·me·ti·tis
des·ce·met·o·cele
Des·ce·met's mem·brane
de·scen·sus
de·sen·si·ti·za·tion
de·sen·si·tize
de·sen·si·tized
de·sen·si·tiz·ing
de·sen·si·tiz·er
de·sex
de·sex·u·al·ize
de·sex·u·al·ized
de·sex·u·al·iz·ing
des·ic·cant
des·ic·cate
des·ic·cat·ed
des·ic·cat·ing
des·ic·ca·tion
de·sic·ca·tive
des·ic·ca·tor
des·ic·ca·to·ry
de·si·pra·mine
des·mo·cra·ni·um
pl des·mo·cra·ni·ums *or* des·mo·cra·nia
des·moids
des·mo·lase
des·mo·pla·sia
des·mo·plas·tic
des·mo·some
des·mot·o·my
pl des·mot·o·mies
des·oxy·cor·ti·co·ste·rone
des·qua·mate
des·qua·mat·ed
des·qua·mat·ing
des·qua·ma·tion
des·qua·ma·tive
des·qua·ma·to·ry
des·thio·bi·o·tin
de·stru·do
de·ter·gent
de·te·ri·o·rate
de·te·ri·o·rat·ed
de·te·ri·o·rat·ing
de·te·ri·o·ra·tion
de·ter·mi·nant
de·ter·mi·nate
de·ter·mi·na·tion
de·ter·mi·na·tive
de·ter·mine
de·ter·mined
de·ter·min·ing
de·ter·min·ism
de·ter·sive
de·tor·sion
de·tox·i·cant
de·tox·i·cate
de·tox·i·cat·ed
de·tox·i·cat·ing
de·tox·i·ca·tion
de·tox·i·ca·tor
de·tox·i·fi·ca·tion
de·tox·i·fi·er
de·tox·i·fy
de·tox·i·fied
de·tox·i·fy·ing
de·tri·tal
de·tri·tion
de·tri·tus
pl de·tri·tus
de·tru·sor
de·tru·sor uri·nae
de·tu·ba·tion
de·tu·mes·cence

de·tu·mes·cent
deu·ter·anom·a·lous
deu·ter·anom·a·ly
pl deu·ter·anom·a·lies
deu·ter·an·ope
deu·ter·an·opia
deu·ter·an·opic
deu·te·ri·um
deu·ter·on
deu·ter·op·a·thy
pl deu·ter·op·a·thies
deu·tero·pro·te·ose
deu·ter·ot·o·ky
pl deu·ter·ot·o·kies
deu·tero·tox·in
deu·tom·er·ite
deu·to·plas·mol·y·sis
pl deu·to·plas·mol·y·ses
de·vas·cu·lar·iza·tion
dev·il's-grip
pl dev·il's-grips
de·vi·om·e·ter
dew·claw
dew·lap
dew·lapped
de·worm
dexa·meth·a·sone
dex·ter
dex·trad
dex·tral
dex·tral·i·ty
pl dex·tral·i·ties
dex·tral·ly
dex·tran
dex·tran·ase
dex·trase
dex·trau·ral
dex·trin
also dex·trine
dex·trin·ogen·ic
dex·trin·uria
dex·tro·am·phet·amine
dex·tro·car·dia
dex·tro·car·di·al
dex·tro·car·dio·gram
dex·tro·cer·e·bral
dex·troc·u·lar
dex·troc·u·lar·i·ty
pl dex·troc·u·lar·i·ties
dex·tro·duc·tion
dex·tro·glu·cose
dex·tro·man·u·al
dex·tro·ped·al
dex·tro·po·si·tion
dex·tro·ro·ta·tion
dex·tro·ro·ta·to·ry
also dex·tro·ro·ta·ry
dex·trose
dex·tro·si·nis·tral
dex·tros·uria
dex·tro·tor·sion
dex·tro·ver·sion
di·a·be·tes
pl di·a·be·tes
di·a·be·tes in·sip·i·dus
di·a·be·tes mel·li·tus
di·a·bet·ic
di·a·be·to·gen·ic
di·ace·tyl·mor·phine
di·ac·la·sis
or di·acla·sia
pl di·ac·la·ses
or di·acla·sias
di·a·coele
di·ad
var of dyad
dia·der·mal
or dia·der·ma·tic
or dia·der·mic
di·ad·ic
var of dyadic
di·ad·o·cho·ki·ne·sia
or di·ad·o·ko·ki·ne·sia
di·ad·o·cho·ki·ne·sis
pl di·ad·o·cho·ki·ne·ses
di·ad·o·cho·ki·net·ic
di·ag·nos·able
or di·ag·nose·able
di·ag·nose
di·ag·nosed
di·ag·nos·ing
di·ag·no·sis
pl di·ag·no·ses
di·ag·nos·tic

di·ag·nos·ti·cal·ly
di·ag·nos·ti·cian
dia·ki·ne·sis
pl dia·ki·ne·ses
di·al·y·sance
di·al·y·sate
or di·al·y·zate
di·al·y·sis
pl di·al·y·ses
di·a·lyt·ic
di·a·lyz·able
di·a·lyze
di·a·lyzed
di·a·lyz·ing
di·a·lyz·er
di·a·pe·de·sis
pl di·a·pe·de·ses
di·a·pe·det·ic
di·a·per
di·aph·a·nom·e·ter
di·aph·a·no·met·ric
di·aph·a·no·scope
di·aph·a·nos·co·py
pl di·aph·a·nos·co·pies
di·aph·o·rase
di·a·pho·re·sis
pl di·a·pho·re·ses
di·a·pho·ret·ic
di·a·phragm
di·a·phrag·mat·ic
di·aph·y·se·al
or di·a·phys·i·al
di·aph·y·sec·to·my
pl di·aph·y·sec·to·mies
di·aph·y·sis
pl di·aph·y·ses
di·a·plas·tic
di·apoph·y·sis
pl di·apoph·y·ses
di·ar·rhea
or di·ar·rhoea
di·ar·rhe·al
or di·ar·rhe·ic
also di·ar·rhoe·al
or di·ar·rhoe·ic
di·ar·thric
di·ar·thro·sis
pl di·ar·thro·ses
di·ar·tic·u·lar
di·as·chi·sis
pl di·as·chi·ses
dia·scope
dia·scop·ic
di·as·co·py
pl di·as·co·pies
di·a·stal·sis
pl di·a·stal·ses
di·as·ta·sis
pl di·as·ta·ses
di·a·ste·ma
pl di·a·ste·ma·ta
di·a·ste·mat·ic
di·a·ste·ma·to·my·e·lia
di·as·to·le
di·a·stol·ic
di·a·tax·ia
dia·ther·mo·co·ag·u·la·tion
dia·ther·my
pl dia·ther·mies
di·ath·e·sis
pl di·ath·e·ses
di·a·thet·ic
di·ax·on
also di·ax·one
di·ax·on·ic
di·az·e·pam
di·a·zine
Di·both·rio·ceph·a·lus
di·bu·caine
di·ceph·a·lus
pl di·ceph·a·li
di·chlo·ra·mine
di·chlo·ro·ben·zene
di·chlo·ro·di·eth·yl sul·fide
di·chlo·ro·di·flu·o·ro·meth·ane
di·chlo·ro·eth·yl
also di·chlor·eth·yl
di·chlo·ro·hy·drin
or di·chlor·hy·drin
di·chlo·ro·phen·ar·sine
di·chlo·ro·phen·oxy·ace·tic
di·chog·a·mous
or di·cho·gam·ic
di·chog·a·my
pl di·chog·a·mies
di·cho·ri·al

di·cho·ri·on·ic
dich·otic
dich·oti·cal·ly
di·chro·ic
also di·chro·it·ic

di·chro·ism
di·chro·mat
di·chro·mate
di·chro·mat·ic
di·chro·ma·tism
di·chro·ma·top·sia
di·chro·mic
di·chro·mo·phil
di·cli·dot·o·my
pl di·cli·dot·o·mies

Dick test
di·co·phane
di·cou·ma·rin
Di·cro·coe·li·um
di·crot·ic
also di·cro·tal
or di·cro·tous

di·cro·tism
Dic·tyo·cau·lus
di·dac·tyl
or di·dac·tyle
also di·dac·ty·lous

di·dac·ty·lism
di·del·phic
Di·del·phis
did·y·mi·tis
di·dym·i·um
diel·drin
di·en·ce·phal·ic
di·en·ceph·a·lon
die·ner
di·en·es·trol
also di·en·oes·trol
Di·ent·amoe·ba
di·er·e·sis
pl di·er·e·ses

di·es·ter
di·es·trous
or di·es·tru·al
also di·oes·trous
or di·oes·tru·al

di·es·trus
or di·es·trum
also di·oes·trus
or di·oes·trum

di·et
di·etary
pl di·etar·ies

di·et·er
di·etet·ic
di·etet·i·cal·ly
di·etet·ics
di·eth·yl·am·ide
di·eth·yl·amine
di·eth·yl·car·bam·azine
di·eth·yl·ene
di·eth·yl·stil·bes·trol
di·eti·tian
or di·eti·cian

Die·tl's cri·sis
di·eto·ther·a·py
pl di·eto·ther·a·pies

dif·fer·en·tial
dif·fer·en·tial·ly
dif·fer·en·ti·ate
dif·fer·en·ti·at·ed
dif·fer·en·ti·at·ing
dif·fer·en·ti·a·tion
dif·flu·ence
also dif·lu·ence

dif·flu·ent
dif·frac·tion
dif·fu·sate
dif·fuse
dif·fused
dif·fus·ing
dif·fus·ible
dif·fu·sion
di·ga·met·ic
di·gas·tric
Di·ge·nea
di·ge·ne·ous
di·gen·e·sis
pl di·gen·e·ses

di·ge·net·ic
di·gest
di·ges·tant
di·gest·er
di·ges·tion
di·ges·tive
di·ges·tive·ly
di·ges·tive·ness
dig·i·lan·ide
or dig·i·lan·id

dig·it
dig·i·tal
dig·i·tal·in
dig·i·tal·is
dig·i·ta·li·za·tion
dig·i·ta·lize
dig·i·ta·lized
dig·i·ta·liz·ing

dig·i·tal·ly
dig·i·tal·ose
dig·i·tate
also dig·i·tat·ed

dig·i·tate·ly
dig·i·ta·tion
dig·i·ti·grade
dig·i·to·nin
dig·i·toxi·gen·in
digi·tox·in
digi·tox·ose
dig·i·tus
pl di·gi·ti

di·glos·sia
di·gox·in
di·hy·drate
di·hy·dro·er·go·cor·nine
di·hy·dro·er·got·a·mine
di·hy·dro·strep·to·my·cin
di·hy·dro·ta·chys·ter·ol
di·hy·droxy·alu·mi·num
di·hy·droxy·phen·yl·al·a·nine
di·io·do·hy·droxy·quin·o·line
or di·io·do·hy·droxy·quin

di·iso·pro·pyl flu·o·ro·phos·phate
di·lac·er·a·tion
di·la·ta·tion
di·la·ta·tion·al
di·la·ta·tor
di·la·tion
di·la·tor
di·men·hy·dri·nate
di·mer·cap·rol
di·meth·yl·ni·tro·sa·mine
di·meth·yl phthal·ate
di·meth·yl·sulf·ox·ide
di·meth·yl·trypt·amine
di·meth·yl·tu·bo·cu·ra·rine
di·me·tria
di·mor·phic
di·mor·phism
di·mor·phous
di·ni·tro-or·tho-cre·sol
di·ni·tro·phe·nol
di·nu·cle·o·tide
Di·oc·to·phy·ma
Di·oc·to·phy·me
di·oes·trous, di·oes·tru·al
vars of diestrous

di·oes·trus
di·oes·trum
vars of diestrus

di·op·ter
di·op·tom·e·ter
di·op·tric
di·op·trics
di·op·try
pl di·op·tries

di·ose
di·os·gen·in
di·otic
di·ovu·lar
di·ox·ane
di·ox·ide
di·ox·in
di·pen·tene
di·pep·ti·dase
di·pep·tide
Di·pet·a·lo·ne·ma
di·phen·an
di·phen·hydr·amine
di·phe·nyl·amine
di·phe·nyl·chlo·ro·ar·sine
also di·phe·nyl·chlor·ar·sine

di·phe·nyl·hy·dan·to·in
di·phos·gene
di·phos·phate
di·phos·pho·gly·cer·ic
di·phos·pho·pyr·i·dine nu·cle·o·tide
di·phos·pho·thi·a·mine
also di·phos·pho·thi·a·min

diph·the·ria

diph·the·ri·al
or diph·the·ri·an
diph·the·ria·phor
diph·ther·ic
diph·the·rin
diph·the·rit·ic
diph·the·ri·tis
diph·the·roid
diph·the·ro·tox·in
di·phyl·lo·both·ri·a·sis
Di·phyl·lo·both·ri·i·dae
Di·phyl·lo·both·ri·um
di·phy·odont
dip·la·cu·sis
pl dip·la·cu·ses
di·ple·gia
dip·lo·al·bu·min·uria
dip·lo·ba·cil·lus
pl dip·lo·ba·cil·li
dip·lo·blas·tic
dip·lo·car·dia
dip·lo·coc·cal
dip·lo·coc·cic
dip·lo·coc·coid
dip·lo·coc·cus
pl dip·lo·coc·ci
dip·lo·co·ria
dip·loe
dip·lo·et·ic
dip·lo·gen·e·sis
pl dip·lo·gen·e·ses
di·plo·ic
dip·loid
dip·loi·dy
pl dip·loi·dies
di·plo·mate
dip·lo·neu·ral
dip·lo·pia
dip·lo·sis
pl dip·lo·ses
dip·lo·some
dip·lo·tene
di·pole
di·po·tas·si·um
di·pro·so·pus
dip·so·ma·nia
dip·so·ma·ni·ac
dip·so·ma·ni·a·cal
Dip·ter·yx
di·pus
di·py·gus
Di·py·lid·i·um
di·pyr·i·dam·ole
di·rhin·ic
Di·ro·fi·lar·ia
dis·abil·i·ty
pl dis·abil·i·ties
dis·able
dis·abled
dis·abling
dis·able·ment
di·sac·cha·ri·dase
di·sac·cha·ride
dis·ag·gre·ga·tion
dis·ar·tic·u·late
dis·ar·tic·u·lat·ed
dis·ar·tic·u·lat·ing
dis·ar·tic·u·la·tion
dis·as·sim·i·late
dis·as·sim·i·lat·ed
dis·as·sim·i·lat·ing
dis·as·sim·i·la·tion
dis·as·sim·i·la·tive
disc
var of disk
dis·charge
dis·ci·form
dis·cis·sion
dis·co·blas·tic
dis·co·blas·tu·la
pl dis·co·blas·tu·las
or dis·co·blas·tu·lae
dis·co·gas·tru·la
pl dis·co·gas·tru·las
or dis·co·gas·tru·lae
dis·cog·ra·phy
pl dis·cog·ra·phies
dis·coid
dis·cop·a·thy
pl dis·cop·a·thies
dis·co·pla·cen·ta
pl dis·co·pla·cen·tas
or dis·co·pla·cen·tae
dis·co·pla·cen·tal
dis·cus
pl dis·cus·es
also dis·ci
dis·cus pro·lig·er·us
dis·cu·tient
dis·ease

dis·eased
dis·equi·lib·ri·um
pl dis·equi·lib·ri·ums *or* dis·equi·lib·ria
dis·func·tion
var of dysfunction
dis·gen·ic
var of dysgenic
dis·in·fect
dis·in·fec·tant
dis·in·fec·tion
dis·in·fest
dis·in·fes·tant
dis·in·fes·ta·tion
dis·in·hi·bi·tion
dis·in·sec·tion
dis·in·ser·tion
dis·in·te·grate
dis·in·te·grat·ed
dis·in·te·grat·ing
dis·in·te·gra·tion
dis·in·te·gra·tive
dis·in·tox·i·cate
dis·in·tox·i·cat·ed
dis·in·tox·i·cat·ing
dis·in·tox·i·ca·tion
dis·in·vag·i·na·tion
dis·joint·ed
disk
or disc
dis·lo·cate
dis·lo·cat·ed
dis·lo·cat·ing
dis·lo·ca·tion
dis·mem·ber
dis·mem·ber·ment
dis·or·der
dis·or·ga·ni·za·tion
dis·or·ga·nize
dis·or·ga·nized
dis·or·ga·niz·ing
dis·ori·ent
dis·ori·en·ta·tion
dis·pen·sa·ry
pl dis·pen·sa·ries
dis·pen·sa·to·ry
pl dis·pen·sa·to·ries
dis·pense
dis·pensed
dis·pens·ing
di·sper·my
pl di·sper·mies
dis·per·sant
di·spi·reme
also di·spi·rem
dis·place
dis·placed
dis·plac·ing
dis·place·ment
dis·sect
dis·sec·tion
dis·sec·tor
dis·sep·i·ment
dis·sep·i·men·tal
dis·sim·i·late
dis·sim·i·lat·ed
dis·sim·i·lat·ing
dis·sim·i·la·tion
dis·sim·u·late
dis·sim·u·lat·ed
dis·sim·u·lat·ing
dis·sim·u·la·tion
dis·so·ciant
dis·so·ci·ate
dis·so·ci·at·ed
dis·so·ci·at·ing
dis·so·ci·a·tion
dis·so·lu·tion
dis·solve
dis·solved
dis·solv·ing
dis·so·nance
dis·tad
dis·tal
dis·tem·per
dis·tem·per·oid
dis·ten·si·bil·i·ty
pl dis·ten·si·bil·i·ties
dis·ten·si·ble
dis·ten·sion
or dis·ten·tion
dis·til·late
dis·til·la·tion
dis·to·clu·sion
Dis·to·ma
di·sto·ma·to·sis
pl di·sto·ma·to·ses
dis·to·mi·a·sis
pl dis·to·mi·a·ses
Dis·to·mum
dis·to-oc·clu·sal

dis•tor•tion
dis•tract•i•bil•i•ty
pl dis•tract•i•bil•i•ties
dis•trac•tion
dis•trac•tive
dis•trib•ute
dis•trib•ut•ed
dis•trib•ut•ing
dis•tri•bu•tion
dis•turb
dis•tur•bance
dis•turbed
di•sul•fate
di•sul•fide
di•sul•fi•ram
di•thra•nol
di•ure•sis
pl di•ure•ses
di•uret•ic
di•va•ga•tion
di•va•lent
di•var•i•ca•tion
di•ver•gence
di•ver•gent
di•ver•tic•u•lar
di•ver•tic•u•lec•to•my
pl di•ver•tic•u•lec•to•mies
di•ver•tic•u•li•tis
di•ver•tic•u•lo•sis
di•ver•tic•u•lum
pl di•ver•tic•u•la
di•vi-di•vi
pl di•vi-di•vi
or di•vi-di•vis
di•vi•sion
di•vulse
di•vulsed
di•vuls•ing
di•vul•sion
di•vul•sor
di•zy•got•ic
diz•zi•ness
diz•zy
diz•zi•er
diz•zi•est
djen•kol•ic
DN•ase
also DNA•ase
Do•bell's so•lu•tion
doc•i•mas•tic
doc•i•ma•sy
or doc•i•ma•sia
pl doc•i•ma•sies
or doc•i•ma•sias
doc•o•sa•no•ic
doc•tor
doc•trine
do•deca•no•ic
dog•ma•tist
dog•tooth
dol
dol•i•cho•ce•phal•ic
also dol•i•cho•ceph•a•lous
dol•i•cho•ceph•a•lism
dol•i•cho•ceph•a•ly
pl dol•i•cho•ceph•a•lies
dol•i•cho•cra•ni•al
dol•i•cho•cra•ny
pl dol•i•cho•cra•nies
dol•i•cho•fa•cial
dol•i•cho•pel•lic
dol•i•cho•pro•sop•ic
dol•i•cho•uran•ic
do•lor
do•lo•rif•ic
do•lo•ri•met•ric
do•lo•rim•e•try
pl do•lo•rim•e•tries
dom•i•nance
dom•i•nant
dom•i•na•tor
do•nee
Don Juan
pl Don Juans
don•nan equi•lib•ri•um
do•nor
Don•o•van body
do•pa
do•pa•mine
Dopp•ler ef•fect
Dopp•ler shift
do•ra•pho•bia
dor•nase
do•ro•ma•nia
dor•sad
dor•sal
dor•sal•gia
dor•sa•lis
pl dor•sa•les
dor•si•duct
dor•si•flex
dor•si•flex•ion

dor·si·flex·or
dor·si·spi·nal
dor·so·ceph·a·lad
dor·so·lat·er·al
also dor·si·lat·er·al

dor·so·lum·bar
also dor·si·lum·bar

dor·so·ven·trad
dor·so·ven·tral
dor·so·ven·tral·ly
dor·sum
pl dor·sa

dos·age
do·sim·e·ter
also dose·me·ter

do·si·met·ric
do·sim·e·try
pl do·sim·e·tries

dou·ble-blind
dou·ble-joint·ed
dou·blet
douche
douched
douch·ing
Doug·las
doug·las·itis
dou·rine
Do·ver's pow·der
dove·tail
Down's syn·
drome
dox·y·cy·cline
dox·yl·amine
drachm
drac·on·ti·a·sis
pl drac·on·ti·a·ses

dra·cun·cu·li·a·
sis
pl dra·cun·cu·li·a·
ses

dra·cun·cu·lo·sis
pl dra·cun·cu·lo·ses

Dra·cun·cu·lus
dra·gée
drag·on's blood
drain·age
drap·e·to·ma·nia
dras·tic
draw·sheet
dream·work
drench
drep·a·no·cyte
drep·a·no·cy·to·
sis
pl drep·a·no·cy·to·
ses

Drink·er res·pi·
ra·tor
drom·o·graph
drom·o·ma·nia
drom·o·trop·ic
drop·let
drop·per
drop·si·cal
drop·sy
pl drop·sies

dro·soph·i·la
drug
drugged
drug·ging
drug-fast
drug·gist
drug·mak·er
drug·store
drum·head
drunk·ard
drunk·en
drunk·en·ly
drunk·en·ness
drunk·o·me·ter
druse
pl dru·sen

dry-nurse
verb
dry-nursed
dry-nurs·ing
dry nurse
noun

D.T.'s
du·al·ism
Du·boi·sia
Du Bois-Rey·
mond's law
or Du Bois-Rey·
mond's prin·ci·ple

Du·chenne-Erb
pa·ral·y·sis
duck·foot·ed
Du·crey's ba·cil·
lus
duc·tal
duc·til·i·ty
pl duc·til·i·ties

duct·less
duct·ule
duc·tus
pl duc·tus

duc·tus ar·te·ri·o·
sus

duc·tus cho·le·do·chus
duc·tus de·fer·ens
duc·tus ve·no·sus
Duf·fy an·ti·gen
also Duf·fy fac·tor
dul·ca·ma·ra
dul·ci·tol
Du·long and Pe·tit's law
dump·ing syn·drome
du·o·de·nal
du·o·de·nec·to·my
pl du·o·de·nec·to·mies
du·o·de·ni·tis
du·o·de·no·en·ter·os·to·my
pl du·o·de·no·en·ter·os·to·mies
du·o·de·nor·rha·phy
pl du·o·de·nor·rha·phies
du·o·de·nos·co·py
pl du·o·de·nos·co·pies
du·o·de·num
pl du·o·de·na
or du·o·de·nums
du·plic·i·tas
Du·puy·tren's con·trac·ture
Du·puy·tren's frac·ture
du·ra ma·ter
also du·ra
du·ral
du·ra·plas·ty
pl du·ra·plas·ties
du·ri·tis
du·ro·ar·ach·ni·tis
dwarf·ism
dy·ad
also di·ad
dy·ad·ic
also di·ad·ic
dy·nam·ics
dy·na·mo·gen·e·sis
pl dy·na·mo·gen·e·ses
dy·na·mo·gen·ic
also dy·na·mog·e·nous
dy·na·mog·e·ny
pl dy·na·mog·e·nies
dy·na·mo·graph
dy·na·mom·e·ter
dy·na·mo·met·ric
dy·na·mom·e·try
pl dy·na·mom·e·tries
dy·na·mo·neure
dy·na·mo·scope
dy·na·therm
dyne
dys·acou·sia
also dys·acou·sis
pl dys·acou·sias
or dys·acou·ses
dys·ad·ap·ta·tion
dys·an·ti·graph·ia
dys·aphia
dys·ap·ta·tion
dys·ar·te·ri·ot·o·ny
pl dys·ar·te·ri·ot·o·nies
dys·ar·thria
dys·ar·thric
dys·ar·thro·sis
pl dys·ar·thro·ses
dys·au·to·no·mia
dys·au·to·nom·ic
dys·ba·rism
dys·ba·sia
dys·bu·lia
dys·che·zia
also dys·che·sia
dys·che·zic
dys·chi·ria
dys·chon·dro·pla·sia
dys·chroia
dys·chro·ma·top·sia
dys·chro·ma·top·tic
dys·chro·mia
dys·co·ria
dys·cra·sia
dys·cri·nism
dys·di·ad·o·cho·ki·ne·sia
dys·en·ter·ic
dys·en·tery
pl dys·en·ter·ies

dys•er•gia
also dys•er•gy
pl dys•er•gias
also dys•er•gies

dys•es•the•sia
dys•es•thet•ic
dys•func•tion
also dis•func•tion

dys•gen•e•sis
pl dys•gen•e•ses

dys•gen•ic
also dis•gen•ic

dys•gen•ics
dys•ger•mi•no•ma
pl dys•ger•mi•no•mas
or dys•ger•mi•no•ma•ta

dys•geu•sia
dys•gno•sia
dys•gon•ic
dys•graph•ia
dys•hi•dro•sis
or dys•idro•sis
pl dys•hi•dro•ses
or dys•idro•ses

dys•ker•a•to•sis
pl dys•ker•a•to•ses

dys•ker•a•tot•ic
dys•ki•ne•sia
dys•ki•net•ic
dys•la•lia
dys•lec•tic
dys•lex•ia
dys•lex•i•ac
dys•lex•ic
dys•lo•gia
dys•men•or•rhea
also dys•men•or•rhoea

dys•men•or•rhe•al
or dys•men•or•rhe•ic

dys•met•ria
dys•mne•sia
dys•mor•pho•pho•bia
dys•on•to•ge•net•ic
dys•os•mia
dys•os•to•sis
pl dys•os•to•ses

dys•pa•reu•nia
dys•pep•sia
dys•pep•tic
also dys•pep•ti•cal

dys•pep•ti•cal•ly
dys•pha•gia
dys•phag•ic
dys•pha•sia
dys•pha•sic
dys•phe•mia
dys•pho•nia
dys•phon•ic
dys•pho•ria
dys•phor•ic
dys•phra•sia
dys•pla•sia
dys•plas•tic
dys•pnea
also dys•pnoea

dys•pne•ic
or dys•pnoe•ic

dys•prax•ia
dys•pro•si•um
dys•rhyth•mia
dys•rhyth•mic
dys•se•ba•cia
dys•sta•sia
dys•syn•er•gia
also dys•syn•er•gy
pl dys•syn•er•gias
also dys•syn•er•gies

dys•syn•er•gic
dys•tax•ia
dys•thy•mia
dys•thy•mic
dys•to•cia
or dys•to•kia

dys•to•cial
dys•to•nia
dys•ton•ic
dys•to•pia
dys•tro•phic
dys•tro•phy
also dys•tro•phia
pl dys•tro•phies
also dys•tro•phi•as

dys•uria
dys•uric

E

ear•ache
ear•drum
ear•lobe
ear pick
ear•piece
ear•plug
ear•wax
Eb•er•thel•la
ebri•e•ty
pl ebri•e•ties

eb•ul•lism
eb•ur•na•tion
ebur•ne•ous

ecau·date
ec·bol·ic
ec·cen·tric
ec·cen·tri·cal·ly
ec·chy·mosed
ec·chy·mo·sis
pl ec·chy·mo·ses

ec·chy·mot·ic
ec·co·pro·ti·co·phor·ic
ec·crine
ec·cri·nol·o·gy
pl ec·cri·nol·o·gies

ec·cy·e·sis
pl ec·cy·e·ses

ec·dem·ic
ec·dys·i·al
ec·dy·sis
pl ec·dy·ses

ec·dy·sone
ec·go·nine
echi·nate
also echi·nat·ed

echi·no·coc·co·sis
pl echi·no·coc·co·ses

echi·no·coc·cus
pl echi·no·coc·ci

Echi·no·der·ma·ta
Ech·i·noi·dea
Echi·no·rhyn·chus
echi·nu·late
also echi·nu·lat·ed

Ech·is
echo
pl ech·oes

echo·en·ceph·a·log·ra·phy
pl echo·en·ceph·a·log·ra·phies

echo·ki·ne·sia
or echo·ki·ne·sis
pl echo·ki·ne·sias
or echo·ki·ne·ses

echo·la·lia
echo·lo·ca·tion
echo·mim·ia
ec·chon·dro·ma
echo·prax·ia
echo·vi·rus
Eck fis·tu·la
eclamp·sia
eclamp·tic
eclec·tic
eclec·ti·cism
eclipse
ecoid
or oe·coid

eco·phys·i·ol·o·gist
écor·ché
ec·pho·ria
pl ec·pho·ri·as
or ec·pho·ri·ae

ec·pho·rize
ec·pho·rized
ec·pho·riz·ing
ec·sta·sy
also ec·sta·cy
pl ec·sta·sies
also ec·sta·cies

ec·stat·ic
ec·tad
ec·tal
ec·ta·sia
ec·ta·sis
pl ec·ta·ses

ec·tat·ic
ect·eth·moid
also ect·eth·moi·dal
or ec·to·eth·moid

ec·thy·ma
ec·thym·a·tous
ec·to·blast
ec·to·car·dia
ec·to·cor·nea
ec·to·crine
ec·to·cyst
ec·to·derm
ec·to·der·mal
or ec·to·der·mic

ec·to·en·tad
ec·to·eth·moid
var of ectethmoid

ec·to·gen·ic
ec·tog·e·nous
ec·to·hor·mon·al
ec·to·hor·mone
ec·to·loph
ec·to·mere
ec·to·morph
ec·to·my
pl ec·to·mies

ec·to·par·a·site
ec·to·phyte
ec·to·pia
ec·to·pic
ec·to·pla·cen·tal
ec·to·plasm
ec·to·plas·mat·ic

ec·to·plas·mic
ect·os·te·al
ect·os·to·sis
pl ect·os·to·ses

ec·to·thrix
ec·to·zo·on
pl ec·to·zoa

ec·tro·dac·tyl·ia
ec·tro·dac·tyl·ism
ec·tro·dac·ty·ly
pl ec·tro·dac·ty·lies

ec·tro·me·lia
ec·tro·me·lic
ec·tro·pi·on
ec·tro·pi·um
ec·ze·ma
ec·ze·ma·ti·za·tion
ec·ze·ma·tous
ede·ma
also oe·de·ma
pl ede·mas
or ede·ma·ta
also oe·de·mas
or oe·de·ma·ta

edem·a·tous
eden·tate
eden·tu·late
eden·tu·lous
educt
educ·tion
ef·fect
ef·fec·tor
ef·fem·i·na·tion
ef·fer·ent
conducting outward from a center (*see* afferent)

ef·fer·vesce
ef·fer·vesced
ef·fer·vesc·ing
ef·fer·ves·cence
the process of giving off gas bubbles (*see* efflorescence)

ef·fer·ves·cent
ef·fleu·rage
ef·flo·resce
ef·flo·resced
ef·flo·resc·ing
ef·flo·res·cence
a rash, also *the process of forming a powdery chemical crust* (*see* effervescence)

ef·flo·res·cent
ef·flu·vi·um
also ef·flu·via
pl ef·flu·via
or ef·flu·vi·ums
also ef·flu·vias

eges·ta
ego
pl egos

ego·cen·tric
ego·cen·tric·i·ty
pl ego·cen·tric·i·ties

ego-dys·ton·ic
ego·ism
ego·ist
ego·is·tic
also ego·is·ti·cal

ego·is·ti·cal·ly
ego·ma·nia
ego·ma·ni·ac
ego·ma·ni·a·cal
ego·ma·ni·a·cal·ly

egoph·o·ny
also ae·goph·o·ny
pl egoph·o·nies
also ae·goph·o·nies

ego-syn·ton·ic
ego-syn·to·ny
pl ego-syn·to·nies

ego·tism
ego·tist
ego·tis·tic
or ego·tis·ti·cal

ego·tis·ti·cal·ly
ei·det·ic
Eijk·man test
ei·ko·nom·e·ter
Ei·me·ria
Ei·me·ri·id·ae
ejac·u·late
ejac·u·lat·ed
ejac·u·lat·ing
ejac·u·la·tion
ejac·u·la·to·ry
ejec·ta
ejec·tor
el·a·pid
Elap·i·dae
elas·tase
elas·ti·ca
elas·tic·i·ty
pl elas·tic·i·ties

elas·tin
elas·tom·e·ter
elas·to·sis
pl elas·to·ses

ela·tion
el·bow
Elec·tra com·plex

elec·tro·bi·ol·o·gy
pl elec·tro·bi·ol·o·gies

elec·tro·car·dio·gram

elec·tro·car·dio·graph

elec·tro·car·di·og·ra·phy
pl elec·tro·car·di·og·ra·phies

elec·tro·cau·ter·i·za·tion

elec·tro·cau·tery
pl elec·tro·cau·ter·ies

elec·tro·co·ag·u·la·tion

elec·tro·con·trac·til·i·ty
pl elec·tro·con·trac·til·i·ties

elec·tro·con·vul·sive

elec·tro·cor·ti·co·gram

elec·tro·cor·ti·co·graph·ic

elec·tro·cor·ti·co·graph·i·cal·ly

elec·tro·cute
elec·tro·cut·ed
elec·tro·cut·ing

elec·tro·cu·tion

elec·trode

elec·tro·der·mal

elec·tro·des·ic·ca·tion

elec·tro·di·al·y·sis
pl elec·tro·di·al·y·ses

elec·tro·en·ceph·a·lo·gram

elec·tro·en·ceph·a·lo·graph

elec·tro·en·ceph·a·lo·graph·ic

elec·tro·en·ceph·a·log·ra·phy
pl elec·tro·en·ceph·a·log·ra·phies

elec·tro·end·os·mo·sis
also elec·tro·end·os·mose
pl elec·tro·end·os·mo·ses

elec·tro·gen·e·sis
pl elec·tro·gen·e·ses

elec·tro·gen·ic

elec·tro·gram

elec·trog·ra·phy
pl elec·trog·ra·phies

elec·tro·hys·tero·graph

elec·tro·ky·mo·graph

elec·tro·ky·mog·ra·phy
pl elec·tro·ky·mog·ra·phies

elec·trol·o·gist

elec·trol·y·sis
pl elec·trol·y·ses

elec·tro·lyt·ic

elec·tro·lyte

elec·tro·lyze
elec·tro·lyzed
elec·tro·lyz·ing

elec·tro·mag·net

elec·tro·myo·gram

elec·tro·myo·graph

elec·tro·my·og·ra·phy
pl elec·tro·my·og·ra·phies

elec·tro·nar·co·sis
pl elec·tro·nar·co·ses

elec·tro·neg·a·tive

elec·tro·oc·u·lo·gram

elec·tro·oc·u·log·ra·phy
pl elec·tro·oc·u·log·ra·phies

elec·tro·os·mo·sis
also elec·tro·os·mose
or elec·tros·mo·sis
pl elec·tro·os·mo·ses
also elec·tros·mo·ses

elec·tro·pho·rese
elec·tro·pho·resed
elec·tro·pho·res·ing

elec·tro·pho·re·sis
pl elec·tro·pho·re·ses

elec·tro·pho·ret·ic

elec·tro·pho·reto·gram

elec·tro·phren·ic

elec·tro·phys·i·ol·o·gy
pl elec·tro·phys·i·ol·o·gies

elec·tro·plexy
pl elec·tro·plex·ies

elec·tro·pos·i·tive
elec·tro·ret·ino·gram
elec·tro·ret·i·no·graph
elec·tro·ret·i·no·graph·ic
elec·tro·ret·i·nog·ra·phy
pl elec·tro·ret·i·nog·ra·phies

elec·tro·shock
elec·tro·sleep
elec·tro·sur·gery
pl elec·tro·sur·ger·ies

elec·tro·tax·is
pl elec·tro·tax·es

elec·tro·ther·a·py
pl elec·tro·ther·a·pies

elec·tro·tome
elec·tro·ton·ic
elec·trot·o·nus
elec·trot·ro·pism
elec·tu·ary
pl elec·tu·ar·ies

el·e·doi·sin
el·eo·stear·ic
or el·aeo·stear·ic

el·e·phan·ti·a·sis
pl el·e·phan·ti·a·ses

el·e·va·tor
elim·i·nant
elim·i·nate
elim·i·nat·ed
elim·i·nat·ing
elim·i·na·tion
elim·i·na·tive
elix·ir
el·lip·sis
pl el·lip·ses

el·lip·soid
el·lip·to·cyte
el·lip·to·cy·to·sis
pl el·lip·to·cy·to·ses

el·u·ant
or el·u·ent

el·u·ate
elute
elut·ed
elut·ing
elu·tion
ema·ci·ate
ema·ci·at·ed
ema·ci·at·ing
e·ma·ci·a·tion
em·a·na·tion
e·man·ci·pa·tion
emas·cu·late
emas·cu·lat·ed
emas·cu·lat·ing
emas·cu·la·tion
emas·cu·la·tor
Em·ba·dom·o·nas
em·balm
em·bar·rass
em·bar·rass·ment

em·bed
or im·bed
em·bed·ded
or im·bed·ded
em·bed·ding
or im·bed·ding

em·be·lia
em·bo·le
var of emboly
em·bo·lec·to·my
pl em·bo·lec·to·mies

em·bol·ic
em·bo·lism
em·bo·li·za·tion
em·bo·lo·la·lia
also em·bo·la·lia

em·bo·lo·phra·sia
em·bo·lus
pl em·bo·li

em·bo·ly
also em·bo·le
pl em·bo·lies
also em·bo·les

em·bouche·ment
em·bra·sure
em·bro·cate
em·bro·cat·ed
em·bro·cat·ing
em·bro·ca·tion
em·bryo
pl em·bry·os

em·bryo·car·dia
em·bryo·gen·e·sis
pl em·bryo·gen·e·ses

em·bryo·ge·net·ic
em·bryo·gen·ic
em·bry·og·e·ny
pl em·bry·og·e·nies

em·bry·oid
em·bry·ol·o·gist
em·bry·ol·o·gy
pl em·bry·ol·o·gies
em·bry·o·ma
pl em·bry·o·mas
or em·bry·o·ma·ta
em·bry·o·nal
em·bry·o·nate
em·bry·o·nat·ed
em·bry·o·nat·ing
em·bry·on·ic
em·bry·op·a·thy
pl em·bry·op·a·thies
em·bryo·phore
em·bryo·tome
em·bry·ot·o·my
pl em·bry·ot·o·mies
em·bryo·troph
or em·bryo·trophe
em·bry·ot·ro·phy
pl em·bry·ot·ro·phies
em·e·sis
pl em·e·ses
emet·ic
em·e·tine
em·i·nence
em·i·nen·tia
emis·sion
em·men·a·gog·ic
em·men·a·gogue
em·me·trope
em·me·tro·pia
em·o·din
emol·li·ent
emo·tion
emo·tion·al
em·path·ic
em·pa·thize
em·pa·thized
em·pa·thiz·ing
em·pa·thy
pl em·pa·thies
em·phy·se·ma
em·phy·sem·a·tous
em·pir·ic
em·pir·i·cal
em·pir·i·cism
em·plas·tic
em·pros·thot·o·nos
em·py·ema
pl em·py·em·a·ta
or em·py·emas
em·py·e·mic
em·py·reu·ma
pl em·py·reu·ma·ta
em·py·reu·mat·ic
or em·py·reu·mat·i·cal
emul·gent
emul·si·ble
emul·si·fi·er
emul·si·fy
emul·si·fied
emul·si·fy·ing
emul·sin
emul·sion
emul·sive
emul·soid
emunc·to·ry
pl emunc·to·ries
enam·el
en·an·them
or en·an·the·ma
pl en·an·thems
or en·an·the·ma·ta
en·an·them·a·tous
en·ar·thro·di·al
en·ar·thro·sis
pl en·ar·thro·ses
en·cap·su·lant
en·cap·su·late
en·cap·su·lat·ed
en·cap·su·lat·ing
en·cap·su·la·tion
en·cap·sule
en·cap·suled
en·cap·sul·ing
en·ceinte
en·ceph·a·lal·gia
en·ce·phal·ic
en·ceph·a·lit·ic
en·ceph·a·li·tis
pl en·ceph·a·lit·i·des
en·ceph·a·li·to·gen·ic
also en·ceph·a·li·tog·e·nous
en·ceph·a·li·to·zo·on
pl en·ceph·a·li·to·zoa
en·ceph·a·lo·cele
also en·ceph·a·lo·coele
en·ceph·a·lo·gram

en·ceph·a·lo·graph
en·ceph·a·log·ra·phy
pl en·ceph·a·log·ra·phies
en·ceph·a·loid
en·ceph·a·lo·ma·la·cia
en·ceph·a·lo·men·in·gi·tis
pl en·ceph·a·lo·men·in·git·i·des
en·ceph·a·lo·mere
en·ceph·a·lo·my·eli·tis
pl en·ceph·a·lo·my·elit·i·des
en·ceph·a·lon
pl en·ceph·a·la
en·ceph·a·lop·a·thy
pl en·ceph·a·lop·a·thies
en·ceph·a·lo·sis
pl en·ceph·a·lo·ses
en·chon·dral
en·chon·dro·ma
pl en·chon·dro·mas
or en·chon·dro·ma·ta
en·clave
en·clit·ic
en·cop·re·sis
pl en·cop·re·ses
en·coun·ter group
en·crus·ta·tion
var of incrustation
en·cyst
en·cys·ta·tion
en·cyst·ment
end·amoe·ba
also end·ame·ba
end·aor·ti·tis
end·ar·ter·ec·to·my
pl end·ar·ter·ec·to·mies
end·ar·te·ri·al
end·ar·te·ri·tis
end·ar·te·ri·tis ob·lit·er·ans
end·ar·te·ri·um
pl end·ar·te·ria
end·au·ral
end·brain
en·dem·ic
en·der·mic
en·do·bi·ot·ic
en·do·blast
en·do·bron·chi·al
en·do·car·di·ac
en·do·car·di·al
en·do·car·di·tis
en·do·car·di·um
pl en·do·car·dia
en·do·cer·vi·cal
en·do·cer·vi·ci·tis
en·do·chon·dral
en·do·cra·ni·al
en·do·cra·ni·um
pl en·do·cra·nia
en·do·crine
en·do·crin·ic
en·do·cri·no·log·ic
or en·do·cri·no·log·i·cal
en·do·cri·nol·o·gy
pl en·do·cri·nol·o·gies
en·do·cri·no·path·ic
en·do·cri·nop·a·thy
pl en·do·cri·nop·a·thies
en·doc·ri·nous
en·do·cyst
en·do·cy·to·sis
en·do·derm
end·odon·tia
end·odon·tic
end·odon·ti·cal·ly
end·odon·tics
end·odon·tist
en·do·en·zyme
en·do·eryth·ro·cyt·ic
en·dog·a·my
pl en·dog·a·mies
en·do·gas·tric
en·do·gen·ic
en·dog·e·nous
en·do·gna·thi·on
En·do·li·max
en·do·lymph
en·do·me·tri·al
en·do·me·tri·o·ma
pl en·do·me·tri·o·mas
or en·do·me·tri·o·ma·ta

en•do•me•tri•o•sis
pl en•do•me•tri•o•ses
en•do•me•tri•tis
en•do•me•tri•um
pl en•do•me•tria
en•do•mi•to•sis
pl en•do•mi•to•ses
en•do•mix•is
en•do•morph
en•do•mor•phic
en•do•my•si•um
pl en•do•my•sia
en•do•neu•ri•um
pl en•do•neu•ria
en•do•nu•cle•ase
en•do•par•a•site
en•do•par•a•sit•ism
en•do•pep•ti•dase
en•do•phle•bi•tis
pl en•do•phle•bit•i•des
en•do•phyte
en•do•phyt•ic
en•do•plasm
en•do•plas•mic
en•do•plas•mic re•tic•u•lum
en•do•plast
en•do•plas•tic
en•do•poly•ploid
en•do•poly•ploi•dy
pl en•do•poly•ploi•dies
en•do•ra•dio•sonde
en•do•sarc
en•do•scope
en•do•scop•ic
en•do•scop•i•cal•ly
en•dos•co•py
pl en•dos•co•pies
en•do•sep•sis
pl en•do•sep•ses
en•do•skel•e•ton
end•os•mom•e•ter
end•os•mo•sis
pl end•os•mo•ses
end•os•mot•ic
en•do•some
en•do•spore
end•os•te•al
end•os•te•i•tis
or end•os•ti•tis
end•os•te•um
pl end•os•tea
end•os•to•ma
pl end•os•to•mas
or end•os•to•ma•ta
en•do•the•li•al
en•do•the•lio•cho•ri•al
en•do•the•lio•cyte
en•do•the•li•o•ma
pl en•do•the•li•o•mas
or en•do•the•li•o•ma•ta
en•do•the•li•um
pl en•do•the•lia
en•do•ther•my
pl en•do•ther•mies
en•do•thrix
pl en•do•thri•ces
en•do•tox•in
en•do•tra•che•al
en•do•ve•nous
en•dy•ma
en•e•ma
pl en•e•mas
also en•e•ma•ta
en•er•get•ic
en•er•get•i•cal•ly
en•er•get•ics
en•er•gid
en•er•giz•er
en•er•gy
pl en•er•gies
en•er•vate
en•er•vat•ed
en•er•vat•ing
en•er•va•tion
weakening (*see* innervation)
en•globe
en•globed
en•glob•ing
en•globe•ment
en•gorge
en•gorged
en•gorg•ing
en•gorge•ment
en•graft
en•gram
also en•gramme
en•large
en•larged
en•larg•ing
en•large•ment
eno•lase
eno•li•za•tion
enol•o•gy
or oe•nol•o•gy
pl enol•o•gies
or oe•nol•o•gies

en·oph·thal·mos
also en·oph·thal·mus

en·or·gan·ic

en·os·to·sis
pl en·os·to·ses

en·sheathe
also in·sheathe

en·sheathed
also in·sheathed

en·sheath·ing
also in·sheathing

en·si·form

en·tad

en·tal

ent·ame·bi·a·sis
or ent·amoe·bi·a·sis
pl ent·ame·bi·a·ses
or ent·amoe·bi·a·ses

ent·amoe·ba
also ent·ame·ba

en·ter·al

en·ter·al·gia

en·ter·ec·to·my
pl en·ter·ec·to·mies

en·ter·ic

en·ter·it·i·dis

en·ter·i·tis
pl en·ter·it·i·des
or en·ter·i·tis·es

En·tero·bac·te·ri·a·ce·ae

en·tero·bac·te·ri·al

en·tero·bac·te·ri·um
pl en·tero·bac·te·ria

en·ter·o·bi·a·sis
pl en·ter·o·bi·a·ses

En·ter·o·bi·us

en·tero·cele
hernia (*see* entero-coele)

en·tero·coc·cus
pl en·tero·coc·ci

en·tero·coele
or en·tero·coel
coelom (*see* entero-cele)

en·tero·coe·lic

en·tero·coe·lous

en·tero·co·li·tis

en·tero·cyst

en·tero·cys·to·cele

en·tero·en·ter·os·to·my
pl en·tero·en·ter·os·to·mies

en·tero·gas·trone

en·ter·og·e·nous

en·tero·hep·a·ti·tis
pl en·tero·hep·a·tit·i·des

en·tero·ki·nase

en·tero·lith

en·ter·ol·y·sis
pl en·ter·ol·y·ses

en·ter·on

en·tero·patho·gen·ic

en·ter·op·a·thy
pl en·ter·op·a·thies

en·tero·pex·y
pl en·tero·pex·ies

en·tero·plas·ty
pl en·tero·plas·ties

en·ter·op·to·sis
pl en·ter·op·to·ses

en·ter·op·tot·ic

en·ter·or·rha·gia

en·ter·or·rha·phy
pl en·ter·or·rha·phies

en·ter·os·to·my
pl en·ter·os·to·mies

en·ter·ot·o·my
pl en·ter·ot·o·mies

en·tero·tox·emia

en·tero·tox·in

en·tero·vi·ral

en·tero·vi·rus

en·tero·zoa

en·tero·zo·an

en·to·blast

en·to·coele
or en·to·coel

en·to·cone

en·to·co·nid

en·to·cor·nea

en·to·derm

en·to·mol·o·gy
pl en·to·mol·o·gies

En·to·moph·tho·ra

en·top·ic

en·to·plasm

ent·op·tic

ent·op·tos·co·py
pl ent·op·tos·co·pies

en·to·ret·i·na

en·to·sarc

en·to·zoa
sing en·to·zo·on

en·to·zo·ic

en·tro·pi·on
en·ty·py
pl en·ty·pies
enu·cle·ate
enu·cle·at·ed
enu·cle·at·ing
enu·cle·a·tion
en·ure·sis
pl en·ure·ses
en·ven·om·ation
en·ven·om·iza·tion
en·vi·ron·ment
en·vi·ron·men·tal
en·vi·ron·men·tal·ism
en·vi·ron·men·tal·ist
en·vi·ron·men·tal·ly
en·zo·ot·ic
en·zy·got·ic
en·zy·mat·ic
also en·zy·mic
en·zy·mat·i·cal·ly
also en·zy·mi·cal·ly
en·zyme
en·zy·mol·o·gist
en·zy·mol·o·gy
pl en·zy·mol·o·gies
eon·ism
eo·sin
or eo·sine
eo·sin·o·cyte
eo·sin·o·pe·nia
eo·sin·o·phil
or eo·sin·o·phile

eo·sin·o·phil·ia
eo·sin·o·phil·ic
epac·tal
ep·ar·te·ri·al
ep·ax·i·al
also ep·ax·on·ic
ep·en·ceph·a·lon
pl ep·en·ceph·a·la
ep·en·dy·ma
ep·en·dy·mal
ep·en·dy·mi·tis
pl ep·en·dy·mit·i·des
ep·en·dy·mo·ma
pl ep·en·dy·mo·mas
also ep·en·dy·mo·ma·ta
ep·eryth·ro·zo·on
pl ep·eryth·ro·zoa
ep·eryth·ro·zo·on·o·sis
pl ep·eryth·ro·zo·on·o·ses
ephe·bic
ephe·dra
ephed·rine
ephe·lis
pl ephe·li·des
epi·blast
epi·blas·tic
epi·bol·ic
epib·o·ly
also epib·o·le
pl epib·o·lies
also epib·o·les
epi·can·thic
epi·can·thus
epi·car·dia
epi·car·di·al

epi·car·di·um
pl epi·car·dia
epi·chord·al
epi·con·dyle
epi·con·dyl·i·an
epi·con·dyl·ic
epi·con·dy·li·tis
epi·cor·a·coid
also epi·cor·a·coi·dal
epi·cra·ni·al
epi·cra·ni·um
pl epi·cra·ni·ums
or epi·cra·nia
epi·cri·sis
pl epi·cri·ses
epi·crit·ic
epi·cys·ti·tis
epi·cyte
ep·i·dem·ic
ep·i·de·mic·i·ty
pl ep·i·de·mic·i·ties
ep·i·de·mi·o·log·ic
or ep·i·de·mi·o·log·i·cal
ep·i·de·mi·o·log·i·cal·ly
ep·i·de·mi·ol·o·gist
ep·i·de·mi·ol·o·gy
pl ep·i·de·mi·ol·o·gies
epi·derm
epi·der·mal
also epi·der·mic
epi·der·mat·ic
epi·der·mi·dal·i·za·tion

epi·der·mis
epi·der·mi·za·tion
epi·der·moid
also epi·der·moid·al
epi·der·mol·y·sis
pl epi·der·mol·y·ses
epi·der·mo·my·co·sis
pl epi·der·mo·my·co·ses
Ep·i·der·moph·y·ton
epi·der·moph·y·to·sis
pl epi·der·moph·y·to·ses
ep·i·did·y·mal
ep·i·did·y·mis
pl ep·i·did·y·mi·des
ep·i·did·y·mi·tis
epi·du·ral
epi·fol·lic·u·li·tis
epi·gas·tric
or epi·gas·tri·cal
or epi·gas·tri·al
also epi·gas·tral
epi·gas·tri·um
also epi·gas·trae·um
pl epi·gas·tria
also epi·gas·traea
epi·gen·e·sis
pl epi·gen·e·ses
epi·gen·e·tic
epi·glot·tal
also epi·glot·tic
epi·glot·tid·e·an
epi·glot·tis
epi·glot·ti·tis
epi·hy·al
epi·la·mel·lar
epi·i·la·tion
epi·lem·ma
epi·lem·mal
ep·i·lep·sy
pl ep·i·lep·sies
ep·i·lep·tic
ep·i·lep·ti·form
ep·i·lep·to·gen·ic
ep·i·lep·toid
ep·i·loia
epi·mere
epi·mer·ic
epim·er·ite
epi·mor·pho·sis
pl epi·mor·pho·ses
epi·my·si·um
pl epi·my·sia
epi·neph·rine
also epi·neph·rin
epi·neu·ral
epi·neu·ri·um
epi·nych·i·um, epi·onych·i·um
vars of eponychium
epi·ot·ic
epi·phar·ynx
epi·phe·nom·e·nal·ism
epi·phe·nom·e·non
pl epi·phe·nom·e·na
epiph·o·ra
epiph·y·se·al
also ep·i·phys·i·al
ep·i·phys·io·de·sis
pl ep·i·phys·io·de·ses
ep·i·phys·io·ly·sis
pl ep·i·phys·io·ly·ses
epiph·y·sis
pl epiph·y·ses
e·piph·y·si·tis
epi·pi·al
ep·i·plo·ic
epip·lo·on
pl epip·loa
epi·pter·ic
epi·sclera
epi·scler·al
epi·si·ot·o·my
pl epi·si·ot·o·mies
epi·som·al
epi·som·al·ly
epi·some
epi·spa·di·as
epi·spas·tic
epis·ta·sis
pl epis·ta·ses
ep·i·stat·ic
ep·i·stax·is
epis·te·mo·phil·ia
epis·te·mo·phil·i·ac
epi·ster·nal
epi·ster·num
pl epi·ster·na
ep·i·stro·phe·us
ep·i·taxy
pl ep·i·tax·ies
epi·ten·din·e·um
ep·i·thal·a·mus
pl ep·i·thal·a·mi
ep·i·the·li·al

ep·i·the·li·oid
ep·i·the·li·o·ma
pl ep·i·the·li·o·mas
or ep·i·the·li·o·ma·ta

ep·i·the·li·o·ma·tous
ep·i·the·li·um
pl ep·i·the·lia
also ep·i·the·li·ums

ep·i·the·li·za·tion
or ep·i·the·li·al·i·za·tion

ep·i·the·lize
also ep·i·the·li·al·ize

ep·i·the·lized
also ep·i·the·li·al·ized

ep·i·the·liz·ing
also ep·i·the·li·al·iz·ing

ep·i·trich·i·um
epi·troch·lea
epi·troch·le·ar
epi·tu·ber·cu·lo·sis
pl epi·tu·ber·cu·lo·ses

epi·tym·pan·ic
epi·tym·pa·num
pl epi·tym·pa·ni
also epi·tym·pa·nums

epi·typh·li·tis
epi·vag·i·ni·tis
epi·zo·ic
epi·zo·on
pl epi·zoa

epi·zo·ot·ic
epi·zo·ot·i·ol·o·gy
or epi·zo·ot·ol·o·gy
or epi·zo·ol·o·gy
pl epi·zo·ot·i·ol·o·gies
or epi·zo·ot·ol·o·gies
or epi·zo·ol·o·gies

ep·onych·i·um
also epi·nych·i·um
or epi·onych·i·um

ep·ooph·o·ron
ep·or·nit·ic
Ep·som salts
or Ep·som salt

Ep·stein-Barr vi·rus
epu·lis
pl epu·li·des

ep·u·loid
equa·tion
equa·tion·al
equa·tion·al·ly
equa·tor
equa·to·ri·al
equi·len·in
equi·lib·ri·um
pl equi·lib·ri·ums
or equi·lib·ria

eq·ui·lin
equi·po·tent
equiv·a·lence
equiv·a·len·cy
pl equiv·a·len·cies

equiv·a·lent
equiv·a·lent·ly
era·sion
erec·tile
erec·til·i·ty
pl erec·til·i·ties

erec·tion
erec·tor
er·e·ma·cau·sis
er·e·thism
er·e·this·mic
er·ga·sia
er·gas·tic
er·gas·to·plasm
er·go·cal·cif·er·ol
er·go·cor·nine
er·go·cris·tine
er·go·gen·ic
er·go·graph
er·go·graph·ic
er·gom·e·ter
er·go·met·ric
er·go·met·rine
er·go·nom·ic
er·go·nom·ics
er·gon·o·mist
er·go·no·vine
er·gos·ter·ol
er·got
er·got·a·mine
er·go·ther·a·py
pl er·go·ther·a·pies

er·go·thi·o·ne·ine
er·got·i·nine
er·got·ism
er·got·ized
er·i·o·dic·ty·on
Er·len·mey·er flask
erog·e·nous
also er·o·gen·ic

erose
erose·ly

ero·sion
ero·sive
eros·ive·ness
ero·siv·i·ty
pl ero·siv·i·ties
erot·ic
also erot·i·cal
erot·i·cal·ly
erot·i·cism
erot·i·cist
erot·i·ci·za·tion
erot·i·cize
erot·i·cized
erot·i·ciz·ing
er·o·tism
er·o·ti·za·tion
er·o·tize
er·o·tized
er·o·tiz·ing
ero·to·gen·e·sis
pl ero·to·gen·e·ses
ero·to·gen·ic
ero·to·ma·nia
ero·to·path
er·o·top·a·thy
pl er·o·top·a·thies
er·rat·ic
er·rhine
er·u·bes·cent
eru·cic
eruct
eruc·tate
eruc·tat·ed
eruc·tat·ing
eruc·ta·tion
erup·tion
erup·tive
Erys·i·mum
ery·sip·e·las
ery·si·pel·a·tous
ery·sip·e·loid
ery·sip·e·lo·thrix
er·y·the·ma
er·y·the·mal
er·y·them·a·tous
er·y·thor·bate
er·y·thor·bic
er·y·thras·ma
eryth·re·de·ma
er·y·thre·mia
also er·y·thrae·mia
er·y·thrism
er·y·thris·tic
eryth·ri·tol
eryth·ro·blast
eryth·ro·blas·te·mia
eryth·ro·blas·to·sis
pl eryth·ro·blas·to·ses
eryth·ro·blas·to·sis fe·tal·is
eryth·ro·blas·tot·ic
eryth·ro·cru·or·in
eryth·ro·cyte
eryth·ro·cy·the·mia
eryth·ro·cy·tom·e·ter
eryth·ro·cy·to·poi·e·sis
pl eryth·ro·cy·to·poi·e·ses
eryth·ro·cy·to·sis
pl eryth·ro·cy·to·ses
eryth·ro·der·ma
pl eryth·ro·der·mas
or eryth·ro·der·ma·ta
eryth·ro·der·mia
eryth·ro·dex·trin
also eryth·ro·dex·trine
eryth·ro·gen·e·sis
pl eryth·ro·gen·e·ses
eryth·ro·gen·ic
eryth·ro·gone
also eryth·ro·go·ni·um
ery·throid
er·y·thro·i·dine
eryth·ro·leu·co·sis
or eryth·ro·leu·ko·sis
eryth·ro·leu·ke·mia
eryth·ro·me·lal·gia
eryth·ro·my·cin
er·y·thron
eryth·ro·phage
eryth·ro·pha·gia
eryth·ro·pha·go·cy·to·sis
pl eryth·ro·pha·go·cy·to·ses
er·y·throph·i·lous
also eryth·ro·phile
eryth·ro·phle·ine
eryth·ro·phore
er·y·thro·pia
or er·y·throp·sia
eryth·ro·pla·sia

eryth·ro·poi·e·sis
eryth·ro·poi·et·ic
eryth·ro·poi·e·tin
er·y·throse
eryth·ru·lose
es·cape
es·caped
es·cap·ing
es·cap·ism
es·cap·ist
es·char
es·cha·rot·ic
Esch·e·rich·ia
es·cu·le·tin
or aes·cu·le·tin
es·cu·lin
or aes·cu·lin
es·cutch·eon
es·er·ine
Es·march bandage
es·od·ic
esoph·a·ge·al
also esoph·a·gal
or oe·soph·a·ge·al
esoph·a·gi·tis
esoph·a·go·gas·tros·to·my
pl esoph·a·go·gas·tros·to·mies
esoph·a·go·scope
esoph·a·gus
also oe·soph·a·gus
pl esoph·a·gi
also oe·soph·a·gi
eso·pho·ria
eso·tro·pia
eso·tro·pic

es·pun·dia
es·sence
es·sen·tial
es·ter
es·ter·ase
es·ter·i·fi·ca·tion
es·ter·i·fy
es·ter·i·fied
es·ter·i·fy·ing
es·the·sia
also aes·the·sia
es·the·si·om·e·ter
es·the·si·om·e·try
pl es·the·si·om·e·tries
es·the·sio·phys·i·ol·o·gy
pl es·the·sio·phys·i·ol·o·gies
es·the·sis
pl es·the·ses
es·thet·ics
var of aesthetics
es·thi·o·mene
es·tra·di·ol
also oes·tra·di·ol
es·tral
also oes·tral
es·trin
also oes·trin
es·trin·iza·tion
es·tri·ol
also oes·tri·ol
es·tro·gen
also oes·tro·gen
es·tro·gen·ic
also oes·tro·gen·ic

es·tro·ge·nic·i·ty
pl es·tro·ge·nic·i·ties
es·trone
also oes·trone
es·trous
or oes·trous
es·tru·al
or oes·tru·al
es·trus
or es·trum
or oes·trus
or oes·trum
eth·am·bu·tol
etha·mi·van
eth·a·nol
eth·a·nol·amine
ether
ethe·re·al
also ethe·ri·al
ether·i·fi·ca·tion
ether·i·fy
ether·i·fied
ether·i·fy·ing
ether·iza·tion
ether·ize
ether·ized
ether·iz·ing
eth·i·cal
eth·i·cal·i·ty
pl eth·i·cal·i·ties
eth·i·cal·ly
eth·i·cal·ness
eth·ics
eth·i·on·amide
ethis·ter·one
eth·moid
eth·moi·dal

eth·moid·i·tis
eth·mo·tur·bi·nal
etho·hexa·di·ol
ethol·o·gy
pl ethol·o·gies
eth·o·sux·i·mide
eth·yl
eth·yl·ene
eth·yl·ene·di·amine
eth·yl·ene·di·amine·tet·ra·ace·tic
eth·yl·mor·phine
eti·o·late
eti·o·lat·ed
eti·o·lat·ing
eti·o·la·tion
eti·o·log·ic
or eti·o·log·i·cal
eti·ol·o·gy
or ae·ti·ol·o·gy
also ai·ti·ol·o·gy
pl eti·ol·o·gies
or ae·ti·ol·o·gies
also ai·ti·ol·o·gies
etio·patho·gen·e·sis
pl etio·patho·gen·e·ses
etio·por·phy·rin
or ae·tio·por·phy·rin
Eu·bac·te·ri·um
eu·caine
eu·ca·lyp·tole
or eu·ca·lyp·tol
eu·ca·lyp·tus
pl eu·ca·lyp·ti
euc·at·ro·pine
Eu·ces·to·da
eu·chro·mat·ic
eu·chro·ma·tin
eu·cra·sia
eu·di·om·e·ter
eu·gen·ic
also eu·gen·i·cal
eu·gen·i·cist
eu·gen·ics
eu·gen·ism
eu·ge·nol
Eu·gle·na
eu·glob·u·lin
eu·gon·ic
eu·mor·phic
eu·my·cete
Eu·my·ce·tes
eu·nuch
eu·nuch·ism
eu·nuch·oid
eu·nuch·oi·dal
eu·nuch·oid·ism
eu·pa·to·rin
eu·pa·to·ri·um
eu·pep·sia
eu·pep·tic
eu·phen·ic
eu·phen·ics
eu·pho·ria
eu·pho·ri·ant
eu·phor·ic
eu·phor·i·cal·ly
eu·plas·tic
eu·ploid
eu·ploi·dy
pl eu·ploi·dies
eup·nea
also eup·noea
eu·prax·ia
Eu·ro·ti·a·les
eu·ry·ce·phal·ic
also eu·ry·ceph·a·lous
eu·ryg·nath·ic
eu·ryg·na·thism
eu·ryg·na·thous
eu·ry·on
eu·ry·some
also eu·ry·so·mat·ic
or eu·ry·so·mic
eu·sta·chian
eu·tec·tic
eu·tha·na·sia
eu·tha·na·sic
eu·then·ics
eu·ther·mic
eu·thy·roid
eu·thy·roid·ism
eu·to·cia
en·tro·phic
eu·tro·phy
pl eu·tro·phies
evac·u·ant
evac·u·ate
evac·u·at·ed
evac·u·at·ing
evac·u·a·tion
evag·i·na·tion
ev·a·nes·cent
even·tra·tion
ever·sion
ev·i·rate
ev·i·ra·tion

evis·cer·ate
evis·cer·at·ed
evis·cer·at·ing
evis·cer·a·tion
evo·ca·tion
evo·ca·tor
evo·lu·tion
evul·sion
ewe-neck
ewe-necked
Ew·ing's sar·co·ma
also Ew·ing's tu·mor
ex·am·i·na·tion
ex·am·ine
ex·am·ined
ex·am·in·ing
ex·am·in·er
ex·an·them
also ex·an·the·ma
pl ex·an·thems
also ex·an·them·a·ta
or ex·an·the·mas
ex·an·them·a·tous
ex·ca·vate
ex·ca·vat·ed
ex·ca·vat·ing
ex·ca·va·tion
ex·ca·va·tor
ex·cip·i·ent
ex·cise
ex·cised
ex·cis·ing
ex·ci·sion
ex·cit·abil·i·ty
pl ex·cit·abil·i·ties
ex·cit·able
ex·cit·ant
ex·ci·ta·tion
ex·cit·ato·ry
ex·cite·ment
ex·ci·tor
ex·clave
ex·clu·sion
ex·co·ri·ate
ex·co·ri·at·ed
ex·co·ri·at·ing
ex·co·ri·a·tion
ex·cre·ment
ex·cre·men·tal
ex·cre·men·ti·tious
ex·cres·cence
ex·cre·ta
ex·cre·tal
ex·crete
ex·cret·ed
ex·cret·ing
ex·cret·er
ex·cre·tion
ex·cre·to·ry
ex·cur·sion
ex·cys·ta·tion
ex·cyst·ment
ex·en·ter·ate
ex·en·ter·at·ed
ex·en·ter·at·ing
ex·en·ter·a·tion
ex·er·e·sis
pl ex·er·e·ses
ex·flag·el·la·tion
ex·fo·li·ate
ex·fo·li·at·ed
ex·fo·li·at·ing
ex·fo·li·a·tion
ex·fo·li·a·tive
ex·ha·la·tion
ex·hale
ex·haled
ex·hal·ing
ex·haust
ex·haus·tion
ex·hi·bi·tion·ist
ex·hil·a·rant
ex·hu·ma·tion
ex·hume
ex·humed
ex·hum·ing
ex·i·tus
pl ex·i·tus
exo·cho·ri·on
pl exo·cho·ria
exo·crine
ex·o·cri·nol·o·gy
pl ex·o·cri·nol·o·gies
ex·od·ic
exo·don·tia
exo·don·tist
exo·en·zyme
exo·eryth·ro·cyt·ic
ex·og·a·my
pl ex·og·a·mies
exo·gas·tru·la
ex·og·e·nous
exo·nu·cle·ase
exo·pep·ti·dase
exo·pho·ria
ex·oph·thal·mic
ex·oph·thal·mos
also ex·oph·thal·mus

exo·phyt·ic
exo·skel·e·ton
ex·os·mo·sis
pl ex·os·mo·ses
exo·spore
exo·spo·ri·um
pl exo·spo·ria
ex·os·to·sis
pl ex·os·to·ses
ex·o·ter·ic
ex·o·ter·i·cal·ly
exo·tox·ic
exo·tox·in
exo·tro·pia
ex·pec·tant
ex·pec·to·rant
ex·pec·to·rate
ex·pec·to·rat·ed
ex·pec·to·rat·ing
ex·pec·to·ra·tion
ex·per·i·ment
ex·pi·ra·tion
ex·pi·ra·to·ry
ex·pire
ex·pired
ex·pir·ing
ex·plant
ex·plo·ra·tion
ex·plor·ato·ry
ex·plore
ex·plored
ex·plor·ing
ex·plor·er
ex·plo·sion
ex·pose
ex·posed
ex·pos·ing
ex·po·sure
ex·san·gui·nate
ex·san·gui·nat·ed
ex·san·gui·nat·ing
ex·san·gui·na·tion
ex·san·guine
ex·sect
ex·sec·tion
ex·sic·cate
ex·sic·cat·ed
ex·sic·cat·ing
ex·sic·ca·tion
ex·sic·co·sis
pl ex·sic·co·ses
ex·stro·phy
pl ex·stro·phies
ex·ten·sion
ex·ten·sor
ex·te·ri·or
ex·te·ri·or·ize
ex·te·ri·or·ized
ex·te·ri·or·iz·ing
ex·tern
ex·ter·nal
ex·tero·cep·tive
ex·tero·cep·tor
ex·tero·fec·tive
ex·ti·ma
pl ex·ti·mae
or ex·ti·mas
ex·tinc·tion
ex·tin·guish
ex·tir·pate
ex·tir·pat·ed
ex·tir·pat·ing
ex·tir·pa·tion
ex·tor·sion
ex·tra-ar·tic·u·lar
ex·tra·buc·cal
ex·tra·bul·bar
ex·tra·cap·su·lar
ex·tra·cel·lu·lar
ex·tra·chro·mo·som·al
ex·tract·ant
ex·trac·tion
ex·trac·tive
ex·trac·tor
ex·tra·cys·tic
ex·tra·du·ral
ex·tra·em·bry·on·ic
also ex·tra·em·bry·o·nal
ex·tra·gen·i·tal
ex·tra·he·pat·ic
ex·tra·med·ul·lary
ex·tra·mi·to·chon·dri·al
ex·tra·mu·ral
ex·tra·nu·cle·ar
ex·tra·oc·u·lar
ex·tra·py·ra·mi·dal
ex·tra·re·nal
ex·tra·sen·so·ry
ex·tra·sys·to·le
ex·tra·tub·al

ex·tra·uter·ine
ex·tra·vag·i·nal
ex·trav·a·sate
ex·trav·a·sat·ed
ex·trav·a·sat·ing
ex·trav·a·sa·tion
ex·tra·vas·cu·lar
ex·tra·ven·tric·u·lar
ex·tra·ver·sion
or ex·tro·ver·sion
ex·tra·ver·sive
or ex·tro·ver·sive
ex·tra·vert
or ex·tro·vert
ex·tra·vert·ed
or ex·tro·vert·ed
ex·trem·i·ty
pl ex·trem·i·ties
ex·trin·sic
ex·tro·spec·tion
ex·trude
ex·trud·ed
ex·trud·ing
ex·tru·sion
ex·tu·bate
ex·tu·bat·ed
ex·tu·bat·ing
ex·tu·ba·tion
ex·u·date
ex·u·da·tion
ex·u·da·tive
ex·u·vi·ae
ex·u·vi·al
ex·u·vi·ate
ex·u·vi·at·ed
ex·u·vi·at·ing
ex·u·vi·a·tion
eye·ball
eye·brow
eye·cup
eyed·ness
eye·drop·per
eye·drop·per·ful
eye·glass·es
eye·lash
eye·lid
eye·sight
eye·strain
eye·wash

F

fa·bel·la
pl fa·bel·lae
Fa·bi·ana
fab·ri·ca·tion
Fa·bry's dis·ease
fab·u·la·tion
face·bow
face-lift·ing
fac·et
also fa·cette
fa·cia
var of fascia
fa·cial
of the face (*see* fascial)
fa·cial·ly
fa·cies
pl fa·cies
fa·cil·i·ta·tion
fac·ti·tious
fac·to·ri·al
fac·ul·ta·tive
fae·cal
var of fecal
fae·ca·lith
var of fecalith
fae·ces
var of feces
fago·py·rism
Fahr·en·heit
fail·ure
fal·cate
fal·cial
fal·ci·form
fal·cu·la
fal·cu·lar
Fal·lo·pi·an
Fal·lot's te·tral·o·gy
falx
pl fal·ces
fa·mes
fa·mil·ial
fam·i·ly
pl fam·i·lies
fan·go
pl fan·gos
Fan·nia
fan·ta·size
fan·ta·sized
fan·ta·siz·ing
fan·tasm
var of phantasm
fan·tast
or phan·tast
fan·ta·sy
fan·ta·sied
fan·ta·sy·ing

fan·ta·sy
also phan·ta·sy
pl fan·ta·sies
also phan·ta·sies

fan·tom
var of phantom

fa·rad·ic
or far·a·da·ic

far·a·dism
far·a·di·za·tion
far·a·dize
far·a·dized
far·a·diz·ing
far·cy
pl far·cies

far·i·na·ceous
far·sight·ed
far·sight·ed·ness
fas·cia
or fa·cia
pl fas·ci·ae
or fas·cias
or fa·cias

fas·cial
of a sheet of connective tissue (*see* facial)

fas·ci·cle
fas·ci·cled
fas·cic·u·lar
fas·cic·u·late
or fas·cic·u·lat·ed

fas·cic·u·la·tion
fas·cic·u·lus
pl fas·cic·u·li

fas·ci·ec·to·my
pl fas·ci·ec·to·mies

fas·ci·o·la
pl fas·ci·o·lae
or fas·ci·o·las

Fas·ci·o·la
fas·ci·o·lar
fas·ci·o·li·a·sis
pl fas·ci·o·li·a·ses

Fas·ci·o·loi·des
fas·ci·o·lop·si·a·sis
pl fas·ci·o·lop·si·a·ses

Fas·ci·o·lop·sis
fas·ci·tis
fas·tid·i·um
fas·tig·i·um
fast·ness
fa·tal
fa·tal·i·ty
pl fa·tal·i·ties

fa·ti·ga·bil·i·ty
also fa·tigu·abil·i·ty
pl fa·ti·ga·bil·i·ties
also fa·tigu·abil·i·ties

fa·ti·ga·ble
also fa·tigu·able

fa·tigue
fa·tigued
fa·tigu·ing
fat-sol·u·ble
fat·ty
fat·ti·er
fat·ti·est
fau·ces
fau·cial
fa·ve·o·late
fa·ve·o·lus
pl fa·ve·o·li

fa·vism
fa·vus

fe·bric·u·la
feb·ri·fa·cient
fe·brif·ic
feb·rif·u·gal
feb·ri·fuge
fe·brile
fe·bris
fe·cal
also fae·cal

fe·ca·lith
also fae·ca·lith

fe·ca·loid
fe·ces
also fae·ces

Fech·ner's law
fec·u·la
pl fec·u·lae

fec·u·lent
fe·cun·date
fe·cun·dat·ed
fe·cun·dat·ing
fe·cun·da·tion
fe·cun·di·ty
pl fe·cun·di·ties

fee·ble·mind·ed
fee·ble·mind·ed·ness
feed·back
Feh·ling's so·lu·tion
or Feh·ling so·lu·tion

Fe·li·dae
fe·line
fel·late
fel·lat·ed
fel·lat·ing

fel·la·tio
also fel·la·tion
pl fel·la·tios
also fel·la·tions

fel·la·tor
felo-de-se
pl fe·lo·nes-de-se
or felo-de-se

fel·on
felt·work
fe·male
fem·i·nism
fem·i·ni·za·tion
fem·i·nize
fem·i·nized
fem·i·niz·ing
fem·o·ral
fem·o·ro·tib·i·al
fe·mur
pl fe·murs
or fem·o·ra

fe·nes·tra
pl fe·nes·trae

fe·nes·trate
or fen·es·trat·ed

fen·es·tra·tion
fen·tan·yl
fenu·greek
also foenu·greek

fer·ment
fer·men·ta·tion
fer·men·ta·tive
fer·re·dox·in
fer·ric
fer·ri·he·mo·glo·bin
fer·ri·por·phy·rin
fer·ri·pro·to·por·phy·rin
fer·ri·tin
fer·ro·por·phy·rin
fer·ro·pro·to·por·phy·rin
fer·rous
fer·ru·gi·nous
also fer·ru·gin·e·ous

fer·rule
fer·tile
fer·til·i·ty
pl fer·til·i·ties

fer·ti·li·za·tion
fer·til·ize
fer·til·ized
fer·til·iz·ing
fer·til·i·zin
fes·cue foot
fes·ter
fes·ti·na·tion
fes·toon
fe·tal
also foe·tal

fe·ta·tion
fe·ti·cide
also foe·ti·cide

fe·tish
also fe·tich

fe·tish·ism
also fe·tich·ism

fet·lock
fe·tol·o·gist
fe·tol·o·gy
pl fe·tol·o·gies

fe·tom·e·try
pl fe·tom·e·tries

fe·tor
also foe·tor

fe·tus
also foe·tus
pl fe·tus·es
also foe·tus·es
or foe·ti

Feul·gen re·ac·tion
fe·ver
fe·ver·ous
fi·ber
or fi·bre

fi·ber-op·tic
fi·ber op·tics
fi·ber·scope
fi·bril
fi·bril·la
pl fi·bril·lae

fi·bril·lar
fi·bril·lary
fi·bril·late
fi·bril·lat·ed
fi·bril·lat·ing
fi·bril·la·tion
fi·brin
fi·brin·o·gen
fi·brino·geno·pe·nia
fi·bri·noid
fi·bri·no·ly·sin
fi·bri·no·ly·sis
pl fi·bri·no·ly·ses

fi·bri·no·lyt·ic
fi·bri·no·pu·ru·lent
fi·bri·nous

fi·bro·ad·e·no·ma
pl fi·bro·ad·e·no·mas
or fi·bro·ad·e·no·ma·ta

fi·bro·blast
fi·bro·blas·tic
fi·bro·car·ti·lage
fi·bro·car·ti·lag·i·nous
fi·bro·cel·lu·lar
fi·bro·cyte
fi·bro·elas·tic
fi·broid
fi·bro·in
fi·bro·ma
pl fi·bro·mas
also fi·bro·ma·ta

fi·bro·ma·toid
fi·bro·ma·to·sis
pl fi·bro·ma·to·ses

fi·bro·ma·tous
fi·bro·mus·cu·lar
fi·bro·my·o·ma
pl fi·bro·my·o·mas
also fi·bro·my·o·ma·ta

fi·bro·myo·si·tis
fi·bro·myx·o·ma
pl fi·bro·myx·o·mas
or fi·bro·myx·o·ma·ta

fi·bro·pla·sia
fi·bro·plas·tic
fi·bro·sar·co·ma
pl fi·bro·sar·co·mas
or fi·bro·sar·co·ma·ta

fi·brose
fi·bro·sis
pl fi·bro·ses

fi·bro·si·tis
fi·brot·ic
fi·brous
fib·u·la
pl fib·u·lae
or fib·u·las

fib·u·lar
fib·u·lo·cal·ca·ne·al
fi·cin
field of vi·sion
fi·la·ceous
fil·a·ment
fi·lar
fi·lar·ia
pl fi·lar·i·ae

fi·lar·i·al
fil·a·ri·a·sis
also fi·lar·i·o·sis
pl fil·a·ri·a·ses
also fi·lar·i·o·ses

fi·lar·i·cide
fi·lar·i·form
fi·lar·i·id
Fi·lar·i·oi·dea
fil·ial
fi·lic·ic
fi·li·form
fil·let
fill·ing
fi·lo·po·di·um
also fi·lo·pod
pl fi·lo·po·dia
also fi·lo·pods

fil·ter
fil·ter·abil·i·ty
pl fil·ter·abil·i·ties

fil·ter·able
or fil·tra·ble

fil·trate
fil·trat·ed
fil·trat·ing
fil·tra·tion
fil·trum
fi·lum
pl fi·la

fim·bri·a
pl fim·bri·ae

fim·bri·ate
or fim·bri·at·ed

fim·bri·a·tion
fin·ger
fin·gered
fin·ger·nail
fin·ger·print
fin·ger·tip
fire·bug
fire·damp
first aid
first-de·gree
fish·skin dis·ease
or fish-scale dis·ease

fis·sion
fis·sip·a·rous
fis·su·ra
pl fis·su·rae

fis·sur·al
fis·su·ra·tion
fis·sure
fis·sured
fis·sur·ing
fis·tu·la
pl fis·tu·las
or fis·tu·lae

fis·tu·li·za·tion
fis·tu·lize

fis·tu·lized
fis·tu·liz·ing
fis·tu·lot·o·my
pl fis·tu·lot·o·mies
fis·tu·lous
fix·ate
fix·at·ed
fix·at·ing
fix·a·tion
fix·a·tive
fix·ing
fla·bel·lum
pl fla·bel·la
flac·cid
flac·cid·i·ty
pl flac·cid·i·ties
fla·gel·lar
Flag·el·la·ta
Flag·el·la·tae
flag·el·late
verb
flag·el·lat·ed
flag·el·lat·ing
fla·gel·late
adjective or noun
flag·el·la·tion
flag·el·lo·sis
pl flag·el·lo·ses
fla·gel·lum
pl fla·gel·la
also fla·gel·lums
flat·foot
flat-foot·ed
flat·u·lence
or flat·u·len·cy
pl flat·u·lenc·es
or flat·u·len·cies
flat·u·lent
fla·tus
flat·worm
fla·va·none
fla·ve·do
pl fla·ve·dos
fla·vi·an·ic
fla·vin
fla·vine
Fla·vo·bac·te·ri·um
fla·vone
fla·vo·noid
fla·vo·nol
fla·vo·pro·tein
fla·vor
flea·bite
flea-bit·ten
Fletch·er·ism
fletch·er·ize
fletch·er·ized
fletch·er·iz·ing
flex·im·e·ter
flex·ion
or flec·tion
flex·or
flex·ur·al
flex·ure
floc
flocced
floc·cing
floc·cil·la·tion
floc·cose
floc·cu·lar
floc·cu·late
floc·cu·lat·ed
floc·cu·lat·ing
floc·cu·la·tion
floc·cule
floc·cu·lence
floc·cu·lent
floc·cu·lus
pl floc·cu·li
Flor·ence flask
floss
flo·ta·tion
also floa·ta·tion
flow·me·ter
fluc·tu·ant
flu·id
flu·id·ex·tract
flu·id·glyc·er·ate
flu·id·i·ty
pl flu·id·i·ties
flu·id·ounce
flu·idram
or flu·idrachm
fluke
flu·o·cin·o·lone ac·e·to·nide
flu·or
flu·or·ap·a·tite
flu·o·rene
flu·o·res·ce·in
flu·o·res·cence
flu·o·res·cent
flu·o·ri·date
flu·o·ri·dat·ed
flu·o·ri·dat·ing
flu·o·ri·da·tion
flu·o·ride
flu·o·ri·di·za·tion
flu·o·ri·dize
flu·o·ri·dized
flu·o·ri·diz·ing

flu•o•ri•nate
flu•o•ri•nat•ed
flu•o•ri•nat•ing
flu•o•ri•na•tion
flu•o•rine
flu•o•ro•chrome
flu•o•rom•e•ter
or flu•o•rim•e•ter

flu•o•rom•e•try
or flu•o•rim•e•try
pl flu•o•rom•e•tries
or flu•o•rim•e•tries

flu•o•ro•roent•gen•og•ra•phy
pl flu•o•ro•roent•gen•og•ra•phies

flu•o•ro•scope
flu•o•ro•scop•ic
flu•o•ro•scop•i•cal•ly
flu•o•ros•co•pist
flu•o•ros•co•py
pl flu•o•ros•co•pies

flu•o•ro•sis
flu•o•ro•ura•cil
fluo•sil•i•cate
flu•phen•azine
flut•ter
fly•belt
fo•cal
fo•cal•ize
fo•cal•ized
fo•cal•iz•ing
fo•cim•e•ter
also fo•com•e•ter

fo•cus
pl fo•cus•es
or fo•ci

foenu•greek
var of fenugreek

foe•tal
var of fetal

foe•ti•cide
var of feticide

foe•tor
var of fetor

foe•tus
var of fetus

fo•la•cin
fo•late
fo•li•a•ceous
fo•li•ate
fo•lic
fo•lie
fo•lie à deux
pl fo•lies à deux

fo•lin•ic
fo•li•ose
or fo•li•ous

fo•li•um
pl fo•lia

fol•li•cle
fol•lic•u•lar
fol•lic•u•late
or fol•lic•u•lat•ed

fol•lic•u•lin
fol•lic•u•li•tis
fol•lic•u•lo•ma
pl fol•lic•u•lo•mas
or fol•lic•u•lo•ma•ta

fol•lic•u•lus
pl fol•lic•u•li

fol•low-up
fo•ment
fo•men•ta•tion

fomi•tes
fon•ta•nel
also fon•ta•nelle

foot-and-mouth dis•ease
foot•bath
foot•sore
foot•sore•ness
fo•ra•men
pl fo•ram•i•na
or fo•ra•mens

fo•ra•men mag•num
fo•ra•men ova•le
fo•ra•mi•nif•er•ous
for•ceps
pl for•ceps
also for•ceps•es
or for•ci•pes

for•ci•pate
also for•ci•pat•ed

for•ci•pres•sure
For•dyce dis•ease
fore•arm
fore•brain
fore•con•scious
fore•fin•ger
fore•foot
pl fore•feet

fore•gut
fore•head
fore•leg
fore•limb
fore•milk
fo•ren•sic
fo•ren•si•cal•ly

fore·paw
fore·play
fore·plea·sure
fore·skin
fore·stom·ach
fore·top
fore·wa·ters
form·al·de·hyde
for·ma·lin
for·ma·lin·ize
  for·ma·lin·ized
  for·ma·lin·iz·ing
for·mate
for·ma·tion
for·ma·tive
forme fruste
  pl formes frustes
for·mic
for·mi·ca·tion
for·mol·ize
  for·mol·ized
  for·mol·iz·ing
for·mu·la
  pl for·mu·las
  or for·mu·lae
for·mu·lary
  pl for·mu·lar·ies
for·mu·la·tion
for·myl
for·ni·cate
  for·ni·cat·ed
  for·ni·cat·ing
for·ni·ca·tion
for·ni·ca·tor
for·ni·ca·trix
  pl for·ni·ca·tri·ces
for·nix
  pl for·ni·ces
fos·sa
  pl fos·sae
fos·sette
fos·su·la
  pl fos·su·lae
fos·su·late
fou·droy·ant
foun·der
four·chette
fo·vea
  pl fo·ve·ae
fo·vea cen·tra·lis
fo·ve·ate
  or fo·ve·at·ed
fo·ve·a·tion
fo·ve·iform
fo·ve·o·la
  pl fo·ve·o·lae
  or fo·ve·o·las
fo·ve·o·lar
fo·ve·o·late
fox·glove
frac·tion·ate
  frac·tion·at·ed
  frac·tion·at·ing
frac·tion·ation
frac·ture
  frac·tured
  frac·tur·ing
fra·gil·i·tas os·si·um
fra·gil·i·ty
  pl fra·gil·i·ties
fra·gil·o·cyte
fra·gil·o·cy·to·sis
  pl fra·gil·o·cy·to·ses
fraise
fram·be·sia
  also fram·boe·sia
frame·work
fran·ci·um
fra·ter·nal
freckle
  freck·led
  freck·ling
free-as·so·ci·ate
free-float·ing
free-liv·ing
free·mar·tin
freeze-dry
  freeze-dried
  freeze-dry·ing
freeze-etch·ing
frem·i·tus
fre·nal
fren·u·lum
  pl fren·u·la
fre·num
  pl fre·nums
  or fre·na
fren·zied
fren·zy
  pl fren·zies
fre·tum
  pl fre·ta
Freud·ian
Freund's ad·ju·vant
fri·a·bil·i·ty
  pl fri·a·bil·i·ties
fri·a·ble

fri·a·ble·ness
Fried·länd·er's ba·cil·lus
also Fried·länd·er ba·cil·lus
Fried·man test
also Fried·man's test
Fried·reich's atax·ia
also Fried·reich's dis·ease
frig·id
fri·gid·i·ty
pl fri·gid·i·ties
frig·o·rif·ic
Fröh·lich's syn·drome
or Froeh·lich's syn·drome
frons
pl fron·tes
front·ad
fron·tal
fron·ta·lis
fron·tal·ly
front·let
fron·to·oc·cip·i·tal
fron·to·pa·ri·e·tal
fron·to·tem·po·ral
frost·bite
frost·bit
frost·bit·ten
frost·bit·ing
frot·tage
fruc·to·san
fruc·tose
fruc·to·side
fru·giv·o·rous
frus·trate
frus·trat·ed
frus·trat·ing
frus·tra·tion
fuch·sine
or fuch·sin
fuch·sin·o·phil
fuch·sin·o·phil·ic
fu·cose
fu·gac·i·ty
pl fu·gac·i·ties
fu·gi·tive
fugue
ful·crum
pl ful·crums
or ful·cra
ful·gu·rant
ful·gu·rate
ful·gu·rat·ed
ful·gu·rat·ing
ful·gu·ra·tion
full-blood·ed
full·mouthed
ful·mi·nant
ful·mi·nate
ful·mi·nat·ed
ful·mi·nat·ing
fu·ma·gil·lin
fu·ma·rase
fu·ma·rate
fu·mar·ic
fu·mig·a·cin
func·tion
func·tion·al
func·tion·al·ly
fun·dal
fun·da·ment
fun·dec·to·my
pl fun·dec·to·mies
fun·dic
fun·du·lus
pl fun·du·lus
fun·dus
pl fun·di
fun·du·scop·ic
also fun·do·scop·ic
fun·dus·co·py
also fun·dos·co·py
pl fun·dus·co·pies
also fun·dos·co·pies
fun·gal
fun·gate
fun·gat·ed
fun·gat·ing
fun·gi·cid·al
fun·gi·cid·al·ly
fun·gi·cide
fun·gi·ci·din
fun·gi·form
Fun·gi Im·per·fec·ti
fun·gi·stat·ic
fun·gi·tox·ic
fun·gi·tox·ic·i·ty
pl fun·gi·tox·ic·i·ties
fun·goid
fun·gos·i·ty
pl fun·gos·i·ties
fun·gous
fun·gus
pl fun·gi
also fun·gus·es
fu·nic
fu·ni·cle

fu·nic·u·lar
fu·nic·u·li·tis
fu·nic·u·lus
pl fu·nic·u·li

fu·nis
fu·ra·nose
fu·ra·zol·i·done
fur·cal
fur·co·cer·cous
fur·cu·la
pl fur·cu·lae

fur·fur
fur·fu·ra·ceous
fur·fu·ral
fur·fu·ryl
fu·ro·se·mide
fur·se·mide
fu·run·cle
boil (*see* carbuncle, caruncle)

fu·run·cu·lar
fu·run·cu·loid
fu·run·cu·lo·sis
pl fu·run·cu·lo·ses

fu·run·cu·lous
fu·run·cu·lus
pl fu·run·cu·li

fu·sar·i·um
pl fu·sar·ia

fu·si·form
Fu·si·for·mis
fu·sion
fu·sion·al
fu·so·bac·te·ri·um
pl fu·so·bac·te·ria

fu·so·cel·lu·lar
fu·so·spi·ro·chet·al
fus·ti·ga·tion

G

G ac·id
gad·fly
pl gad·flies

Gad·i·dae
gad·ole·ic
Ga·dus
ga·lac·ta·gogue
or ga·lac·to·gogue

ga·lac·tan
ga·lac·tic
ga·lac·tin
ga·lac·to·cele
ga·lac·to·lip·id
also ga·lac·to·lip·ide
or ga·lac·to·lip·in

ga·lac·to·phore
gal·ac·toph·o·ri·tis
gal·ac·toph·o·rous
ga·lac·to·poi·e·sis
pl ga·lac·to·poi·e·ses

ga·lac·to·poi·et·ic
ga·lac·tor·rhea
or ga·lac·tor·rhoea

ga·lac·tos·amine
ga·lac·to·scope
ga·lac·tose
ga·lac·to·se·mia
ga·lac·tos·emic
ga·lac·to·si·dase
ga·lac·to·side
gal·ac·to·sis
pl gal·ac·to·ses

ga·lac·tos·uria
ga·lac·to·ther·a·py
pl ga·lac·to·ther·a·pies

ga·lea
ga·lea apo·neu·ro·ti·ca
ga·len·ic
or ga·len·i·cal
adjective
relating to a galenical

Ga·len·ic
also Ga·len·i·cal
adjective
of Galen

ga·len·i·cal
noun
medicinal preparation

Ga·len·ism
gal·la
gal·la·mine
gal·late
gall·blad·der
gal·lein
gal·lic
Gal·li·for·mes
gal·li·na·ceous
gal·li·um
gall·stone
gal·van·ic
gal·va·nism
gal·va·ni·za·tion
gal·va·nize
gal·va·nized

gal•va•niz•ing
gal•va•no•cau•tery
pl gal•va•no•cau•ter•ies
gal•va•nom•e•ter
gal•va•no•sur•gery
pl gal•va•no•sur•ger•ies
gal•va•no•tax•is
pl gal•va•no•tax•es
gal•va•no•trop•ic
gal•va•not•ro•pism
gam•boge
gam•etan•gium
pl gam•etan•gia
ga•mete
ga•met•ic
ga•met•i•cal•ly
ga•me•to•cide
ga•me•to•cyte
ga•me•to•gen•e•sis
pl ga•me•to•gen•e•ses
ga•me•to•gen•ic
or gam•e•tog•e•nous
gam•etog•e•ny
pl gam•etog•e•nies
ga•me•to•go•ni•um
pl ga•me•to•go•nia
gam•e•tog•o•ny
pl gam•e•tog•o•nies
gam•e•toid
ga•me•to•ki•net•ic
gam•ic
gam•ma-ben•zene hexa•chlo•ride
gam•ma•cism
also gam•ma•cis•mus
gam•ma glob•u•lin
gamo•gen•e•sis
pl gamo•gen•e•ses
gam•o•ge•net•ic
gam•o•ge•net•i•cal•ly
gam•one
gam•ont
gan•gli•al
gan•gli•at•ed
also gan•gli•ate
gan•gli•form
gan•gli•o•blast
gan•gli•o•cyte
gan•gli•o•ma
pl gan•gli•o•mas
or gan•gli•o•ma•ta
gan•gli•on
pl gan•glia
also gan•gli•ons
gan•gli•on•at•ed
also gan•gli•on•ate
gan•glio•nec•to•my
pl gan•glio•nec•to•mies
gan•glio•neu•ro•ma
gan•gli•on•ic
gan•gli•on•it•is
gan•gli•o•side
gan•glio•si•do•sis
pl gan•glio•si•do•ses
gan•go•sa
gan•grene
gan•gre•nous
Gan•ser syn•drome
gape•worm
gar•get
gar•goyl•ism
gar•ru•li•ty
pl gar•ru•li•ties
Gart•ner's duct
gas•eous
gas•kin
gas•se•ri•an
gas•ter
Gas•ter•oph•i•lus
gas•tral
gas•tral•gia
gas•tral•gic
gas•trec•to•my
pl gas•trec•to•mies
gas•tric
gas•trin
gas•tri•tis
pl gas•trit•i•des
gas•tro•aceph•a•lus
pl gas•tro•aceph•a•li
gas•tro•anas•to•mo•sis
pl gas•tro•anas•to•mo•ses
gas•tro•cele
gas•troc•ne•mi•al

gas·troc·ne·mi·us
pl gas·troc·ne·mii

gas·tro·coel
also gas·tro·coele

gas·tro·col·ic
gas·tro·co·lot·o·my
pl gas·tro·co·lot·o·mies

gas·tro·di·a·phane
gas·tro·di·aph·a·nos·co·py
pl gas·tro·di·aph·a·nos·co·pies

Gas·tro·dis·coi·des
gas·tro·du·o·de·nal
gas·tro·du·o·de·ni·tis
gas·tro·du·o·de·nos·to·my
pl gas·tro·du·o·de·nos·to·mies

gas·tro·en·ter·ic
gas·tro·en·ter·i·tis
pl gas·tro·en·ter·it·i·des
or gas·tro·en·ter·i·tis·es

gas·tro·en·ter·ol·o·gist
gas·tro·en·ter·ol·o·gy
pl gas·tro·en·ter·ol·o·gies

gas·tro·en·ter·op·a·thy
pl gas·tro·en·ter·op·a·thies

gas·tro·en·ter·os·to·my
pl gas·tro·en·ter·os·to·mies

gas·tro·ep·i·plo·ic
gas·tro·esoph·a·ge·al
gas·tro·esoph·a·gi·tis
gas·tro·ga·vage
gas·tro·gen·ic
gas·tro·graph
gas·tro·he·pat·ic
gas·tro·in·tes·ti·nal
gas·tro·je·ju·nos·to·my
pl gas·tro·je·ju·nos·to·mies

gas·tro·lav·age
gas·tro·li·enal
gas·tro·lith
gas·trol·o·gist
gas·trol·o·gy
pl gas·trol·o·gies

gas·trol·y·sis
pl gas·trol·y·ses

gas·tro·pexy
pl gas·tro·pex·ies

Gas·troph·i·lus
gas·tro·pho·tor
gas·tro·phren·ic
gas·tro·pli·ca·tion

Gas·trop·o·da
gas·trop·o·dous
gas·trop·to·sis
pl gas·trop·to·ses

gas·tror·rha·phy
pl gas·tror·rha·phies

gas·tros·chi·sis
pl gas·tros·chi·ses

gas·tro·scope
gas·tro·scop·ic
gas·tros·co·py
pl gas·tros·co·pies

gas·tro·splen·ic
gas·tros·to·my
pl gas·tros·to·mies

gas·trot·o·my
pl gas·trot·o·mies

gas·tru·la
pl gas·tru·las
or gas·tru·lae

gas·tru·la·tion
gas·tru·late
gas·tru·lat·ed
gas·tru·lat·ing
Gatch bed
Gau·cher's dis·ease
gaul·the·ria
gaul·the·rin
gaunt·let
ga·vage
geel·dik·kop
Gei·ger count·er
or Gei·ger-Mül·ler count·er

gel
gelled

gel·ling
gel·ate
gel·at·ed
gel·at·ing
gel·a·tin
also gel·a·tine
ge·la·ti·ni·za·tion
ge·lat·i·nize
ge·la·tin·ized
ge·la·tin·iz·ing
ge·lat·i·nous
ge·la·tion
gel·ose
gel·se·mine
ge·mel·lus
pl ge·mel·li
also ge·mel·lus·es
gem·i·nate
gem·i·nat·ed
gem·i·nat·ing
gem·i·nate·ly
gem·i·na·tion
gem·i·nous
gem·ma
pl gem·mae
gem·mate
gem·ma·tion
gem·mu·la·tion
gem·mule
ge·na
pl ge·nae
ge·nal
gen·der
ge·ne·al·o·gy
pl ge·ne·al·o·gies
gen·era
pl of genus

gen·er·a·tion
gen·er·a·tive
gen·er·a·tive·ly
ge·ner·ic
ge·net·ic
ge·net·i·cist
ge·net·ics
ge·net·o·tro·phic
ge·ni·al
gen·ic
gen·i·cal·ly
ge·nic·u·late
or ge·nic·u·lat·ed
ge·nic·u·late·ly
ge·nic·u·lum
pl ge·nic·u·la
ge·nio·glos·sus
pl ge·nio·glos·si
ge·nio·hy·oid
ge·ni·on
ge·ni·o·plas·ty
pl ge·nio·plas·ties
gen·i·tal
gen·i·ta·lia
gen·i·tal·i·ty
pl gen·i·tal·i·ties
gen·i·tals
gen·i·to·cru·ral
gen·i·to·fem·o·ral
gen·i·to·uri·nary
geno·der·ma·to·sis
pl geno·der·ma·to·ses
ge·nome
or ge·nom
ge·nom·ic

ge·no·type
ge·no·typ·i·cal
gen·ta·mi·cin
gen·tian
gen·ti·o·bi·ose
gen·ti·o·pic·rin
gen·tis·ic
gen·ti·sin
genu
pl gen·ua
ge·nus
pl gen·era
genu val·gum
genu va·rum
geny·plas·ty
pl geny·plas·ties
geo·med·i·cine
geo·pa·thol·o·gy
pl geo·pa·thol·o·gies
ge·oph·a·gism
ge·oph·a·gy
or geo·pha·gia
pl ge·oph·a·gies
or geo·pha·gi·as
Ge·oph·i·lus
geo·tax·is
or geo·taxy
pl geo·tax·es
or geo·tax·ies
ge·ot·ri·cho·sis
geo·tro·pic
geo·tro·pi·cal·ly
ge·ot·ro·pism
ge·ra·ni·ol
ge·rat·ic
ger·a·tol·o·gy
pl ger·a·tol·o·gies

ger·bil
also ger·bille

ge·ri·at·ric
ger·i·a·tri·cian
ge·ri·at·rics
ge·ri·a·trist
ger·ma·nin
ger·ma·ni·um
Ger·man mea·sles
germ cell
germ·free
ger·mi·cid·al
ger·mi·cide
ger·mi·nal
ger·mi·no·ma
germ lay·er
germ plasm
germ·proof
germy
germ·i·er
germ·i·est
ger·o·der·ma
or ger·o·der·mia

ge·ron·tal
ger·on·tol·o·gy
pl ger·on·tol·o·gies

ge·ron·to·phil·ia
ge·ron·to·ther·a·py
pl ge·ron·to·ther·a·pies

ge·stalt
pl ge·stalt·en
or ge·stalts

ges·tate
ges·tat·ed
ges·tat·ing
ges·ta·tion
ges·to·sis
pl ges·to·ses

gi·ant·ism
giar·dia
giar·di·a·sis
also giar·di·o·sis
pl giar·di·a·ses
also giar·di·o·ses

gib·ber·el·lic
gib·ber·el·lin
gib·ber·ish
gib·bon
gib·bos·i·ty
pl gib·bos·i·ties

gib·bous
adjective
humpbacked (*see* gibbus)

gib·bus
noun
spinal deformity (*see* gibbous)

gib·lets
gi·gan·tism
gil·bert
gill arch
gill cleft
Gill·more nee·dles
gill slit
gilt
or yilt

Gim·ber·nat's lig·a·ment
gin·gi·va
pl gin·gi·vae
gin·gi·val
gin·gi·vec·to·my
pl gin·gi·vec·to·mies

gin·gi·vi·tis
gin·gi·vo·la·bi·al
gin·gi·vo·plas·ty
pl gin·gi·vo·plas·ties

gin·gi·vo·sto·ma·ti·tis
pl gin·gi·vo·sto·ma·tit·i·des
or gin·gi·vo·sto·ma·ti·tis·es

gin·gly·form
gin·gly·mo·ar·thro·dia
gin·gly·mo·ar·thro·di·al
gin·gly·moid
gin·gly·mus
pl gin·gly·mi

Gi·rard re·agent
or Gi·rard's re·agent

gir·dle
gi·tal·in
gi·tog·e·nin
gi·tox·i·gen·in
giz·zard
gla·bel·la
pl gla·bel·lae

gla·brous
glad·i·ate
glad·i·o·lus
pl glad·i·o·li

glairy
glair·i·er
glair·i·est
glan·dered

glan·der·ous
glan·ders
gland of Bar·
  tho·lin
glan·du·la
  pl glan·du·lae
glan·du·lar
glan·du·lous
glans
  pl glan·des
glans cli·to·ri·dis
glans pe·nis
Gla·se·ri·an fis·
  sure
Glas·ser's dis·
  ease
glass·es
Glau·ber's salt
  also Glau·ber salt
glau·co·ma
glau·co·ma·to·
  cy·clit·ic
glau·co·ma·tous
gleety
  gleet·i·er
  gleet·i·est
gle·no·hu·mer·al
gli·a·cyte
gli·a·din
gli·al
glio·blas·to·ma
  pl glio·blas·to·mas
  or glio·blas·to·ma·ta
gli·o·ma
  pl gli·o·mas
  or gli·o·ma·ta
gli·o·ma·to·sis
  pl gli·o·ma·to·ses

gli·o·ma·tous
gli·o·sis
  pl gli·o·ses
glio·tox·in
Glis·son's cap·
  sule
Glo·bid·i·um
glo·bin
glo·bose
glo·bose·ly
glo·bos·i·ty
  pl glo·bos·i·ties
glob·u·lar
glob·ule
glob·u·lin
glo·bus hys·ter·i·
  cus
glo·bus pal·li·dus
glo·mal
glo·man·gi·o·ma
  pl glo·man·gi·o·mas
  or glo·man·gi·o·ma·
    ta
glome
glo·mec·to·my
  pl glo·mec·to·mies
glom·er·ate
glo·mer·u·lar
glo·mer·u·li·tis
glo·mer·u·lo·ne·
  phri·tis
  pl glo·mer·u·lo·ne·
    phrit·i·des
glo·mer·u·lo·scle·
  ro·sis
  pl glo·mer·u·lo·scle·
    ro·ses

glo·mer·u·lose
glo·mer·u·lus
  pl glo·mer·u·li
glo·mus
  pl glom·era
  also glo·mi
glo·mus ca·rot·i·
  cum
glos·sa
  pl glos·sae
  also glos·sas
glos·sal
glos·sal·gia
glos·san·thrax
glos·si·na
glos·si·tis
glos·so·dy·na·
  mom·e·ter
gloss·odyn·ia
glos·so·graph
glos·so·hy·al
glos·so·kin·es·
  thet·ic
glos·so·la·lia
glos·sol·o·gy
  pl glos·sol·o·gies
glos·so·pal·a·ti·
  nus
  pl glos·so·pal·a·ti·ni
glos·sop·a·thy
  pl glos·sop·a·thies
glos·so·pha·ryn·
  geal
glot·tal
glot·tic
glot·tis
  pl glot·tis·es
  or glot·ti·des

glot·tol·o·gy
pl glot·tol·o·gies

glu·ca·gon
glu·car·ic
glu·cide
glu·co·ascor·bic
glu·co·cor·ti·coid
glu·co·ki·nase
glu·co·kin·in
glu·co·lip·id
also glu·co·lip·ide

glu·col·y·sis
pl glu·col·y·ses

glu·co·neo·gen·e·sis
pl glu·co·neo·gen·e·ses

glu·con·ic
glu·co·pro·tein
glu·co·py·ra·nose
glu·co·san
glu·cose
glu·cose-1-phos·phate
glu·cose-6-phos·phate
glu·co·si·dase
glu·co·side
glu·co·sid·ic
glu·co·sid·i·cal·ly
glu·co·sone
glu·cos·uria
gluc·uron·ic
gluc·uron·i·dase
gluc·uro·nide
glu·ta·mate
glu·tam·ic
glu·ta·min·ase
glu·ta·mine
glu·ta·min·ic
glu·tar·al·de·hyde
glu·tar·ic
glu·ta·thi·one
glu·te·al
glu·te·lin
glu·ten
glu·te·nin
glu·teo·fem·o·ral
glu·teth·i·mide
glu·te·us
pl glu·tei

glu·ti·nous
glu·tose
gly·can
gly·ce·mia
also gly·cae·mia

gly·ce·mic
glyc·er·al·de·hyde
gly·cer·ic
glyc·er·ide
glyc·er·id·ic
glyc·er·in
or glyc·er·ine

glyc·er·ite
glyc·er·ol
glyc·ero·phos·phate
glyc·ero·phos·pho·ric
glyc·er·ose
gly·cine
gly·cin·uria
gly·co·chol·ate
gly·co·chol·ic
gly·co·coll
gly·co·cy·amine
gly·co·gen
gly·co·gen·e·sis
pl gly·co·gen·e·ses

gly·co·ge·net·ic
gly·co·gen·ic
gly·co·ge·nol·y·sis
pl gly·co·ge·nol·y·ses

gly·cog·e·nous
gly·col
gly·col·al·de·hyde
gly·co·late
gly·col·ic
also gly·col·lic

gly·co·lip·id
also gly·co·lip·ide

gly·col·y·sis
pl gly·col·y·ses

gly·co·lyt·ic
gly·co·neo·gen·e·sis
pl gly·co·neo·gen·e·ses

gly·co·pep·tide
gly·co·pro·tein
gly·co·pty·a·lism
gly·cor·rhea
gly·co·si·a·lia
gly·co·si·dase
gly·co·side
gly·co·sid·ic
gly·cos·uria
gly·cos·u·ric
gly·co·tro·pic
also gly·co·tro·phic

glyc·ure·sis
pl glyc·ure·ses

glyc·uron·ic
glyc·yr·rhi·zic
glyc·yr·rhi·zin
gly·ox·al
gly·ox·a·lase
gly·ox·a·line
gly·ox·yl·ic
gnath·al·gia
gnath·ic
or gna·thal

gna·thi·on
Gna·thos·to·ma
gna·thos·to·mi·a·sis
pl gna·thos·to·mi·a·ses

gno·to·bi·ol·o·gy
pl gno·to·bi·ol·o·gies

gno·to·bi·ote
gno·to·bi·ot·ic
gno·to·bi·ot·i·cal·ly
gno·to·bi·ot·ics
gob·let cell
goi·ter
also goi·tre

goi·tro·gen
goi·tro·gen·ic
also goi·ter·o·gen·ic

goi·tro·ge·nic·i·ty
pl goi·tro·ge·nic·i·ties

Gol·gi ap·pa·ra·tus
also Gol·gi com·plex

Gol·gi body
gom·pho·sis
pl gom·pho·ses

go·nad
go·nad·al
go·nad·ec·to·my
pl go·nad·ec·to·mies

go·nad·ec·to·mize
go·nad·ec·to·mized
go·nad·ec·to·miz·ing
go·nad·o·tro·phic
or go·nad·o·tro·pic

go·nad·o·tro·phin
or go·nad·o·tro·pin

go·nal·gia
gon·ar·throc·ace
gon·ar·throt·o·my
pl gon·ar·throt·o·mies

gon·e·cys·to·lith
gon·e·poi·e·sis
pl gon·e·poi·e·ses

go·nio·cra·ni·om·e·try
pl go·nio·cra·ni·om·e·tries

go·ni·om·e·ter
go·ni·on
pl go·nia

go·nio·scope
go·nio·scop·ic
go·ni·os·co·py
pl go·ni·os·co·pies

go·ni·tis

gono·coc·cal
or gon·o·coc·cic

gono·coc·cus
pl gono·coc·ci

gono·cyte
gono·duct
also gon·a·duct

gono·gen·e·sis
pl gono·gen·e·ses

go·nom·ery
pl go·nom·er·ies

gono·phore
gon·or·rhea
gon·or·rhe·al
go·ny·au·lax
Gooch cru·ci·ble
or Gooch fil·ter

goose bumps
goose·flesh
goose pim·ples
gorge
gorged
gorg·ing
gor·get
gos·sy·pol
goun·dou
pl goun·dous

gout·i·ness
gouty
gout·i·er
gout·i·est
Gow·er's tract
Graaf·ian fol·li·cle
grac·i·lis

gra•di•ent
Gra•ham's law
gram•i•ci•din
gram•i•niv•o•rous
gram•mol•e•cule
or gram-mo•lec•u•lar weight

gram-neg•a•tive
gram-pos•i•tive
Gram's meth•od
Gram's so•lu•tion
Gram stain
also Gram's stain

gram-vari•able
gra•na
pl of granum

gra•na•tum
gran•di•ose
grand mal
gran•ule
gran•u•lar
gran•u•late
gran•u•lat•ed
gran•u•lat•ing
gran•u•la•tion
gran•u•lo•blast
gran•u•lo•blas•tic
gran•u•lo•blas•to•sis
pl gran•u•lo•blas•to•ses

gran•u•lo•cyte
gran•u•lo•cy•to•pe•nia
gran•u•lo•cy•to•pe•nic
gran•u•lo•cy•to•poi•e•sis
pl gran•u•lo•cy•to•poi•e•ses

gran•u•lo•cy•to•sis
pl gran•u•lo•cy•to•ses

gran•u•lo•ma
pl gran•u•lo•mas
or gran•u•lo•ma•ta

gran•u•lo•ma in•gui•na•le
or gran•u•lo•ma ve•ne•re•um

gran•u•lo•ma py•o•gen•i•cum
gran•u•lo•ma•to•sis
pl gran•u•lo•ma•to•ses

gran•u•lom•a•tous
gran•u•lo•pe•nia
gran•u•lo•plas•tic
gran•u•lo•poi•e•sis
pl gran•u•lo•poi•e•ses

gran•u•lo•sa
gran•u•lo•sis
pl gran•u•lo•ses

gra•num
pl gra•na

graph•ite
gra•phit•ic
graph•o•log•i•cal
gra•phol•o•gy
pl gra•phol•o•gies

grapho•mo•tor
graph•or•rhea
grapho•spasm
grat•tage
grav•el
grav•el-blind
Graves' dis•ease
grav•id
grav•i•da
pl grav•i•das
or grav•i•dae

gra•vid•ic
gra•vid•i•ty
pl gra•vid•i•ties

grav•id•ness
grav•i•do•car•di•ac
gra•vi•me•ter
grav•i•met•ric
also grav•i•met•ri•cal

grav•i•met•ri•cal•ly
gra•vim•e•try
pl gra•vim•e•tries

grav•i•ty
pl grav•i•ties

gray•out
green•sick•ness
green soap
green•stick frac•ture
gref•fo•tome
greg•a•loid
Greg•a•ri•na
greg•a•rine
greg•a•rin•i•an
Greg•a•rin•i•da
greg•a•ri•no•sis
pl greg•a•ri•no•ses

Greg•o•ry's pow•der

grin·de·lia
grind·ing
gripp·al
grippe
gris·eo·ful·vin
gris·tle
gro·cer's itch
group prac·tice
group ther·a·py
or group psy·cho·ther·a·py
grow
grew
grown
grow·ing
growth
gru·el
grunt·ing
gry·po·sis
pl gry·po·ses
guai·a·col
guai·a·cum
or guai·ac
gua·nase
gua·neth·i·dine
gua·ni·dine
gua·nine
gua·no·phore
gua·no·sine
gua·nyl·ic
gua·ra·na
gu·ber·nac·u·lum
pl gu·ber·nac·u·la
Guil·lain-Bar·ré syn·drome
guil·lo·tine
guin·ea pig
guin·ea worm
gu·lar
gul·let
gu·lose
gum ar·a·bic
gum·boil
gum·ma
pl gum·mas
also gum·ma·ta
gum·ma·tous
gum·my
gum·mi·er
gum·mi·est
gur·ney
pl gur·neys
gus·ta·tion
gus·ta·tive
gus·ta·to·ri·al
gus·ta·to·ri·al·ly
gus·ta·to·ri·ly
gus·ta·to·ry
gut·ta
pl gut·tae
gut·ta-per·cha
gut·tate
gut·tie
gut·tur·al
Gut·zeit test
gyn·an·drism
gyn·an·droid
gyn·an·dro·morph
gyn·an·dro·mor·phism
gyn·an·dro·mor·phous
gyn·atre·sia
gy·ne·co·gen·ic
gy·ne·cog·ra·phy
pl gy·ne·cog·ra·phies
gy·ne·coid
gy·ne·co·log·ic
gy·ne·col·o·gy
pl gy·ne·col·o·gies
gy·ne·co·mas·tia
gy·no·gam·one
gy·no·gen·e·sis
pl gy·no·gen·e·ses
gyre
gy·rec·to·my
pl gy·rec·to·mies
gyr·en·ceph·a·late
also gyr·en·ce·phal·ic
or gyr·en·ceph·a·lous
gy·rose
gy·ro·spasm
gy·rus
pl gy·ri

H

ha·ben·u·la
pl ha·ben·u·lae
hab·it
hab·it-form·ing
ha·bit·u·ate
ha·bit·u·at·ed
ha·bit·u·at·ing
ha·bit·u·a·tion
hab·i·tus
pl hab·i·tus
Hab·ro·ne·ma

hab·ro·ne·mi·a·sis
also hab·ro·ne·mo·sis
haem
var of heme
Hae·ma·dip·sa
Hae·ma·moe·ba
Hae·ma·phy·sa·lis
Hae·ma·to·pi·nus
hae·ma·tox·y·lon
hae·min
var of he·min
hae·mo·bar·ton·el·la
pl hae·mo·bar·ton·el·lae
hae·mo·glo·bin
var of hemoglobin
Hae·mo·greg·a·ri·na
hae·mo·greg·a·rine
or he·mo·greg·a·rine
Hae·mon·chus
Hae·mo·pro·te·us
haem·or·rha·gia
Hae·mo·spo·rid·ia
hae·mo·spo·rid·ian
ha·la·tion
hal·a·zone
half-blood·ed
half-bred
half-breed
half-caste
half-life
hal·i·but-liv·er oil
ha·lide
hal·i·ste·re·sis
hal·i·ste·ret·ic
hal·i·to·sis
pl hal·i·to·ses
hal·lu·ci·nate
hal·lu·ci·nat·ed
hal·lu·ci·nat·ing
hal·lu·ci·na·tion
hal·lu·ci·na·tive
hal·lu·ci·na·to·ry
hal·lu·ci·no·gen
hal·lu·ci·no·gen·ic
hal·lu·ci·no·sis
pl hal·lu·ci·no·ses
hal·lux
pl hal·lu·ces
hal·o·ge·ton
ha·lom·e·ter
halo·per·i·dol
halo·phil
halo·phile
halo·phil·ic
or ha·loph·i·lous
halo·thane
hal·zoun
Ham·a·me·lis
ha·mar·tia
ham·ar·to·ma
pl ham·ar·to·mas
or ham·ar·to·ma·ta
ham·ar·to·ma·tous
ha·mate
ha·ma·tum
pl ha·ma·ta
or ha·ma·tums
ham·mer
ham·mer·toe
ham·string
ham·u·lar
ham·u·lus
pl ham·u·li
hand·ed·ness
hand·i·cap
hand·piece
Hand-Schül·ler-Chris·tian dis·ease
hang·nail
hang·over
hang-up
han·sen·osis
han·sen·ot·ic
Han·sen's ba·cil·lus
pl Han·sen's ba·cil·li
Han·sen's dis·ease
hap·lo·dont
hap·lo·don·ty
pl hap·lo·don·ties
hap·loid
hap·loi·dy
pl hap·loi·dies
hap·lol·o·gy
pl hap·lol·o·gies
hap·lont

hap·lon·tic
hap·lo·scope
hap·lo·scop·ic
hap·lo·type
hap·lo·typ·ic
hap·ten
  also hap·tene
hap·ten·ic
hap·tic
  or hap·ti·cal
hap·to·glo·bin
hap·to·phore
hard·en·ing
hard-of-hear·ing
Har·dy-Wein·berg law
  also Har·dy-Wein·berg prin·ci·ple
hare·lip
hare·lipped
har·ma·line
har·ma·lol
har·mine
har·mo·nia
har·mon·ic
har·mo·ny
  pl har·mo·nies
har·poon
harts·horn
hash·ish
haus·to·ri·um
  pl haus·to·ria
haus·tral
haus·trat·ed
haus·tra·tion
haus·trum
  pl haus·tra
haus·tus
  pl haus·tus
ha·ver·sian
head·ache
head·achy
head·lock
head·shrink·er
health·ful
healthy
  health·i·er
  health·i·est
heart·beat
heart·burn
heart-lung
heart·wa·ter
heart·worm
heat·stroke
heavy chain
he·be·phre·nia
he·be·phre·nic
Heb·er·den's node
he·bet·ic
heb·e·tude
hec·tic
hec·ti·cal·ly
hede·o·ma
he·don·ic
he·don·i·cal·ly
he·do·nism
he·do·nist
he·do·nis·tic
he·li·an·thin
  also he·li·an·thine
hel·i·coid
  or hel·i·coi·dal
hel·i·co·ru·bin
hel·i·co·tre·ma
he·lio·phobe
he·li·o·sis
  pl he·li·o·ses
he·lio·tax·is
  pl he·lio·tax·es
he·lio·ther·a·py
  pl he·lio·ther·a·pies
he·lio·tro·pic
he·lio·tro·pi·cal·ly
he·li·ot·ro·pin
he·li·ot·ro·pism
He·lio·zoa
he·lio·zo·an
he·lio·zo·ic
he·li·um
he·lix
  pl he·li·ces
  also he·lix·es
he·lix·in
hel·le·bore
hel·le·bo·rine
hel·minth
  pl hel·minths
hel·min·thi·a·sis
  pl hel·min·thi·a·ses
hel·min·thic
hel·min·thoid
hel·min·thol·o·gy
  pl hel·min·thol·o·gies
He·lo·der·ma
he·lo·ma
  pl he·lo·mas
  or he·lo·ma·ta
he·lot·o·my
  pl he·lot·o·mies

he·ma·cy·tom·e·ter
or he·mo·cy·tom·e·ter

he·mad

he·ma·dy·na·mom·e·ter

hem·ag·glu·ti·nate
hem·ag·glu·ti·nat·ed
hem·ag·glu·ti·nat·ing

hem·ag·glu·ti·na·tion

hem·ag·glu·ti·nin
or he·mo·ag·glu·ti·nin

he·mal

he·man·gi·ec·ta·sis
pl he·man·gi·ec·ta·ses

he·man·gio·blas·to·ma
pl he·man·gio·blas·to·mas
or he·man·gio·blas·to·ma·ta

he·man·gio·en·do·the·li·o·ma
pl he·man·gio·en·do·the·li·o·mas
or he·man·gio·en·do·the·li·o·ma·ta

hem·an·gi·o·ma
pl hem·an·gi·o·mas
also hem·an·gi·o·ma·ta

hem·an·gi·o·ma·to·sis
pl hem·an·gi·o·ma·to·ses

hem·an·gio·sar·co·ma
pl hem·an·gio·sar·co·mas
or hem·an·gio·sar·co·ma·ta

he·ma·poi·e·sis
or he·mo·poi·e·sis
pl he·ma·poi·e·ses
or he·mo·poi·e·ses

hem·ar·thro·sis
pl hem·ar·thro·ses

he·ma·tein

he·ma·therm

he·ma·ther·mal
or he·ma·ther·mous

he·mat·ic

he·ma·tid

he·ma·ti·dro·sis

he·ma·tim·e·ter

he·ma·tin

he·ma·ti·ne·mia

he·ma·tin·ic

he·ma·tin·om·e·ter

he·ma·tin·o·met·ric

he·ma·ti·nu·ria

he·ma·to·blast

he·ma·to·blas·tic

he·ma·to·cele

he·ma·to·chy·lu·ria

he·ma·to·col·pos
or he·ma·to·col·pus

he·ma·to·crit

he·ma·to·cry·al

he·ma·to·cyst

he·ma·to·cyte

he·ma·tog·e·nous

he·ma·to·gone
or he·ma·to·go·nia

he·ma·toid

he·ma·toi·din

he·ma·to·log·ic
or he·ma·to·log·i·cal

he·ma·tol·o·gist

he·ma·tol·o·gy
pl he·ma·tol·o·gies

he·ma·to·lymph·an·gi·o·ma
pl he·ma·to·lymph·an·gi·o·mas
or he·ma·to·lymph·an·gi·o·ma·ta

he·ma·tol·y·sis
pl he·ma·tol·y·ses

he·ma·to·lyt·ic

he·ma·to·ma
pl he·ma·to·mas
also he·ma·to·ma·ta

he·ma·tom·e·ter

he·ma·to·me·tra

he·ma·to·my·e·lia

he·ma·to·my·eli·tis
pl he·ma·to·my·eli·tis·es
also he·ma·to·my·elit·i·des

he·ma·toph·a·gous

he·ma·to·poi·e·sis
pl he·ma·to·poi·e·ses

he•ma•to•poi•et•ic
he•ma•to•poi•et•i•cal•ly
he•ma•to•por•phy•rin
he•ma•to•por•phy•ri•ne•mia
he•ma•tor•rha•chis
he•ma•to•sal•pinx
pl he•ma•to•sal•pin•ges

he•ma•to•scope
hem•a•to•sper•mato•cele
he•ma•to•ther•mal
he•ma•tox•y•lin
he•ma•to•zo•an
he•ma•to•zo•on
pl he•ma•to•zoa

he•ma•tu•ria
hem•au•to•graph
hem•au•to•graph•ic
hem•au•tog•ra•phy
heme
also haem

hem•er•a•lo•pia
hem•er•a•lo•pic
hemi•ac•e•tal
hemi•an•al•ge•sia
hemi•an•es•the•sia
hemi•anop•sia
also hemi•ano•pia

hemi•anop•tic
hemi•atax•ia
hemi•at•ro•phy
pl hemi•at•ro•phies

hemi•bal•lism
also hemi•bal•lis•mus

he•mic
hemi•car•dia
hemi•cel•lu•lose
hemi•cel•lu•los•ic
hemi•cen•trum
pl hemi•cen•trums
or hemi•cen•tra

hemi•ce•re•brum
pl hemi•ce•re•brums
or hemi•ce•re•bra

hemi•cho•rea
hemi•co•lec•to•my
pl hemi•co•lec•to•mies

hemi•cra•nia
hemi•dys•tro•phy
pl hemi•dys•tro•phies

hemi•fa•cial
hemi•glo•bin
hemi•glos•sec•to•my
pl hemi•glos•sec•to•mies

hemi•hy•per•tro•phy
pl hemi•hy•per•tro•phies

hemi•hyp•es•the•sia
hemi•kar•y•on
hemi•kar•y•ot•ic

hemi•lam•i•nec•to•my
pl hemi•lam•i•nec•to•mies

hemi•lar•yn•gec•to•my
pl hemi•lar•yn•gec•to•mies

hemi•lat•er•al
hemi•man•dib•u•lec•to•my
pl hemi•man•dib•u•lec•to•mies

he•min
also hae•min

hemi•ne•phrec•to•my
pl hemi•ne•phrec•to•mies

hemi•o•pia
or hemi•op•sia

hemi•op•ic
hemi•pa•re•sis
pl hemi•par•e•ses

hemi•pel•vec•to•my
pl hemi•pel•vec•to•mies

hemi•ple•gia
hemi•ple•gic
He•mip•tera
he•mip•ter•an
also he•mip•ter•on

he•mip•ter•ous
hemi•sect
hemi•sec•tion
hemi•sphere

hemi·spher·ec·to·my
pl hemi·spher·ec·to·mies

hemi·spher·ic
or hemi·spher·i·cal

hemi·tho·rax
pl hemi·tho·rax·es
or hemi·tho·ra·ces

hemi·zy·gote
hemi·zy·gous
hem·lock
he·mo·ag·glu·ti·nin
var of hemagglutinin

he·mo·blast
he·mo·chro·ma·to·sis
pl he·mo·chro·ma·to·ses

he·mo·chrome
he·mo·chro·mo·gen
he·mo·clas·tic
he·mo·con·cen·tra·tion
he·mo·co·nia
also he·mo·ko·nia

he·mo·co·ni·o·sis
pl he·mo·co·ni·o·ses

he·mo·cu·pre·in
he·mo·cy·a·nin
he·mo·cyte
he·mo·cy·to·blast
he·mo·cy·to·blas·tic
he·mo·cy·tom·e·ter
var of hemacytometer

he·mo·di·al·y·sis
pl he·mo·di·al·y·ses

he·mo·di·lu·tion
he·mo·dy·nam·ic
he·mo·dy·nam·i·cal·ly
he·mo·dy·nam·ics
he·mo·fla·gel·late
he·mo·fus·cin
he·mo·glo·bin
also hae·mo·glo·bin

he·mo·glo·bi·ne·mia
he·mo·glo·bin·ic
he·mo·glo·bi·nom·e·ter
he·mo·glo·bi·nom·e·try
pl he·mo·glo·bi·nom·e·tries

he·mo·glo·bin·op·a·thy
pl he·mo·glo·bin·op·a·thies

he·mo·glo·bin·ous
he·mo·glo·bin·uria
he·mo·glo·bin·uric
he·mo·gram
he·mo·greg·a·rine
var of haemogregarine

he·mo·his·tio·blast
he·mo·ko·nia
var of hemoconia

he·mo·lymph
he·mo·ly·sin
he·mo·ly·sis
pl he·mo·ly·ses

he·mo·lyt·ic
he·mo·lyze
he·mo·lyzed
he·mo·lyz·ing
he·mom·e·ter
he·mo·met·ric
he·mom·e·try
pl he·mom·e·tries

he·mop·a·thy
pl he·mop·a·thies

he·mo·peri·car·di·um
pl he·mo·peri·car·dia

he·mo·peri·to·ne·um
pl he·mo·peri·to·ne·ums
or he·mo·peri·to·nea

he·mo·phage
he·mo·pha·gia
he·mo·phago·cyte
he·mo·phago·cyt·ic
he·moph·a·gous
he·mo·phile
he·mo·phil·ia
he·mo·phil·i·ac
he·mo·phil·ic

He·moph·i·lus
he·mo·pho·bia
he·mo·pneu·mo·tho·rax
pl he·mo·pneu·mo·tho·rax·es
or he·mo·pneu·mo·tho·ra·ces
he·mo·poi·e·sis
var of hemapoiesis
he·mo·poi·et·ic
he·mo·poi·etin
he·mo·pro·tein
He·mo·pro·te·us
he·mop·ty·sis
pl he·mop·ty·ses
hem·or·rhage
hem·or·rhag·ic
hem·or·rhag·in
hem·or·rhoid
hem·or·rhoid·al
hem·or·rhoid·ec·to·my
pl hem·or·rhoid·ec·to·mies
he·mo·sal·pinx
pl he·mo·sal·pin·ges
he·mo·sid·er·in
he·mo·sid·er·o·sis
pl he·mo·sid·er·o·ses
he·mo·sid·er·ot·ic
He·mo·spo·rid·ia
he·mo·sta·sis
pl he·mo·sta·ses
he·mo·stat
he·mo·stat·ic
he·mo·tho·rax
pl he·mo·tho·rax·es
or he·mo·tho·ra·ces
he·mo·tox·in
he·mot·ro·phe
he·mo·zo·on
pl he·mo·zoa
hen·bane
Hen·le's loop
Hen·le's sheath
he·par
hep·a·rin
hep·a·rin·iza·tion
hep·a·rin·ize
hep·a·rin·ized
hep·a·rin·iz·ing
hep·a·tec·to·mize
hep·a·tec·to·mized
hep·a·tec·to·miz·ing
hep·a·tec·to·my
pl hep·a·tec·to·mies
he·pat·ic
he·pat·i·ca
he·pat·i·co·du·o·de·nos·to·my
pl he·pat·i·co·du·o·de·nos·to·mies
he·pat·i·co·li·thot·o·my
pl he·pat·i·co·li·thot·o·mies
hep·a·ti·tis
pl hep·a·tit·i·des
hep·a·ti·za·tion
hep·a·tize
hep·a·tized
hep·a·tiz·ing
he·pa·to·cel·lu·lar
he·pa·to·cu·pre·in
he·pa·to·cyte
he·pa·to·gen·ic
or hep·a·tog·e·nous
hep·a·to·ma
pl hep·a·to·mas
or hep·a·to·ma·ta
hep·a·to·me·gal·ic
hep·a·to·meg·a·ly
pl hep·a·to·meg·a·lies
hep·a·top·a·thy
pl hep·a·top·a·thies
hep·a·to·pexy
pl hep·a·to·pex·ies
hep·a·to·por·tal
hep·a·tos·co·py
pl hep·a·tos·co·pies
hep·a·to·spleno·meg·a·ly
pl hep·a·to·spleno·meg·a·lies
hep·a·to·tox·ic
hep·a·to·tox·ic·i·ty
pl hep·a·to·tox·ic·i·ties
hep·a·to·tox·in
hep·tad
hep·tose
hep·tu·lose
herb·al
herb·al·ist
her·bi·cid·al
her·bi·cid·al·ly
her·bi·cide
her·biv·o·rous

he·red·i·tar·i·an
he·red·i·tar·i·an·ism
he·red·i·tar·i·ly
he·red·i·tary
he·red·i·ty
pl he·red·i·ties
her·i·ta·bil·i·ty
pl her·i·ta·bil·i·ties
her·i·ta·ble
her·i·tage
her·maph·ro·dism
her·maph·ro·dite
her·maph·ro·dit·ic
her·maph·ro·dit·ism
her·met·ic
also her·met·i·cal
her·met·i·cal·ly
her·nia
pl her·ni·as
or her·ni·ae
her·ni·al
her·ni·ate
her·ni·at·ed
her·ni·at·ing
her·ni·a·tion
her·ni·or·rha·phy
pl her·ni·or·rha·phies
her·ni·ot·o·my
pl her·ni·ot·o·mies
her·o·in
her·o·in·ism
her·pan·gi·na
her·pes
her·pes sim·plex
her·pes·vi·rus
her·pet·ic
her·pet·i·form
Her·pe·tom·o·nas
hes·per·i·din
hes·per·i·tin
also hes·per·e·tin
Het·er·a·kis
het·er·ax·i·al
het·er·ecious
var of heteroecious
het·ero·ag·glu·ti·nin
het·ero·au·to·tro·phic
het·ero·aux·in
het·ero·blas·tic
het·ero·blas·ty
pl het·ero·blas·ties
het·ero·cary·on
var of heterokaryon
het·ero·cary·o·sis
var of heterokaryosis
het·ero·cary·ot·ic
var of heterokaryotic
het·ero·cel·lu·lar
het·ero·chro·mat·ic
het·ero·chro·ma·tin
het·ero·chro·mia
het·ero·chro·mo·some
het·ero·chro·mous
or het·ero·chro·mic
het·er·och·ro·nism
also het·er·och·ro·ny
pl het·er·och·ro·nisms
also het·er·och·ro·nies
het·ero·crine
het·ero·cy·cle
het·ero·cy·clic
het·ero·cyst
het·er·odont
het·er·oe·cious
or het·er·ecious
het·er·oe·cism
het·ero·erot·ic
het·ero·er·o·tism
het·ero·ga·mete
het·ero·ga·met·ic
het·er·og·a·mous
het·er·og·a·my
pl het·er·og·a·mies
het·er·o·ge·ne·ity
pl het·er·o·ge·ne·i·ties
het·er·o·ge·neous
het·er·o·ge·neous·ness
het·ero·gen·e·sis
pl het·ero·gen·e·ses
het·ero·ge·net·ic
het·er·o·gen·ic
het·er·og·e·nous
het·ero·gon·ic
het·er·og·o·ny
pl het·er·og·o·nies

het·ero·graft
het·ero·kary·on
also het·ero·cary·on
het·ero·kary·o·sis
also het·ero·cary·o·sis
het·ero·kary·ot·ic
also het·ero·cary·ot·ic
het·er·ol·o·gous
het·er·ol·o·gy
pl het·er·ol·o·gies
het·ero·ly·sin
het·ero·ly·sis
pl het·ero·ly·ses
het·ero·lyt·ic
het·ero·mas·ti·gote
or het·ero·mas·ti·gate
het·er·om·er·ous
het·ero·mor·phic
or het·ero·mor·phous
het·ero·mor·phism
het·ero·mor·pho·sis
pl het·ero·mor·pho·ses
het·er·on·o·mous
het·er·on·y·mous
het·ero·phe·my
pl het·ero·phe·mies
het·ero·phile
or het·ero·phil
het·ero·pho·ria
het·ero·phor·ic
Het·ero·phy·es
het·ero·phy·id
het·ero·pla·sia
het·ero·plasm
het·ero·plas·tic
het·ero·plas·ti·cal·ly
het·ero·plas·ty
pl het·ero·plas·ties
het·ero·ploid
het·ero·ploi·dy
pl het·ero·ploi·dies
het·ero·pyc·no·sis
also het·ero·pyk·no·sis
het·ero·pyc·not·ic
also het·ero·pyk·not·ic
het·ero·scope
het·er·os·co·py
pl het·er·os·co·pies
het·ero·sex·u·al
het·ero·sex·u·al·i·ty
pl het·ero·sex·u·al·i·ties
het·ero·sex·u·al·ly
het·er·o·sis
pl het·er·o·ses
het·ero·some
het·ero·spo·rous
het·ero·tax·ic
het·ero·tax·is
also het·ero·tax·ia
pl het·ero·tax·es
also het·ero·tax·i·as
het·er·ot·ic
het·ero·to·pia
also het·er·ot·o·py
pl het·ero·to·pias
also het·er·ot·o·pies
het·ero·top·ic
het·er·ot·o·pous
het·ero·trans·plant
het·ero·trans·plan·ta·tion
het·ero·tri·cho·sis
pl het·ero·tri·cho·ses
het·ero·troph
het·ero·tro·phic
het·ero·tro·phi·cal·ly
het·er·ot·ro·phism
het·er·ot·ro·phy
pl het·er·ot·ro·phies
het·ero·tro·pia
het·ero·typ·ic
also het·ero·typ·i·cal
het·ero·xan·thine
also het·ero·xan·thin
het·ero·zy·go·sis
pl het·ero·zy·go·ses
het·ero·zy·gos·i·ty
pl het·ero·zy·gos·i·ties
het·ero·zy·gote
het·ero·zy·got·ic
het·ero·zy·gous
hexa·bi·ose
or hexo·bi·ose
hex·a·canth
or hex·a·can·thous
hexa·chlo·ro·cy·clo·hex·ane

hexa·chlo·ro·eth·ane
or hexa·chlor·eth·ane
hexa·chlo·ro·phene
hexa·chro·mic
hexa·dec·a·no·ic
hexa·me·tho·ni·um
hexa·meth·y·lene·tet·ra·mine
hex·amine
Hex·am·i·ta
hex·am·i·ti·a·sis
hex·a·no·ic
hexa·ploid
hexa·ploi·dy
hex·es·trol
also hex·oes·trol
hexo·bar·bi·tal
hexo·bi·ose
var of hexabiose
hexo·ki·nase
hex·os·amine
hex·o·san
hex·ose
hex·ulose
hex·uron·ic
hex·yl·res·or·cin·ol
hi·a·tal
hi·a·tus
hi·ber·nate
hi·ber·nat·ed
hi·ber·nat·ing
hi·ber·na·tion
hic·cup
also hic·cough
hi·drad·e·ni·tis
hi·drad·e·no·ma
pl hi·drad·e·no·mas
or hi·drad·e·no·ma·ta
hi·dro·sis
pl hi·dro·ses
hi·drot·ic
high-en·er·gy
high-strung
hill·ock
Hill re·ac·tion
hi·lum
pl hi·la
hi·lus
pl hi·li
hind·brain
hind·gut
hip·bone
Hip·pe·la·tes
Hip·po·bos·ca
hip·po·bos·cid
Hip·po·bos·ci·dae
hip·po·cam·pal
hip·po·cam·pus
pl hip·po·cam·pi
Hip·po·crat·ic
Hip·poc·ra·tism
hip·pol·o·gy
pl hip·pol·o·gies
hip·pu·rate
hip·pu·ric
hip·pu·ri·case
hip·pus
hir·sute
hir·sute·ness
hir·su·ti·es
pl hir·su·ti·es
hir·sut·ism
hir·tel·lous
hi·ru·din
Hir·u·din·ea
hir·u·din·e·an
hir·u·di·ni·a·sis
pl hir·u·di·ni·a·ses
Hir·u·din·i·dae
Hi·ru·do
his·ta·mi·nase
his·ta·mine
his·ta·min·er·gic
his·ta·min·ic
his·ti·dase
his·ti·dine
his·tio·cyte
his·tio·cyt·ic
his·tio·cy·to·ma
pl his·tio·cy·to·mas
also his·tio·cy·to·ma·ta
his·tio·cy·to·sis
pl his·tio·cy·to·ses
his·ti·oid
his·to·blast
his·to·chem·i·cal
his·to·chem·i·cal·ly
his·to·chem·is·try
pl his·to·chem·is·tries
his·to·chem·o·graph

his·to·che·mog·ra·phy
pl his·to·che·mog·ra·phies

his·to·com·pat·i·bil·i·ty
pl his·to·com·pat·i·bil·i·ties

his·to·com·pat·i·ble
his·to·cyte
his·to·gen·e·sis
pl his·to·gen·e·ses

his·to·ge·net·ic
his·to·ge·net·i·cal·ly
his·to·gen·ic
his·tog·e·ny
pl his·tog·e·nies

his·to·gram
his·toid
his·to·log·i·cal
or his·to·log·ic

his·to·log·i·cal·ly
his·tol·o·gist
his·tol·o·gy
pl his·tol·o·gies

his·tol·y·sis
pl his·tol·y·ses

his·to·lyt·ic
His·tom·o·nas
his·to·mo·ni·a·sis
his·tone
his·to·path·o·log·ic
or his·to·path·o·log·i·cal

his·to·path·o·log·i·cal·ly
his·to·pa·thol·o·gist
his·to·pa·thol·o·gy
pl his·to·pa·thol·o·gies

his·to·phys·i·o·log·i·cal
or his·to·phys·i·o·log·ic

his·to·phys·i·ol·o·gy
pl his·to·phys·i·ol·o·gies

his·to·plas·ma
his·to·plas·min
his·to·plas·mo·sis
pl his·to·plas·mo·ses

his·to·ry
pl his·to·ries

his·to·tox·ic
his·to·tox·in
his·to·troph
or his·to·trophe

his·tot·ro·pism
his·to·zo·ic
hoarse·ness
Hodg·kin's dis·ease
Hof·meis·ter se·ries
hol·an·dric
hol·an·dry
pl hol·an·dries

ho·lid·ic
ho·lism
ho·lis·tic
ho·lis·ti·cal·ly
ho·lo·blas·tic
ho·lo·blas·ti·cal·ly
ho·lo·crine
ho·lo·en·zyme
ho·log·a·mous
ho·log·a·my
pl ho·log·a·mies

ho·lo·gram
ho·lo·graph
ho·lo·graph·ic
ho·lo·graph·i·cal·ly
ho·log·ra·phy
pl ho·log·ra·phies

ho·lo·gy·nic
ho·log·y·ny
pl ho·log·y·nies

ho·lo·mas·ti·gote
ho·lo·mor·pho·sis
pl ho·lo·mor·pho·ses

ho·lo·phyt·ic
ho·lo·zo·ic
Ho·man's sign
hom·at·ro·pine
hom·ax·i·al
ho·meo·mor·phous
ho·meo·path
ho·meo·path·ic
ho·meo·path·i·cal·ly
ho·me·op·a·thy
pl ho·me·op·a·thies

ho·meo·pla·sia

ho•meo•plas•tic
ho•meo•sta•sis
pl ho•meo•sta•ses
ho•meo•stat•ic
ho•meo•typ•ic
home•sick
home•sick•ness
ho•mi•ci•dal
ho•mi•cid•al•ly
ho•mi•cide
hom•i•nid
also ho•min•ian
Ho•min•i•dae
hom•i•ni•za•tion
hom•i•nized
ho•mo
pl ho•mos
hom•i•noid
Hom•i•noi•dea
ho•mo•blas•tic
ho•mo•cen•tric
ho•moch•ro•nous
ho•mo•cys•te•ine
ho•mo•cys•tine
ho•mo•dont
ho•mo•erot•ic
ho•mo•erot•i•cism
also ho•mo•erot•ism
ho•mo•ga•met•ic
ho•mog•a•mous
or ho•mo•gam•ic
ho•mog•a•my
pl ho•mog•a•mies
ho•mog•e•nate
ho•mo•ge•neous
ho•mo•ge•neous•ly
ho•mo•ge•neous•ness
ho•mo•gen•e•sis
pl ho•mo•gen•e•ses
ho•mo•ge•net•ic
or ho•mo•ge•net•i•cal
ho•mog•e•ni•za•tion
ho•mog•e•nize
ho•mog•e•nized
ho•mog•e•niz•ing
ho•mog•e•nous
ho•mo•gen•tis•ic
ho•mog•e•ny
pl ho•mog•e•nies
ho•mo•graft
ho•moio•therm
ho•moio•ther•mic
or homeo•ther•mic
also ho•moio•ther•mal
ho•mo•lat•er•al
ho•mo•lec•i•thal
ho•mol•o•gize
ho•mol•o•gized
ho•mol•o•giz•ing
ho•mol•o•giz•er
ho•mol•o•gous
ho•mo•logue
or ho•mo•log
ho•mol•o•gy
pl ho•mol•o•gies
ho•mol•y•sis
pl ho•mol•y•ses
ho•mo•lyt•ic
ho•mo•mor•phic
ho•mon•o•mous
hom•on•y•mous
ho•mo•phile
ho•mo•pho•bia
ho•mo•pho•bic
ho•mo•plas•tic
ho•mo•plas•ti•cal•ly
ho•mo•pol•y•mer
hom•or•gan•ic
ho•mo•sex•u•al
ho•mo•sex•u•al•i•ty
pl ho•mo•sex•u•al•i•ties
ho•mo•sex•u•al•ly
ho•mo•spo•rous
ho•mo•spo•ry
pl ho•mo•spo•ries
ho•mo•ther•mous
also ho•mo•ther•mal
or ho•mo•ther•mic
ho•mo•top•ic
ho•mo•trans•plant
ho•mo•trans•plan•ta•tion
ho•mo•typ•al
ho•mo•type
ho•mo•typ•ic
ho•mo•zy•go•sis
pl ho•mo•zy•go•ses
ho•mo•zy•gos•i•ty
ho•mo•zy•gote
ho•mo•zy•got•ic
ho•mo•zy•gous
ho•mo•zy•gous•ly

ho•mun•cu•lus
pl ho•mun•cu•li

hoof-and-mouth dis•ease
hoof•bound
Hooke's law
hook•let
hook•worm
hor•de•nine
hor•de•o•lum
pl hor•de•o•la

Hor•de•um
ho•ri•zon
Hor•mo•den•dron
Hor•mo•den•drum
hor•mon•al
hor•mon•al•ly
hor•mone
Hor•ner's syn•drome
ho•rop•ter
hor•rip•i•la•tion
horse•fly
horse•pox
horse•rad•ish
hos•pi•tal
hos•pi•tal•ism
hos•pi•tal•iza•tion
hos•pi•tal•ize
hos•pi•tal•ized
hos•pi•tal•iz•ing
house•fly
house•maid's knee
Hous•ton's fold
or Hous•ton's valve

Hr fac•tor
Huk•ner test
hu•mate
hu•mec•tant
hu•mec•ta•tion
hu•mer•al
hu•mer•us
pl hu•meri

hu•mic
hu•mid•i•fi•ca•tion
hu•mid•i•fi•er
hu•mid•i•fy
hu•mid•i•fied
hu•mid•i•fy•ing
hu•mid•i•ty
pl hu•mid•i•ties

hu•mid•ly
hu•min
hu•mor
hu•mor•al
hump•back
hump•backed
hu•mu•lus
hunch•back
hunch•backed
hun•ger
Hun•ter's ca•nal
Hun•ting•ton's cho•rea
Hutch•in•so•ni•an teeth
or Hutch•in•so•ni•an in•ci•sors

Hutch•in•son's teeth
Hutch•in•son's tri•ad
Huy•gens eye•piece
or Huy•ghe•ni•an eye•piece
or Huy•ge•ni•an eye•piece

hy•a•line
also hy•a•lin

hy•a•lin•iza•tion
hy•a•li•no•sis
pl hy•a•li•no•ses

hy•a•li•tis
hy•al•o•gen
hy•a•loid
hy•al•o•mere
Hy•a•lom•ma
hy•a•lo•mu•coid
hy•a•lo•plasm
hy•al•uro•nate
hy•al•uron•ic
hy•al•uron•i•dase
hy•brid
hy•brid•ism
hy•brid•iza•tion
hy•brid•ize
hy•brid•ized
hy•brid•iz•ing
hy•dan•to•in
hy•dan•to•in•ate
hy•da•tid
hy•da•tid•i•form
also hy•dat•i•form

hy•da•tid•o•cele
hy•da•tid of Mor•ga•gni

hy·da·tid·o·sis
pl hy·da·tid·o·ses

hyd·no·car·pic
hyd·no·car·pus
hy·dra·gogue
also hy·dra·gog

hy·dral·azine
hy·dran·gea
hy·drar·gyr·ia
also hy·drar·gy·ri·a·sis

hy·drar·gy·rism
hy·drar·gy·rum
hy·drar·thro·sis
pl hy·drar·thro·ses

hy·drase
hy·dras·tine
hy·dras·ti·nine
hy·dras·tis
hy·drate
hy·drat·ed
hy·drat·ing
hy·dra·tion
hy·dra·tor
hy·drau·lic
hy·drau·lics
hy·dra·zide
hy·dra·zone
hy·dre·mia
also hy·drae·mia

hy·dren·ceph·a·lus
also hy·dren·ceph·a·ly
pl hy·dren·ceph·a·li
also hy·dren·ceph·a·lies

hy·dric

hy·dride
hy·droa
hy·dro·bro·mic
hy·dro·car·bon
hy·dro·cele
hy·dro·ce·phal·ic
hy·dro·ceph·a·loid
hy·dro·ceph·a·lus
also hy·dro·ceph·a·ly
pl hy·dro·ceph·a·li
also hy·dro·ceph·a·lies

hy·dro·chlo·ric
hy·dro·chlo·ride
hy·dro·chlo·ro·thi·a·zide
hy·dro·cho·le·re·sis
pl hy·dro·cho·le·re·ses

hy·dro·cho·le·ret·ic
hy·dro·cin·cho·nine
hy·dro·col·loid
hy·dro·col·loi·dal
hy·dro·cor·ti·sone
hy·dro·co·tar·nine
hy·dro·cy·an·ic
hy·dro·gel
hy·dro·gen
hy·drog·e·nase
hy·dro·ge·nate
hy·dro·ge·nat·ed
hy·dro·ge·nat·ing

hy·dro·ge·na·tion
hy·dro·ki·net·ic
hy·dro·ki·net·ics
hy·dro·lase
hy·dro·lymph
hy·dro·ly·sate
also hy·dro·ly·zate

hy·dro·ly·sis
pl hy·dro·ly·ses

hy·dro·lyt·ic
hy·dro·lyz·able
hy·dro·lyze
also hy·dro·lyse

hy·dro·lyzed
also hy·dro·lysed

hy·dro·lyz·ing
also hy·dro·lys·ing

hy·dro·mas·sage
hy·dro·men·in·gi·tis
pl hy·dro·men·in·git·i·des

hy·dro·men·in·go·cele
hy·dro·me·tra
hy·dro·my·e·lia
hy·dro·ne·phro·sis
pl hy·dro·ne·phro·ses

hy·dro·ne·phrot·ic
hy·dro·path·ic
hy·dro·path·i·cal·ly
hy·drop·a·thy
pl hy·drop·a·thies

hy·dro·peri·car·di·um
pl hy·dro·peri·car·dia

hy·dro·peri·to·ne·um
pl hy·dro·peri·to·ne·ums
or hy·dro·peri·to·nea

hy·dro·phil·ic
or hy·dro·phile

hy·droph·i·lous
hy·dro·pho·bia
hy·dro·pho·bic
hy·dro·pho·bic·i·ty
pl hy·dro·pho·bic·i·ties

hy·drop·ic
hy·dro·pneu·mo·tho·rax
pl hy·dro·pneu·mo·tho·rax·es
or hy·dro·pneu·mo·tho·ra·ces

hy·drops
also hy·drop·sy
pl hy·drop·ses
also hy·drop·sies

hy·drops fe·tal·is
hy·dror·rhea
hy·dro·sal·pinx
pl hy·dro·sal·pin·ges

hy·dro·sol
hy·dro·sol·ic
hy·dro·sy·rin·go·my·e·lia
hy·dro·tac·tic
hy·dro·tax·is
pl hy·dro·tax·es

hy·dro·ther·a·peu·tic
or hy·dro·ther·a·peu·ti·cal

hy·dro·ther·a·peu·tics
hy·dro·ther·a·pist
hy·dro·ther·a·py
pl hy·dro·ther·a·pies

hy·dro·ther·mal
hy·dro·ther·mal·ly
hy·dro·tho·rax
pl hy·dro·tho·rax·es
or hy·dro·tho·ra·ces

hy·dro·tro·pic
hy·dro·tro·pi·cal·ly
hy·drot·ro·pism
hy·dro·ure·ter
hy·drous
hy·drox·ide
hy·droxo·co·bal·a·min
hy·droxy
hy·droxy·ap·a·tite
hy·droxy·bu·tyr·ic
hy·droxy·cor·ti·co·ste·rone
hy·drox·yl
hy·drox·yl·amine
hy·drox·y·lase
hy·droxy·pro·line
hy·droxy·quin·o·line

hy·droxy·tryp·ta·mine
hy·droxy·urea
hy·droxy·zine
Hy·dro·zoa
hy·dro·zo·an
hy·dro·zo·on
pl hy·dro·zoa
or hy·dro·zo·ons

hy·dru·ria
hy·ge·ian
hy·giene
hy·gien·ic
also hy·gien·i·cal

hy·gien·i·cal·ly
hy·gien·ics
hy·gien·ist
hy·gric
hy·grine
hy·gro·ma
pl hy·gro·mas
or hy·gro·ma·ta

hy·grom·e·ter
hy·gro·met·ric
hy·grom·e·try
pl hy·grom·e·tries

hy·gro·scop·ic
hy·gro·scop·i·cal·ly
hy·gro·sco·pic·i·ty
pl hy·gro·sco·pic·i·ties

hy·men
hy·men·al
hy·men·oid
Hy·me·nol·e·pis
Hy·me·nop·tera
hy·me·nop·ter·an

hy·me·nop·ter·on
pl hy·me·nop·tera
also hy·me·nop·ter·ons

hy·me·nop·ter·ous

hy·men·ot·o·my
pl hy·men·ot·o·mies

hyo·de·oxy·cho·lic
or hyo·des·oxy·cho·lic

hyo·ep·i·glot·tic
also hyo·ep·i·glot·tid·e·an

hyo·glos·sal

hyo·glos·sus
pl hyo·glos·si

hy·oid
also hy·oi·dal
or hy·oi·de·an

hy·o·scine

hy·o·scy·a·mine

hy·o·scy·a·mus

Hyo·stron·gy·lus

hyo·thy·roid

hyp·acu·sic
or hyp·acou·sic

hyp·al·ge·sia
also hyp·al·gia

hyp·ar·te·ri·al

hyp·ax·i·al
also hyp·ax·on·ic

hy·per·ac·id

hy·per·acid·i·ty
pl hy·per·acid·i·ties

hy·per·ac·tive

hy·per·ac·tiv·i·ty
pl hy·per·ac·tiv·i·ties

hy·per·ad·re·no·cor·ti·cism

hy·per·al·do·ste·ron·ism

hy·per·al·ge·sia

hy·per·al·ge·sic

hy·per·azo·te·mia

hy·per·bar·ic

hy·per·bar·i·cal·ly

hy·per·bil·i·ru·bi·ne·mia

hy·per·brachy·ceph·al

hy·per·brachy·ce·phal·ic

hy·per·brachy·ceph·a·ly
pl hy·per·brachy·ceph·a·lies

hy·per·cal·ce·mia
also hy·per·cal·cae·mia

hy·per·cal·ce·mic

hy·per·cap·nia

hy·per·cap·nic

hy·per·ca·thex·is
pl hy·per·ca·thex·es

hy·per·ce·men·to·sis
pl hy·per·ce·men·to·ses

hy·per·chlo·re·mia

hy·per·chlor·hy·dria

hy·per·cho·les·ter·emia

hy·per·cho·les·ter·e·mic

hy·per·cho·les·ter·ol·emia

hy·per·cho·les·ter·ol·emic

hy·per·chro·mat·ic

hy·per·chro·ma·tism

hy·per·chro·ma·to·sis
pl hy·per·chro·ma·to·ses

hy·per·chro·mia

hy·per·chro·mic

hy·per·cry·al·ge·sia

hy·per·dip·loid

hy·per·dip·loi·dy
pl hy·per·dip·loi·dies

hy·per·dis·ten·tion

hy·per·dy·nam·ic

hy·per·eme·sis
pl hy·per·eme·ses

hy·per·eme·sis grav·i·dar·um

hy·per·emia
also hy·per·ae·mia

hy·per·emic

hy·per·en·dem·ic

hy·per·en·de·mic·i·ty
pl hy·per·en·de·mic·i·ties

hy·per·er·gic

hy·per·er·gy
pl hy·per·er·gies

hy·per·eso·pho·ria
hy·per·es·the·sia
or hy·per·aes·the·sia

hy·per·es·thet·ic
hy·per·es·trin·ism
hy·per·es·tro·gen·ism
hy·per·ex·cit·abil·i·ty
pl hy·per·ex·cit·abil·i·ties

hy·per·exo·pho·ria
hy·per·ex·ten·sion
hy·per·geu·sia
hy·per·glob·u·lin·emia
hy·per·gly·ce·mia
hy·per·gly·ce·mic
hy·per·go·nad·ism
hy·per·he·do·nia
hy·per·hep·a·rin·emia
hy·per·hep·a·rin·emic
hy·per·hi·dro·sis
also hy·per·idro·sis
pl hy·per·hi·dro·ses
also hy·per·idro·ses

hy·per·i·cin
Hy·per·i·cum
hy·per·in·su·lin·ism
hy·per·in·vo·lu·tion
hy·per·ir·ri·ta·bil·i·ty
pl hy·per·ir·ri·ta·bil·i·ties

hy·per·ir·ri·ta·ble
hy·per·ka·le·mia
hy·per·ke·ra·ti·ni·za·tion
hy·per·ker·a·to·sis
pl hy·per·ker·a·to·ses

hy·per·ker·a·tot·ic
hy·per·ki·ne·sia
also hy·per·ki·ne·sis

hy·per·ki·net·ic
hy·per·lac·ta·tion
hy·per·li·pe·mia
hy·per·li·pe·mic
hy·per·lip·id·emia
hy·per·lip·id·emic
hy·per·me·tab·o·lism
hy·per·meta·mor·pho·sis
pl hy·per·meta·mor·pho·ses

hy·per·met·rope
hy·per·me·tro·pia
hy·per·me·tro·pic
hy·perm·ne·sia
hy·perm·ne·sic
hy·per·morph
hy·per·myo·to·nia
hy·per·ne·phro·ma
pl hy·per·ne·phro·mas
or hy·per·ne·phro·ma·ta

hy·per·on·to·morph
hy·per·ope
hy·per·opia
hy·per·opic
hy·per·os·mia
hy·per·os·mic
hy·per·os·to·sis
pl hy·per·os·to·ses

hy·per·par·a·site
hy·per·par·a·sit·ic
hy·per·par·a·sit·ism
hy·per·para·thy·roid·ism
hy·per·path·ia
hy·per·path·ic
hy·per·peri·stal·sis
pl hy·per·peri·stal·ses

hy·per·pha·gia
hy·per·pha·gic
hy·per·pha·lan·gism
hy·per·pi·e·sia
also hy·per·pi·e·sis

hy·per·pi·et·ic
hy·per·pi·tu·ita·rism

hy•per•pi•tu•itary
hy•per•pla•sia
hy•per•plas•tic
hy•per•ploid
hy•per•ploi•dy
pl hy•per•ploi•dies

hy•per•pnea
also hy•per•pnoea

hy•per•pne•ic
hy•per•po•lar•iza•tion
hy•per•po•lar•ize
hy•per•po•lar•ized
hy•per•po•lar•iz•ing
hy•per•pra•gia
hy•per•prax•ia
hy•per•pro•sex•ia
hy•per•pro•tein•emia
hy•per•py•ret•ic
hy•per•py•rex•ia
hy•per•re•flex•ia
hy•per•res•o•nance
hy•per•res•o•nant
hy•per•se•cre•tion
hy•per•sen•si•tive
hy•per•sen•si•tive•ness
hy•per•sen•si•tiv•i•ty
pl hy•per•sen•si•tiv•i•ties

hy•per•sen•si•ti•za•tion
hy•per•sen•si•tize
hy•per•sen•si•tized
hy•per•sen•si•tiz•ing
hy•per•sex•u•al
hyper•sex•u•al•i•ty
pl hy•per•sex•u•al•i•ties

hy•per•som•nia
hy•per•son•ic
hy•per•splen•ic
hy•per•splen•ism
hy•per•sthe•nic
hy•per•sus•cep•ti•bil•i•ty
pl hy•per•sus•cep•ti•bil•i•ties

hy•per•ten•sin
hy•per•ten•sin•ase
hy•per•ten•sin•o•gen
hy•per•ten•sion
hy•per•ten•sive
hy•per•ther•mia
hy•per•ther•mic
hy•per•thy•roid
hy•per•thy•roid•ism
hy•per•thy•ro•sis
also hy•per•thy•re•o•sis
pl hy•per•thy•ro•ses
also hy•per•thy•re•o•ses

hy•per•to•nia
or hy•per•to•ny
pl hy•per•to•ni•as
or hy•per•to•nies
hy•per•ton•ic
hy•per•to•nic•i•ty
pl hy•per•to•nic•i•ties

hy•per•tri•cho•sis
pl hy•per•tri•cho•ses

hy•per•tro•phic
hy•per•tro•phy
pl hy•per•tro•phies

hy•per•uri•ce•mia
hy•per•ven•ti•la•tion
hy•per•vi•ta•min•osis
pl hy•per•vi•ta•min•o•ses

hy•per•vol•emia
hyp•es•the•sia
hy•pha
pl hy•phae

hyp•hi•dro•sis
pl hyp•hi•dro•ses

hy•pho•my•co•sis
pl hy•pho•my•co•ses

hyp•na•gog•ic
or hyp•no•gog•ic

hyp•no•anal•y•sis
pl hyp•no•anal•y•ses

hyp•no•gen•e•sis
pl hyp•no•gen•e•ses

hyp•no•ge•net•ic
hyp•no•ge•net•i•cal•ly
hyp•no•gen•ic
hyp•nog•e•nous
hyp•noid
or hyp•noi•dal

hyp·nol·o·gy
pl hyp·nol·o·gies

hyp·no·pho·bia
or hyp·no·pho·by
pl hyp·no·pho·bias
or hyp·no·pho·bies

hyp·no·pom·pic

hyp·no·sis
pl hyp·no·ses

hyp·no·ther·a·py
pl hyp·no·ther·a·pies

hyp·not·ic

hyp·no·tism

hyp·no·tist

hyp·no·tize
or hyp·no·tise

hyp·no·tized
or hyp·no·tised

hyp·no·tiz·ing
or hyp·no·tis·ing

hyp·no·tox·in

hy·po

hy·po·acid·i·ty
pl hy·po·acid·i·ties

hy·po·ad·re·nal·ism

hy·po·ad·re·nia

hy·po·al·bu·min·emia

hy·po·bar·ic

hy·po·blast

hy·po·blas·tic

hy·po·bran·chi·al

hy·po·bro·mite

hy·po·bro·mous

hy·po·bu·lia

hy·po·bu·lic

hy·po·cal·ce·mia
also hy·po·cal·cae·mia

hy·po·cal·ce·mic
also hy·po·cal·cae·mic

hy·po·cap·nia

hy·po·chlo·re·mia

hy·po·chlo·re·mic

hy·po·chlor·hy·dria

hy·po·chlor·hy·dric

hy·po·chlo·rite

hy·po·chlo·rous

hy·po·chon·dria

hy·po·chon·dri·ac

hy·po·chon·dri·a·cal

hy·po·chon·dri·a·cal·ly

hy·po·chon·dri·a·sis
pl hy·po·chon·dri·a·ses

hy·po·chon·dri·um
pl hy·po·chon·dria

hy·po·chord·al

hy·po·chro·mia

hy·po·chro·mic

hy·po·cone

hy·po·con·id

hy·po·cu·pre·mia
or hy·po·cu·prae·mia

hy·po·cu·pre·mic
also hy·po·cu·prae·mic

hy·po·derm

hy·po·der·ma

hy·po·der·mal

hy·po·der·mat·ic

hy·po·der·mat·i·cal·ly

hy·po·der·mic

hy·po·der·mi·cal·ly

hy·po·der·mis

hy·po·der·moc·ly·sis
pl hy·po·der·moc·ly·ses

hy·po·dip·loid

hy·po·dip·loi·dy
pl hy·po·dip·loi·dies

hy·po·dy·nam·ia

hy·po·dy·nam·ic

hy·po·er·gic

hy·po·er·gy
pl hy·po·er·gies

hy·po·fer·re·mia
also hy·po·fer·rae·mia

hy·po·func·tion

hy·po·ga·lac·tia

hy·po·gas·tric

hy·po·gas·tri·um
pl hy·po·gas·tria

hy·po·gen·e·sis
pl hy·po·gen·e·ses

hy·po·ge·net·ic

hy·po·gen·i·tal·ism

hy·po·glos·sal
hy·po·glos·sus
pl hy·po·glos·si
hy·po·glot·tis
pl hy·po·glot·tis·es
or hy·po·glot·ti·des
hy·po·gly·ce·mia
hy·po·gly·ce·mic
hy·pog·na·thous
hy·po·go·nad·ism
hy·po·hi·dro·sis
pl hy·po·hi·dro·ses
hy·po·ka·le·mia
hy·po·ka·le·mic
hy·po·ki·ne·sia
hy·po·ki·ne·sis
pl hy·po·ki·ne·ses
hy·po·mag·ne·se·mia
hy·po·mag·ne·se·mic
hy·po·ma·nia
hy·po·man·ic
hy·po·mas·tia
hy·po·men·or·rhea
hy·po·me·tab·o·lism
hy·po·morph
hy·po·morph·ic
hy·po·mo·til·i·ty
pl hy·po·mo·til·i·ties
hy·po·na·tre·mia
hy·po·nych·i·al
hy·po·nych·i·um
hy·po·ovar·i·an·ism
hy·po·par·a·thy·roid
hy·po·para·thy·roid·ism
hy·po·pha·lan·gism
hy·po·phar·ynx
pl hy·po·pha·ryn·ges
also hy·po·phar·ynx·es
hy·po·phos·pha·te·mia
hy·po·phre·nia
hy·po·phren·ic
hy·po·phre·no·sis
pl hy·po·phre·no·ses
hy·poph·y·se·al
also hy·po·phys·i·al
hy·poph·y·sec·to·mize
hy·poph·y·sec·to·mized
hy·poph·y·sec·to·miz·ing
hy·poph·y·sec·to·my
pl hy·poph·y·sec·to·mies
hy·poph·y·sis
pl hy·poph·y·ses
hy·poph·y·sis ce·re·bri
hy·po·pi·tu·ita·rism
hy·po·pi·tu·itary
hy·po·pla·sia
hy·po·plas·tic
hy·po·ploid
hy·po·ploi·dy
pl hy·po·ploi·dies
hy·po·po·tas·se·mia
hy·po·po·tas·se·mic
hy·po·pro·sex·ia
hy·po·pro·tein·emia
hy·po·pro·tein·emic
hy·po·pro·throm·bin·emia
hy·po·pro·throm·bin·emic
hy·po·py·on
hy·po·ri·bo·fla·vin·o·sis
pl hy·po·ri·bo·fla·vin·o·ses
hy·po·scler·al
hy·po·se·cre·tion
hy·po·sen·si·tive
hy·po·sen·si·tiv·i·ty
pl hy·po·sen·si·tiv·i·ties
hy·po·sen·si·ti·za·tion
hy·po·sen·si·tize
hy·po·sen·si·tized
hy·po·sen·si·tiz·ing
hy·po·spa·di·ac
hy·po·spa·di·as
or hy·po·spa·dia

hy·pos·ta·sis
pl hy·pos·ta·ses

hy·po·stat·ic
hy·po·sthe·nia
hy·po·sthe·nic
hy·pos·the·nu·ria
hy·pos·the·nu·ric
hy·po·styp·sis
hy·po·styp·tic
hy·po·sul·fite
hy·po·ten·sion
hy·po·ten·sive
hy·po·tha·lam·ic
hy·po·thal·a·mus
pl hy·po·thal·a·mi

hy·po·the·nar
hy·po·ther·mal
hy·po·ther·mia
hy·po·ther·mic
hy·poth·e·sis
pl hy·poth·e·ses

hy·po·thy·roid
hy·po·thy·roid·ism
hy·po·to·nia
or hy·pot·o·ny
pl hy·po·to·nias
or hy·pot·o·nies

hy·po·ton·ic
hy·po·ton·i·cal·ly
hy·po·to·nic·i·ty
pl hy·po·to·nic·i·ties

hy·po·to·nus
hy·po·tri·cho·sis
pl hy·po·tri·cho·ses
or hy·po·tri·cho·sis·es

hy·po·tri·chot·ic

hy·pot·ro·phy
pl hy·pot·ro·phies

hy·po·tym·pa·num
pl hy·po·tym·pa·na
also hy·po·tym·pa·nums

hy·po·vi·ta·min·o·sis
pl hy·po·vi·ta·min·o·ses
or hy·po·vi·ta·min·o·sis·es

hy·po·vi·ta·min·ot·ic
hy·po·vo·le·mia
hy·po·vo·le·mic
hy·po·xan·thine
hy·pox·emia
hy·pox·emic
hy·pox·ia
hy·pox·ic
hyp·si·brachy·ce·phal·ic
hyp·si·brachy·ceph·al·ism
hyp·si·ceph·al
hyp·si·ce·phal·ic
also hyp·si·ceph·a·lous

hyp·si·loid
hyp·so·chro·mic
hyp·so·dont
hyp·so·dont·ism
hys·ter·ec·to·mize
hys·ter·ec·to·mized
hys·ter·ec·to·miz·ing

hys·ter·ec·to·my
pl hys·ter·ec·to·mies

hys·te·ria
hys·ter·ic
or hys·ter·i·cal

hys·ter·i·cal·ly
hys·ter·ics
hys·tero-ep·i·lep·sy
pl hys·tero-ep·i·lep·sies

hys·tero-ep·i·lep·tic
hys·tero·gen·ic
hys·tero·gram
hys·tero·graph
hys·ter·og·ra·phy
pl hys·ter·og·ra·phies

hys·ter·oid
also hys·ter·oi·dal

hys·ter·ol·o·gy
pl hys·ter·ol·o·gies

hys·ter·ol·y·sis
pl hys·ter·ol·y·ses

hys·tero-oo·pho·rec·to·my
pl hys·tero-oo·pho·rec·to·mies

hys·tero·pexy
pl hys·tero·pexies

hys·ter·or·rha·phy
pl hys·ter·or·rha·phies

hys·ter·or·rhex·is
pl hys·ter·or·rhex·es

hys·tero·sal·pin·gec·to·my
pl hys·tero·sal·pin·gec·to·mies

hys·tero·sal·pin·gog·ra·phy
pl hys·tero·sal·pin·gog·ra·phies

hys·tero·sal·pin·go-oo·pho·rec·to·my
pl hys·tero·sal·pin·go-oo·pho·rec·to·mies

hys·tero·scope
hys·tero·scop·ic
hys·ter·os·co·py
pl hys·ter·os·co·pies

hys·tero·sto·mat·o·my
pl hys·tero·sto·mat·o·mies

hys·tero·tely
pl hys·tero·tel·ies

hys·tero·tome

hys·ter·ot·o·my
pl hys·ter·ot·o·mies

hys·tero·trach·e·lec·to·my
pl hys·tero·trach·e·lec·to·mies

hys·tero·trach·e·lor·rha·phy
pl hys·tero·trach·e·lor·rha·phies

hys·tero·tra·che·lot·o·my
pl hys·tero·tra·che·lot·o·mies

hys·tero·trau·ma·tism

I

iat·ric
also iat·ri·cal

iat·ro·chem·i·cal
iat·ro·chem·ist
iat·ro·chem·is·try
pl iat·ro·chem·is·tries

iat·ro·gen·ic
iat·ro·gen·i·cal·ly
iat·ro·ge·nic·i·ty
pl iat·ro·ge·nic·i·ties

iat·ro·math·e·mat·ics
iat·ro·phys·i·cist
iat·ro·phys·ics
I band
ibo·ga·ine
ichor
ichor·ous
ich·tham·nol
ich·thy·ism
or ich·thy·is·mus
pl ich·thy·isms
or ich·thy·is·mus·es

ich·thy·o·col
or ich·thy·o·coll
or ich·thy·o·col·la

ich·thy·oid
ich·thy·oi·dal
ich·thy·oph·a·gous
ich·thyo·sar·co·tox·ism
ich·thy·o·si·form
ich·thy·o·sis
pl ich·thy·o·ses

ich·thy·ot·ic
ich·thyo·tox·ism
ic·tal
ic·ter·ic
ic·ter·i·tious
or ic·ter·i·tous

ic·tero·ane·mia
ic·tero·gen·ic
also ic·ter·og·e·nous

ic·ter·oid
ic·ter·us
ic·ter·us gra·vis
ic·ter·us in·dex
or ic·ter·ic in·dex

ic·tus
ide·ation
ide·ation·al
idée fixe
pl idées fixes

iden·ti·cal
iden·ti·fi·ca·tion
iden·ti·fy
iden·ti·fied
iden·ti·fy·ing
iden·ti·ty
pl iden·ti·ties

ideo·ge·net·ic
ideo·ki·net·ic
ideo·mo·tor
ideo·mus·cu·lar
ideo·pho·bia
ideo·plas·tic
id·i·oc·ra·sy
pl id·i·oc·ra·sies

idio·crat·ic
or idio·crat·i·cal

id·i·o·cy
pl id·i·o·cies

id·io·gen·e·sis
pl id·io·gen·e·ses

id·io·ge·net·ic
id·io·glos·sia
id·io·gram
id·io·la·lia
id·io·mus·cu·lar
id·io·path·ic
id·io·path·i·cal·ly
id·i·op·a·thy
pl id·i·op·a·thies

id·io·plasm
id·io·plas·mat·ic
or id·io·plas·mic

id·io·ret·i·nal
id·io·some
id·io·syn·cra·sy
also id·io·syn·cra·cy
pl id·io·syn·cra·sies
also id·io·syn·cra·cies

id·io·syn·crat·ic
id·io·syn·crat·i·cal·ly
id·i·ot
id·i·ot·ic
also id·i·ot·i·cal

id·i·ot·i·cal·ly
id·i·ot sa·vant
pl id·i·ots sa·vants
or id·i·ot sa·vants

id·i·tol
idose
ig·na·tia
il·e·al
also il·e·ac

ile·ec·to·my
pl ile·ec·to·mies

il·e·itis
pl it·e·it·i·des

il·eo·ce·cal
il·eo·ce·cos·to·my
pl il·eo·ce·cos·to·mies

il·eo·ce·cum
pl il·eo·ce·ca

il·eo·co·lic
il·eo·co·li·tis
il·eo·co·lon·ic
il·eo·co·los·to·my
pl il·eo·co·los·to·mies

il·e·os·to·my
pl il·e·os·to·mies

il·e·um
pl il·ea

il·e·us
il·i·ac
ili·a·cus
pl ili·a·ci

il·io·coc·cy·geal
il·io·cos·ta·lis
il·io·fem·o·ral
il·io·hy·po·gas·tric
il·io·in·gui·nal
il·io·lum·bar
il·io·pec·tin·e·al
il·io·psoas
il·io·pso·at·ic
il·io·tib·i·al
il·i·um
pl il·ia

ill-bred

il·le·git·i·ma·cy
pl il·le·git·i·ma·cies

il·le·git·i·mate
Il·lici·um
il·lin·i·um
ill·ness
il·lu·mi·nance
il·lu·mi·na·tion
il·lu·mi·nism
il·lu·sion
il·lu·sion·al
il·lu·sion·ary
im·ag·ery
pl im·ag·er·ies

imag·i·nal
imag·i·na·tion
imag·i·na·tive
imag·ine
imag·ined
imag·in·ing
ima·go
pl ima·goes
or ima·gi·nes

im·bal·ance
im·be·cile
im·be·cil·ic
im·be·cil·i·ty
pl im·be·cil·i·ties

im·bed
var of embed

im·bibe
im·bibed
im·bib·ing
im·bi·bi·tion
im·bri·cate
im·bri·cat·ed
im·bri·cat·ing

im·bri·ca·tion
im·id·az·ole
im·id·az·o·lyl
im·ide
im·i·do
im·in·az·ole
im·ine
im·i·no
imip·ra·mine
im·ma·ture
im·ma·tu·rity
pl im·ma·tu·ri·ties
im·me·di·ate
im·med·i·ca·ble
im·merse
im·mersed
im·mers·ing
im·mer·sion
im·mis·ci·ble
im·mis·ci·bly
im·mo·bil·i·ty
pl im·mo·bil·i·ties
im·mo·bi·li·za·tion
im·mo·bi·lize
im·mo·bi·lized
im·mo·bi·liz·ing
im·mor·tal
im·mor·tal·i·ty
pl im·mor·tal·i·ties
im·mune
im·mu·ni·ty
pl im·mu·ni·ties
im·mu·ni·za·tion
im·mu·nize
im·mu·nized
im·mu·niz·ing

im·mu·no·as·say
im·mu·no·as·say·able
im·mu·no·chem·is·try
pl im·mu·no·chem·is·tries
im·mu·no·com·pe·tence
im·mu·no·com·pe·tent
im·mu·no·cy·to·chem·i·cal
im·mu·no·cy·to·chem·i·cal·ly
im·mu·no·cy·to·chem·is·try
pl im·mu·no·cy·to·chem·is·tries
im·mu·no·de·fi·cien·cy
pl im·mu·no·de·fi·cien·cies
im·mu·no·dif·fu·sion
im·mu·no·elec·tro·pho·re·sis
pl im·mu·no·elec·tro·pho·re·ses
im·mu·no·elec·tro·pho·ret·ic
im·mu·no·elec·tro·pho·ret·i·cal·ly
im·mu·no·flu·o·res·cence
im·mu·no·flu·o·res·cent

im·mu·no·gen
im·mu·no·gen·e·sis
pl im·mu·no·gen·e·ses
im·mu·no·ge·net·ic
im·mu·no·ge·net·i·cal·ly
im·mu·no·ge·net·ics
im·mu·no·gen·ic
im·mu·no·glob·u·lin
im·mu·no·he·ma·to·log·ic
or im·mu·no·he·ma·to·log·i·cal
im·mu·no·he·ma·tol·o·gist
im·mu·no·he·ma·tol·o·gy
pl im·mu·no·he·ma·tol·o·gies
im·mu·no·his·to·chem·i·cal
im·mu·no·his·to·chem·i·cal·ly
im·mu·no·his·to·chem·is·try
pl im·mu·no·his·to·chem·is·tries
im·mu·no·his·to·log·ic
im·mu·no·his·to·log·i·cal

im·mu·no·his·to·log·i·cal·ly
im·mu·no·his·tol·o·gy
pl im·mu·no·his·tol·o·gies
im·mu·no·log·ic
also im·mu·no·log·i·cal
im·mu·no·log·i·cal·ly
im·mu·nol·o·gist
im·mu·nol·o·gy
pl im·mu·nol·o·gies
im·mu·no·path·o·log·ic
or im·mu·no·path·o·log·i·cal
im·mu·no·pa·thol·o·gist
im·mu·no·pa·thol·o·gy
pl im·mu·no·pa·thol·o·gies
im·mu·no·re·ac·tive
im·mu·no·re·ac·tiv·i·ty
pl im·mu·no·re·ac·tiv·i·ties
im·mu·no·sup·pres·sant
im·mu·no·sup·pres·sion
im·mu·no·sup·pres·sive
im·mu·no·ther·a·peu·tic
im·mu·no·ther·a·py
pl im·mu·no·ther·a·pies
im·mu·no·trans·fu·sion
im·pac·tion
im·pair·ment
im·pal·pa·ble
im·ped·i·ment
im·per·cep·ti·ble
im·per·cep·tion
im·per·fo·rate
im·per·fo·ra·tion
im·per·me·abil·i·ty
pl im·per·me·abil·i·ties
im·per·me·able
im·per·me·ably
im·per·vi·ous
im·pe·tig·i·ni·za·tion
im·pe·tig·i·nized
im·pe·tig·i·nous
im·pe·ti·go
pl im·pe·ti·gos
im·pe·tus
Im·plac·en·ta·lia
im·plant
im·plan·ta·tion
im·po·tence
also im·po·ten·cy
pl im·po·tenc·es
also im·po·ten·cies
im·po·tent
im·po·tent·ly
im·preg·nate
im·preg·nat·ed
im·preg·nat·ing
im·preg·na·tion
im·pres·sion
im·print·ing
im·pulse
im·pul·sion
im·pul·sive
in·ac·tion
in·ac·ti·vate
in·ac·ti·vat·ed
in·ac·ti·vat·ing
in·ac·ti·va·tion
in·ac·tive
in·ac·tiv·i·ty
pl in·ac·tiv·i·ties
in·ad·e·qua·cy
pl in·ad·e·qua·cies
in·ad·e·quate
in·ad·e·quate·ly
in·a·ni·tion
in·ap·par·ent
in·ap·pe·tence
in·ar·tic·u·late
in·ar·tic·u·late·ly
in ar·ti·cu·lo mor·tis
in·as·sim·i·la·ble
in·breathe
in·breathed
in·breath·ing
in·breed
in·bred
in·breed·ing
in·breed·er

Inca bone
in·ca·pac·i·tant
in·ca·pac·i·tate
in·ca·pac·i·tat·ed
in·ca·pac·i·tat·ing
in·ca·pac·i·ta·tion
in·ca·pac·i·ta·tor
in·car·cer·ate
in·car·cer·at·ed
in·car·cer·at·ing
in·car·cer·a·tion
in·cen·di·a·rism
in·cen·di·ary
pl in·cen·di·ar·ies
in·cest
in·ces·tu·ous
in·ces·tu·ous·ly
in·ci·dence
in·ci·sal
in·cise
in·cised
in·cis·ing
in·ci·sion
in·ci·sive
in·ci·sor
in·ci·su·ra
or in·ci·sure
pl in·ci·su·rae
or in·ci·sures
in·cli·na·tion
in·cline
in·cli·nom·e·ter
in·clu·sion
in·co·ag·u·la·ble
in·com·pat·i·bil·i·ty
pl in·com·pat·i·bil·i·ties
in·com·pat·i·ble
in·com·pat·i·bly
in·com·pen·sa·tion
in·com·pe·tence
in·com·pe·ten·cy
pl in·com·pe·ten·cies
in·com·pe·tent
in·con·ti·nence
in·con·ti·nent
in·co·or·di·nate
in·co·or·di·na·tion
in·cor·po·ra·tion
in·cre·to·ry
in·cross
in·cross·bred
in·crus·ta·tion
or en·crus·ta·tion
in·cu·bate
in·cu·bat·ed
in·cu·bat·ing
in·cu·ba·tion
in·cu·ba·tor
in·cu·bus
pl in·cu·bi
also in·cu·bus·es
in·cur·able
in·cur·ably
in·cur·va·tion
in·cus
pl in·cu·des
in·da·mine
In·de·cid·ua
in·den·ta·tion
in·dex
pl in·dex·es
or in·di·ces
in·di·can
in·di·cant
in·di·cate
in·di·cat·ed
in·di·cat·ing
in·di·ca·tion
in·di·ca·tor
in·dig·e·nous
in·di·gest·ibil·i·ty
pl in·di·gest·ibil·i·ties
in·di·gest·ible
in·di·ges·tion
in·di·ru·bin
in·dis·crim·i·nate
in·dis·crim·i·nate·ly
in·dis·posed
in·dis·po·si·tion
in·di·vid·u·a·tion
in·do·cy·a·nine green
in·dole
in·dole·ace·tic
in·dole·bu·tyr·ic
in·do·lence
in·do·lent
in·do·meth·a·cin
in·do·phe·nol
in·duce
in·duced
in·duc·ing
in·duc·er

in·duc·ible
in·duc·tance
in·duc·tion
in·duc·tive
in·duc·tor
in·duc·to·ri·um
in·duc·to·ther·my
pl in·duc·to·ther·mies
in·du·line
also in·du·lin
in·du·rate
in·du·rat·ed
in·du·rat·ing
in·du·ra·tion
in·du·ra·tive
in·du·si·um
pl in·du·sia
in·dwell·ing
ine·bri·ant
ine·bri·ate
ine·bri·at·ed
ine·bri·at·ing
ine·bri·a·tion
in·ebri·ety
pl in·ebri·eties
in·er·tia
pl in·er·tias
also in·er·ti·ae
in ex·tre·mis
in·fan·cy
pl in·fan·cies
in·fant
in·fan·ti·cide
in·fan·tile
in·fan·til·ism
in·farct
in·farct·ed
in·farc·tion
in·fect
in·fec·tion
in·fec·tious
in·fec·tious·ly
in·fec·tive
in·fec·tiv·i·ty
pl in·fec·tiv·i·ties
in·fe·cun·di·ty
pl in·fe·cun·di·ties
in·fe·ri·or
in·fe·ri·or·i·ty
pl in·fe·ri·or·i·ties
in·fer·tile
in·fer·til·i·ty
pl in·fer·til·i·ties
in·fest
in·fes·ta·tion
in·fib·u·la·tion
in·fil·trate
in·fil·trat·ed
in·fil·trat·ing
in·fil·tra·tion
in·firm
in·fir·ma·ry
pl in·fir·ma·ries
in·fir·mi·ty
pl in·fir·mi·ties
in·flame
in·flamed
in·flam·ing
in·flam·ma·tion
in·flam·ma·to·ry
in·fla·tor
or in·flat·er
in·flec·tion
in·flu·en·za
in·fold
in·fra·cla·vic·u·lar
in·frac·tion
in·fra·gle·noid
in·fra·mar·gin·al
in·fra·na·tant
in·fra·or·bit·al
in·fra·son·ic
in·fra·spi·na·tus
pl in·fra·spi·na·ti
in·fra·spi·nous
in·fra·tem·po·ral
in·fun·dib·u·lar
in·fun·dib·u·li·form
in·fun·dib·u·lum
pl in·fun·dib·u·la
in·fuse
in·fused
in·fus·ing
in·fus·ible
in·fu·sion
In·fu·so·ria
in·fu·so·ri·al
in·fu·so·ri·an
in·gest
in·ges·ta
in·ges·tant
in·gest·ible
in·ges·tion
in·ges·tive
in·glu·vi·es
pl in·glu·vi·es
in·gra·ves·cent

in·gre·di·ent
in·grow·ing
in·grown
in·growth
in·guen
pl in·gui·na
in·gui·nal
in·hal·ant
in·ha·la·tion
in·ha·la·tor
in·hale
in·haled
in·hal·ing
in·hal·er
in·her·ent
in·her·ent·ly
in·her·it
in·her·it·abil·i·ty
pl in·her·it·abil·i·ties
in·her·it·able
in·her·i·tance
in·hib·it
in·hi·bi·tion
in·hib·i·tive
in·hib·i·tor
or in·hib·i·ter
in·hib·i·to·ry
in·ho·mo·ge·ne·ity
pl in·ho·mo·ge·ne·ities
in·ho·mo·ge·neous
in·i·ac
also in·i·al
in·i·on
in·ject·able
in·jec·tant
in·jec·tion
in·jec·tor
in·jure
in·jured
in·jur·ing
in·ju·ri·ous
in·ju·ry
pl in·ju·ries
ink·blot
in·nards
in·nate
in·ner ear
in·ner-di·rect·ed
in·ner·vate
in·ner·vat·ed
in·ner·vat·ing
in·ner·va·tion
nerve supply (*see* enervation)
in·ner·va·tion·al
in·no·cent
in·noc·u·ous
in·nom·i·nate
in·nox·ious
in·nu·tri·tion
in·oc·u·la·ble
in·oc·u·lant
in·oc·u·late
in·oc·u·lat·ed
in·oc·u·lat·ing
in·oc·u·la·tion
in·oc·u·la·tive
in·oc·u·la·tor
in·oc·u·lum
pl in·oc·u·la
in·op·er·a·ble
in·or·gan·ic
in·or·gan·i·cal·ly
in·os·cu·late
in·os·cu·lat·ed
in·os·cu·lat·ing
in·os·cu·la·tion
ino·sine
ino·sin·ic
ino·si·tol
ino·tro·pic
in·pa·tient
in·quest
in·qui·line
in·sal·i·vate
in·sal·i·vat·ed
in·sal·i·vat·ing
in·sal·i·va·tion
in·sa·lu·bri·ous
in·sa·lu·bri·ty
pl in·sa·lu·bri·ties
in·sane
in·sane·ly
in·sane·ness
in·san·i·tary
in·san·i·ta·tion
in·san·i·ty
pl in·san·i·ties
in·scrip·tion
in·sect
In·sec·ta
in·sec·ti·cid·al
in·sec·ti·cid·al·ly
in·sec·ti·cide
in·sec·ti·fuge
in·se·cure
in·se·cure·ly

in•se•cu•ri•ty
pl in•se•cu•ri•ties

in•sem•i•nate
in•sem•i•nat•ed
in•sem•i•nat•ing
in•sem•i•na•tion
in•sen•si•ble
in•sen•si•bly
in•ser•tion
in•sheathe
var of ensheathe

in•sight
in si•tu
in•so•bri•ety
pl in•so•bri•eties

in•so•la•tion
in•sol•u•bil•i•ty
pl in•sol•u•bil•i•ties

in•sol•u•ble
in•som•nia
in•som•ni•ac
in•sper•sion
in•spi•ra•tion
in•spi•ra•tor
in•spi•ra•to•ry
in•spire
in•spired
in•spir•ing
in•spi•rom•e•ter
in•spis•sate
in•spis•sat•ed
in•spis•sat•ing
in•spis•sa•tion
in•spis•sa•tor
in•sta•bil•i•ty
pl in•sta•bil•i•ties

in•step
in•still
also in•stil

in•stilled
in•still•ing
in•stil•la•tion
in•stinct
in•stinc•tive
in•stinc•tive•ly
in•stinc•tu•al
in•sti•tutes
in•stru•ment
in•stu•men•tal
in•stru•men•tar•
ium
pl in•stru•men•tar•ia

in•stru•men•ta•
tion
in•suf•fi•cien•cy
pl in•suf•fi•cien•cies

in•suf•fi•cient
in•suf•fi•cient•ly
in•suf•flate
in•suf•flat•ed
in•suf•flat•ing
in•suf•fla•tion
in•suf•fla•tor
in•su•la
pl in•su•lae

in•su•lar
in•su•late
in•su•lat•ed
in•su•lat•ing
in•su•la•tion
in•su•la•tor
in•su•lin
in•su•lin•ase

in•sult
in•sus•cep•ti•bil•i•
ty
pl in•sus•cep•ti•bil•i•
ties

in•sus•cep•ti•ble
in•tact
in•te•grate
in•te•grat•ed
in•te•grat•ing
in•te•gra•tion
in•teg•ri•ty
pl in•teg•ri•ties

in•teg•u•ment
in•teg•u•men•tal
or in•teg•u•men•ta•ry

in•tel•lect
in•tel•lec•tu•al
in•tel•lec•tu•al•
iza•tion
in•tel•lec•tu•al•ize
in•tel•lec•tu•al•
ized
in•tel•lec•tu•al•
iz•ing
in•tel•li•gence
in•tel•li•gence
quo•tient
in•tel•li•gent
in•tem•per•ance
in•tem•per•ate
in•tem•per•ate•ly
in•tem•per•ate•
ness

in•ten•tion
in•ten•tion•al

in·ter·ac·i·nous
also in·ter·ac·i·nar
in·ter·ar·tic·u·lar
in·ter·atri·al
in·ter·brain
in·ter·breed
in·ter·bred
in·ter·breed·ing
in·ter·ca·la·ry
in·ter·ca·late
in·ter·ca·lat·ed
in·ter·ca·lat·ing
in·ter·cap·il·lary
in·ter·ca·rot·id
in·ter·car·pal
in·ter·car·ti·lag·i·nous
in·ter·cav·ern·ous
in·ter·cel·lu·lar
in·ter·cen·tral
in·ter·ce·re·bral
in·ter·clav·i·cle
in·ter·cla·vic·u·lar
in·ter·coc·cy·geal
in·ter·co·lum·nar
also in·ter·co·lum·nal
in·ter·con·dy·lar
in·ter·cos·tal
in·ter·cos·tal·ly
in·ter·cos·to·bra·chi·al
in·ter·course
in·ter·cris·tal
in·ter·cross
in·ter·cru·ral
in·ter·cur·rent
in·ter·cusp·ing
in·ter·den·tal
in·ter·den·ti·um
in·ter·dig·i·tate
in·ter·dig·i·tat·ed
in·ter·dig·i·tat·ing
in·ter·dig·i·ta·tion
in·ter·dis·ci·plin·ary
in·ter·fas·cic·u·lar
in·ter·fer·ence
in·ter·fer·om·e·ter
in·ter·fer·o·met·ric
in·ter·fer·o·met·ri·cal·ly
in·ter·fer·om·e·try
pl in·ter·fer·om·e·tries
in·ter·fer·on
in·ter·fer·tile
in·ter·fer·til·i·ty
pl in·ter·fer·til·i·ties
in·ter·fi·bril·lar
in·ter·fron·tal
in·ter·glob·u·lar
in·ter·grade
in·ter·hemi·spher·ic
in·ter·ki·ne·sis
pl in·ter·ki·ne·ses
in·ter·la·mel·lar
in·ter·lo·bar
in·ter·lob·u·lar
in·ter·mar·riage
in·ter·max·il·la
pl in·ter·max·il·lae
or in·ter·max·il·las
in·ter·max·il·lary
in·ter·me·di·ary
in·ter·me·di·ate
in·ter·me·din
in·ter·me·dio·lat·er·al
in·ter·me·di·us
in·ter·mem·bra·nous
in·ter·men·in·ge·al
in·ter·men·stru·al
in·ter·mi·cel·lar
in·ter·mis·sion
in·ter·mit·tence
in·ter·mit·ten·cy
pl in·ter·mit·ten·cies
in·ter·mit·tent
in·ter·mu·ral
in·ter·mus·cu·lar
in·tern
or in·terne
in·ter·nal
in·ter·nal·iza·tion
in·ter·nal·ize
in·ter·nal·ized
in·ter·nal·iz·ing
in·ter·na·sal
in·ter·na·tion·al unit
in·ter·neu·ral

in·ter·neu·ron
also in·ter·neu·rone
in·ter·neu·ro·nal
in·ter·nist
in·ter·nod·al
in·ter·node
in·ter·nu·cle·ar
in·ter·nun·ci·al
in·tero·cep·tive
in·tero·cep·tor
in·tero·fec·tive
in·ter·or·bit·al
in·ter·os·se·ous
in·ter·os·se·us
pl in·ter·os·sei
in·ter·pa·ri·etal
in·ter·par·ox·ys·mal
in·ter·pe·dun·cu·lar
in·ter·per·son·al
in·ter·pha·lan·ge·al
in·ter·phase
in·ter·po·late
in·ter·po·lat·ed
in·ter·po·lat·ing
in·ter·po·la·tion
in·ter·po·si·tion
in·ter·prox·i·mal
also in·ter·prox·i·mate
in·ter·pu·pil·lary
in·ter·ra·di·al
in·ter·re·nal
in·ter·scap·u·lar
in·ter·sect
in·ter·sec·tion
in·ter·seg·men·tal
in·ter·sen·so·ry
in·ter·sep·tal
in·ter·sex
in·ter·sex·u·al
in·ter·sex·u·al·ism
in·ter·sex·u·al·i·ty
pl in·ter·sex·u·al·i·ties
in·ter·sex·u·al·ly
in·ter·space
in·ter·spi·nal
or in·ter·spi·nous
in·ter·spi·na·lis
pl in·ter·spi·na·les
in·ter·ster·ile
in·ter·ste·ril·i·ty
pl in·ter·ste·ril·i·ties
in·ter·stice
pl in·ter·stic·es
in·ter·sti·tial
also in·ter·sti·cial
in·ter·sti·tium
pl in·ter·sti·tia
in·ter·trans·ver·sa·lis
in·ter·trig·i·nous
in·ter·tri·go
pl in·ter·tri·gos
in·ter·tro·chan·ter·ic
in·ter·tu·ber·cu·lar
in·ter·tu·bu·lar
in·ter·vas·cu·lar
in·ter·ven·tion
in·ter·ven·tric·u·lar
in·ter·ver·te·bral
in·ter·vil·lous
in·tes·ti·nal
in·tes·ti·nal·ly
in·tes·tine
in·ti·ma
pl in·ti·mae
or in·ti·mas
in·ti·mal
in·toed
in·tol·er·ance
in·tor·sion
or in·tor·tion
in·tox·i·cant
in·tox·i·cate
in·tox·i·cat·ed
in·tox·i·cat·ing
in·tox·i·ca·tion
in·tra-ab·dom·i·nal
in·tra·ar·te·ri·al
in·tra·ar·te·ri·al·ly
in·tra·car·di·al·ly
in·tra·car·ti·lag·i·nous
in·tra·cav·i·tary
in·tra·cel·lu·lar
in·tra·ce·re·bral
in·tra·cer·vi·cal
in·tra·cis·ter·nal
in·tra·cis·ter·nal·ly
in·tra·cra·ni·al

in·tra·cra·ni·al·ly
in·trac·ta·ble
in·tra·cu·ta·ne·ous
in·tra·cy·to·plas·mic
in·tra·der·mal
also in·tra·der·mic

in·tra·duct·al
in·tra·du·ral
in·tra·fas·cic·u·lar
in·tra·group
also in·tra·group·al

in·tra·he·pat·ic
in·tra·lo·bar
in·tra·lob·u·lar
in·tra·lu·mi·nal
in·tra·med·ul·lary
in·tra·mem·bra·nous
in·tra·mo·lec·u·lar
in·tra·mu·ral
in·tra·mus·cu·lar
in·tra·na·sal
in·tra·na·tal
in·tra·neu·ral
in·tra·nu·cle·ar
in·tra·oc·u·lar
in·tra·op·er·a·tive
in·tra·op·er·a·tive·ly
in·tra·oral
in·tra·or·bit·al
in·tra·pa·ri·etal
in·tra·par·tum
in·tra·pel·vic
in·tra·peri·car·di·ac
in·tra·per·i·to·ne·al
in·tra·pi·al
in·tra·pleu·ral
in·tra·psy·chic
or in·tra·psy·chi·cal

in·tra·pul·mo·nary
in·tra·pul·mon·ic
in·tra·scro·tal
in·tra·spi·nal
in·tra·stro·mal
in·tra·the·cal
in·tra·tho·rac·ic
in·tra·tra·che·al
in·tra·tub·al
in·tra·uter·ine
in·tra·vag·i·nal
in·trav·a·sa·tion
in·tra·vas·cu·lar
in·tra·vas·cu·lar·ly
in·tra·ve·nous
in·tra·ve·nous·ly
in·tra·ven·tric·u·lar
in·tra·ves·i·cal
in·tra·vi·tal
in·tra·vi·tam
in·tra·vi·tel·line
in·tra·vit·re·ous
in·trin·sic
in·trin·si·cal·ly
in·tro·flex·ion
also in·tro·flec·tion

in·troi·tal
in·troi·tus
pl in·troi·tus

in·tro·ject
in·tro·jec·tion
in·tro·mis·sion
in·tro·mit·tent
in·tro·spect
in·tro·spec·tion
in·tro·spec·tive
in·tro·sus·cep·tion
in·tro·ver·sion
in·tro·ver·sive
in·tro·ver·sive·ly
in·tro·vert
in·tu·bate
in·tu·bat·ed
in·tu·bat·ing
in·tu·ba·tion
in·tu·mesce
in·tu·mesced
in·tu·mesc·ing
in·tu·mes·cence
in·tu·mes·cent
in·tus·sus·cept
in·tus·sus·cep·tion
in·tus·sus·cep·tum
pl in·tus·sus·cep·ta

in·tus·sus·cip·i·ens
pl in·tus·sus·cip·en·tes

in·u·lase
also in·u·lin·ase

in·u·lin
in·unc·tion
in ute·ro
in vac·uo
in·vade
in·vad·ed
in·vad·ing
in·vag·i·nate
in·vag·i·nat·ed
in·vag·i·nat·ing
in·vag·i·na·tion
in·va·lid
in·va·lid·ism
in·va·sion
in·va·sive
in·va·sive·ness
in·ver·sion
in·vert
in·ver·tase
In·ver·te·bra·ta
in·ver·te·brate
in·vert·in
in·ver·tor
in·vest·ment
in·vet·er·ate
in·vi·a·bil·i·ty
pl in·vi·a·bil·i·ties

in·vi·a·ble
in·vis·ca·tion
in vi·tro
in vi·vo
in·vo·lu·cre
in·vo·lu·crum
pl in·vo·lu·cra

in·vol·un·tary
in·vo·lute
in·vo·lu·tion
in·vo·lu·tion·al
Iod·amoe·ba
io·date
io·dide
io·din·ate
io·din·at·ed
io·din·at·ing
io·din·ation
io·dine
also io·din

io·din·oph·i·lous
also io·din·o·phil

io·dism
io·dize
io·dized
io·diz·ing
io·do·ace·tic
io·do·ca·sein
io·do·form
io·do·gor·go·ic
io·dom·e·try
also io·dim·e·try
pl io·dom·e·tries
also io·dim·e·tries

io·do·phile
io·do·phil·ic
io·do·phor
io·do·phtha·lein
io·do·pro·tein
io·dop·sin
io·do·pyr·a·cet
ion ex·change
ion ex·chang·er
io·ni·um

ion·iza·tion
ion·ize
ion·ized
ion·niz·ing
ion·to·pho·re·sis
pl ion·to·pho·re·ses

ion·to·pho·ret·ic
io·ta·cism
ip·e·cac
or ipe·ca·cu·a·nha

ip·o·moea
also ip·o·mea

ipro·ni·a·zid
ip·si·lat·er·al
also ip·so·lat·er·al

ip·si·lat·er·al·ly
iri·dal
iri·dal·gia
iri·dec·tome
iri·dec·to·mize
iri·dec·to·mized
iri·dec·to·miz·ing
iri·dec·to·my
pl iri·dec·to·mies

iri·dec·tro·pi·um
iri·de·mia
iri·den·tro·pi·um
ir·i·des·cence
ir·i·des·cent
irid·i·al
irid·i·an
irid·ic
iri·din
iri·di·za·tion
iri·do·cap·su·li·tis

iri·do·cho·roid·itis
iri·do·cy·clec·to·my
pl iri·do·cy·clec·to·mies
iri·do·cy·cli·tis
iri·do·cy·clo·cho·roid·itis
iri·do·cys·tec·to·my
pl iri·do·cys·tec·to·mies
irid·o·cyte
iri·do·di·al·y·sis
pl iri·do·di·al·y·ses
iri·do·do·ne·sis
pl iri·do·do·ne·ses
iri·do·ki·ne·sia
iri·do·ple·gia
iri·do·scle·rot·o·my
pl iri·do·scle·rot·o·mies
iri·sin
iri·tis
ir·ra·di·ate
ir·ra·di·at·ed
ir·ra·di·at·ing
ir·ra·di·a·tion
ir·ra·tio·nal
ir·ra·tio·nal·i·ty
pl ir·ra·tio·nal·i·ties
ir·ra·tio·nal·ly
ir·re·duc·ibil·i·ty
pl ir·re·duc·ibil·i·ties
ir·re·duc·ible
ir·reg·u·lar
ir·reg·u·lar·i·ty
pl ir·reg·u·lar·i·ties
ir·re·spi·rable
ir·re·sus·ci·ta·ble
ir·ri·gate
ir·ri·gat·ed
ir·ri·gat·ing
ir·ri·ga·tion
ir·ri·ga·tor
ir·ri·ta·bil·i·ty
pl ir·ri·ta·bil·i·ties
ir·ri·ta·ble
ir·ri·tant
ir·ri·tate
ir·ri·tat·ed
ir·ri·tat·ing
ir·ri·ta·tion
ir·ri·ta·tive
ir·ru·ma·tion
is·aux·e·sis
pl is·aux·e·ses
is·aux·et·ic
isch·emia
also isch·aemia
isch·emic
is·chi·ad·ic
is·chi·al
is·chi·at·ic
is·chio·cap·su·lar
is·chio·cav·er·no·sus
is·chio·coc·cy·geus
pl is·chio·coc·cy·gei
is·chio·fe·mo·ral
is·chi·om·e·lus
pl is·chi·om·e·li
is·chio·neu·ral·gia
is·chi·op·a·gus
pl is·chi·op·a·gi
is·chio·pu·bic
is·chio·rec·tal
is·chi·um
pl is·chia
isch·uria
Ishi·ha·ra test
isin·glass
is·land of Lang·er·hans
is·land of Reil
is·let of Lang·er·hans
iso·ag·glu·ti·na·tion
iso·ag·glu·ti·na·tive
iso·ag·glu·ti·nin
iso·ag·glu·tin·o·gen
iso·al·lox·a·zine
iso·am·yl
iso·an·ti·body
pl iso·an·ti·bod·ies
iso·an·ti·gen
iso·bor·nyl
iso·bu·tyl
iso·bu·tyr·ic
iso·cel·lu·lar
iso·chro·mat·ic

iso·chro·mat·o·phil
iso·chro·mo·some
iso·chro·nal
iso·chro·nal·ly
iso·chro·nia
iso·chron·ic
iso·chro·nism
iso·chro·nous
iso·cit·ric
iso·co·ria
iso·cor·tex
pl iso·cor·ti·ces
or iso·cor·tex·es
iso·cy·a·nide
iso·cy·clic
iso·dac·tyl·ism
iso·dont
iso·dose
iso·en·zy·mat·ic
iso·en·zyme
iso·en·zy·mic
iso·flu·ro·phate
iso·ga·mete
iso·ga·met·ic
isog·a·mous
also iso·gam·ic
isog·a·my
pl isog·a·mies
iso·ge·ne·ic
iso·gen·e·sis
pl iso·gen·e·ses
iso·gon·ic
isog·o·ny
pl isog·o·nies
iso·graft
iso·hem·ag·glu·ti·na·tion
iso·hem·ag·glu·ti·nin
iso·he·mo·ly·sin
iso·he·mol·y·sis
pl iso·he·mol·y·ses
iso·hy·dric
iso·im·mu·ni·za·tion
iso·late
iso·lat·ed
iso·lat·ing
iso·la·tion
iso·lec·i·thal
iso·leu·cine
isol·o·gous
iso·logue
or iso·log
iso·malt·ose
iso·mer
isom·er·ase
iso·mer·ic
isom·er·ide
isom·er·ism
isom·er·i·za·tion
isom·er·ize
isom·er·ized
isom·er·iz·ing
isom·er·ous
iso·met·ric
also iso·met·ri·cal
iso·met·rics
iso·me·tro·pia
iso·morph
iso·mor·phic
iso·mor·phism
iso·mor·phous
iso·ni·a·zid
iso·nic·o·ti·no·yl·hy·dra·zine
or iso·nic·o·ti·nyl·hy·dra·zine
iso·ni·trile
isop·a·thy
pl isop·a·thies
iso·pho·ria
iso·pia
iso·plas·tic
iso·pre·cip·i·tin
iso·pren·a·line
iso·prene
iso·pren·oid
iso·pro·pa·nol
iso·pro·pyl
iso·pro·pyl·ar·te·re·nol
iso·pro·ter·e·nol
isop·ter
is·os·mot·ic
Isos·po·ra
iso·spo·rous
iso·spo·ry
pl iso·spo·ries
iso·stere
also iso·ster
isos·the·nu·ria
iso·ton·ic
iso·ton·i·cal·ly
iso·to·nic·i·ty
pl iso·to·nic·i·ties
iso·tope
iso·to·pic

iso·tro·pic
isot·ro·pous
iso·va·le·ric
iso·zyme
iso·zy·mic
isth·mec·to·my
pl isth·mec·to·mies
isth·mi·an
isth·mic
isth·mus
isth·mus of the fau·ces
it·a·con·ic
itch·i·ness
itchy
itch·i·er
itch·i·est
iter
Ix·o·des
ix·o·dic
ix·o·did
Ix·od·i·dae
ix·o·doid
Ix·o·doi·dea

J

jaag·siek·te
or jaag·ziek·te
also jag·siek·te
or jag·ziek·te
jab·o·ran·di
jack·screw
Jack·so·ni·an
Ja·cob·son's car·ti·lage
or Ja·cob·son's tur·bi·nal
Ja·cob·son's nerve
Ja·cob·son's or·gan
jac·ti·tate
jac·ti·tat·ed
jac·ti·tat·ing
jac·ti·ta·tion
jake leg
jal·ap
jala·pin
Ja·mai·ca gin·ger
James·ian
James-Lange the·o·ry
James·town weed
var of jimsonweed
jani·ceps
Ja·nus green
or Ja·nus green B
Ja·risch-Herx·hei·mer re·ac·tion
Jat·ro·pha
ja·troph·ic
jaun·dice
jaun·diced
Ja·velle wa·ter
or Ja·vel wa·ter
ja·vell·iza·tion
jaw·bone
jaw·line
jec·o·rin
jec·o·rize
jec·o·rized
jec·o·riz·ing
je·ju·nal
je·ju·nec·to·my
pl je·ju·nec·to·mies
je·ju·ni·tis
je·ju·no·co·los·to·my
pl je·ju·no·co·los·to·mies
je·ju·no·il·e·itis
pl je·ju·no·il·e·it·i·des
je·ju·no·il·e·os·to·my
pl je·ju·no·il·e·os·to·mies
je·ju·no·je·ju·nos·to·my
pl je·ju·no·je·ju·nos·to·mies
je·ju·nos·to·my
pl je·ju·nos·to·mies
je·ju·not·o·my
pl je·ju·not·o·mies
je·ju·num
pl je·ju·na
Je·kyll and Hyde
jel·ly fish
Jen·ne·ri·an
jet lag
jig·ger
jim·son·weed
or James·town weed
or jimp·son
or jimp·son·weed
jock itch
jock·strap
also jock
or jock·ey strap
Joh·ne's ba·cil·lus

joh·nin
john·ny
pl john·nies
Joule's equiv·a·lent
ju·gal
ju·gal point
also ju·ga·le
jug·u·lar
jug·u·lum
pl jug·u·la
ju·gum
pl ju·ga
or ju·gums
ju·jube
junc·tion
junc·tion·al
junc·tu·ra
pl junc·tu·rae
junc·ture
Jung·ian
ju·ni·per oil
or ju·ni·per-ber·ry oil
ju·ni·per-tar oil
or ju·ni·per tar
ju·ry-mast
jus·to ma·jor
jus·to mi·nor
ju·ve·nile
jux·ta·glo·mer·u·lar
jux·ta·pose
jux·ta·posed
jux·ta·pos·ing
jux·ta·po·si·tion

K

Kahn test
or Kahn re·ac·tion
or Kahn
kak·i·dro·sis
pl kak·i·dro·ses
ka·la azar
ka·li·um
kal·li·din
kal·li·krein
ka·ma·la
also ka·me·la
or ka·mi·la
ka·na·my·cin
ka·olin
also ka·oline
ka·o·lin·osis
pl ka·o·lin·oses
or ka·o·lin·osis·es
ka·ra·ya gum
also ka·ra·ya
Kar·ta·ge·ner's syn·drome
kary·en·chy·ma
pl kary·en·chy·ma·ta
or kary·en·chy·mas
karyo·chrome
kar·yo·clas·ic
or kar·yo·clas·tic
kary·oc·la·sis
or kary·ok·la·sis
pl kary·oc·la·ses
or kary·ok·la·ses
karyo·cyte
karyo·gam·ic
kary·og·a·my
pl kary·og·a·mies
karyo·ki·ne·sis
pl karyo·ki·ne·ses
karyo·ki·net·ic
karyo·lo·bic
kary·ol·o·gy
pl kary·ol·o·gies
karyo·lymph
kary·ol·y·sis
pl kary·ol·y·ses
karyo·lyt·ic
kar·yo·mere
karyo·mi·cro·some
kar·yo·mi·tome
karyo·mi·to·sis
pl karyo·mi·to·ses
karyo·phage
karyo·plasm
also karyo·plas·ma
karyo·plas·mic
or karyo·plas·mat·ic
karyo·pyc·not·ic
karyo·pyk·no·sis
kary·or·rhec·tic
kary·or·rhex·is
pl kary·or·rhex·es
karyo·some
kary·os·ta·sis
pl kary·os·ta·ses
kar·yo·the·ca
karyo·type
karyo·typ·ic
or karyo·typ·i·cal
kat
or khat
or qat
also quat

ka·tab·o·lism
var of catabolism

kata·chro·ma·sis
or cata·chro·ma·sis
pl kata·chro·ma·ses
or cata·chro·ma·ses

kata·ther·mom·e·ter
or cata·ther·mom·e·ter

Ka·ta·ya·ma

ka·thar·sis
var of catharsis

ka·thar·tic
var of ca·thar·tic

kath·i·so·pho·bia

kat·zen·jam·mer

ka·va
or ca·va
also ka·va·ka·va

ked

kef
or kif

kel·lin
var of khellin

ke·loid
or che·loid

ke·loi·dal

ke·lo·ma
pl ke·lo·mas
or ke·lo·ma·ta

Kel·vin scale

Ken·ny meth·od
or Ken·ny treat·ment

keno·pho·bia

keno·tox·in

keph·a·lin
var of cephalin

ker·a·phyl·lo·cele

ker·a·sin

ker·a·tal·gia

ker·a·tec·ta·sia

ker·a·tec·to·my
pl ker·a·tec·to·mies

ke·rat·ic

ker·a·tin
also cer·a·tin

ke·ra·ti·ni·za·tion

ke·ra·tin·ize
ke·ra·tin·ized
ke·ra·tin·iz·ing

ke·ra·ti·no·phil·ic

ke·ra·ti·nous

ker·a·ti·tis
also cer·a·ti·tis
pl ker·a·tit·i·des
also cer·a·tit·i·des

ker·a·to·ac·an·tho·ma
pl ker·a·to·ac·an·tho·mas
or ker·a·to·ac·an·tho·ma·ta

ker·a·to·cele

ker·a·to·cen·te·sis
pl ker·a·to·cen·te·ses

ker·a·to·chro·ma·to·sis
pl ker·a·to·chro·ma·to·ses

ker·a·to·con·junc·ti·vi·tis
or cer·a·to·con·junc·ti·vi·tis

ker·a·to·co·nus

ker·a·to·der·ma

ker·a·to·gen·e·sis
pl ker·a·to·gen·e·ses

ker·a·tog·e·nous

ker·a·to·glo·bus

ker·a·to·hel·co·sis
pl ker·a·to·hel·co·ses

ker·a·to·he·mia

ker·a·to·hy·a·lin

ker·a·toid

ker·a·to·iri·do·scope

ker·a·to·iri·tis

ker·a·to·leu·ko·ma

ker·a·tol·y·sis
pl ker·a·tol·y·ses

ker·a·to·lyt·ic

ker·a·to·ma
pl ker·a·to·mas
or ker·a·to·ma·ta

ker·a·to·ma·la·cia

ker·a·tome

ker·a·tom·e·ter

ker·a·to·my·co·sis
pl ker·a·to·my·co·ses

ker·a·to·nyx·is
pl ker·a·to·nyx·es

ker·a·to·plas·ty
pl ker·a·to·plasties

ker·a·to·rhex·is
pl ker·a·to·rhex·es

ker·a·to·scle·ri·tis

ker·a·to·scope

ker·a·tos·co·py
pl ker·a·tos·co·pies

ker•a•tose
or cer•a•tose

ker•a•to•sis
pl ker•a•to•ses

ker•a•tot•ic

ker•a•tot•o•my
pl ker•a•tot•o•mies

ke•rau•no•pho•bia

ke•ri•on

ker•nic•ter•us

Ker•nig sign
or Ker•nig's sign

ker•o•sine
or ker•o•sene

ke•tal

ke•tene

ke•to

ke•to•ac•i•do•sis
pl ke•to•ac•i•do•ses

ke•to•gen•e•sis
pl ke•to•gen•e•ses

ke•to•gen•ic

ke•to•glu•ta•rate

ke•to•glu•tar•ic

ke•to•hep•tose

ke•to hex•ose

ke•tol•y•sis
pl ke•tol•y•ses

ke•to•lyt•ic

ke•tone

ke•to•ne•mia
or ke•to•nae•mia

ke•to•ne•mic

ke•ton•ic

ke•to•nu•ria

ke•to•re•duc•tase

ke•tose

ke•to•side

ke•to•sis
pl ke•to•ses

ke•to•ste•roid

ke•tot•ic

khat
var of kat

khel•lin
also kel•lin

kid•ney
pl kid•neys

kif
var of kef

kil•u•rane

Kim•mel•stiel-Wilson syn•drome

ki•nase

ki•ne•mat•ic
or ki•ne•mat•i•cal

ki•ne•mat•i•cal•ly

ki•ne•mat•ics
also ci•ne•mat•ics

kin•e•mat•o•graph
var of cinemato-graph

kin•e•plas•ty
var of cineplasty

kin•e•sal•gia

kin•e•scope

ki•ne•sia

ki•ne•si•at•rics

ki•ne•sics

kin•e•sim•e•ter
also ki•ne•si•om•e•ter

ki•ne•si•o•log•ic
or ki•ne•si•o•log•i•cal

ki•ne•si•ol•o•gy
pl ki•ne•si•ol•o•gies

ki•ne•sis
or ci•ne•sis
pl ki•ne•ses
or ci•ne•ses

ki•ne•si•ther•a•py
pl ki•ne•si•ther•a•pies

ki•ne•so•pho•bia

kin•es•the•sia
also kin•aes•the•sia

kin•es•the•si•om•e•ter

kin•es•the•sis
also kin•aes•the•sis
pl kin•es•the•ses
also kin•aes•the•ses

kin•es•thet•ic
also kin•aes•the•ic

ki•net•ic

ki•net•ics

ki•ne•tin

ki•neto•car•dio•gram

ki•net•o•chore

ki•neto•graph

ki•neto•graph•ic

ki•neto•nu•cle•us
pl ki•neto•nu•clei
also ki•neto•nu•cle•us•es

ki•neto•plast
also ci•neto•plast

ki•neto•plas•tic

kin•e•to•sis
pl kin•e•to•ses

ki•neto•some
king's evil
ki•nin
ki•nin•o•gen
ki•nin•o•gen•ic
ki•no
ki•no•cen•trum
pl ki•no•cen•trums
or ki•no•cen•tra

kin•o•mere
kin•o•plasm
also kin•o•plas•ma

kin•ship
ki•ot•o•my
pl ki•ot•o•mies

kiss•ing dis•ease
kiss of life
Kjel•dahl flask
kjel•dahl•iza•tion
kjel•dahl•ize
kjel•dahl•ized
kjel•dahl•iz•ing
Kjel•dahl meth•od
kleb•si•el•la
Klebs-Löff•ler ba•cil•lus
klep•to•lag•nia
kelp•to•ma•nia
or clep•to•ma•nia

klep•to•ma•ni•ac
or clep•to•ma•ni•ac

klep•to•pho•bia
klieg eyes
or kleig eyes

Kline•fel•ter's syn•drome

Kline re•ac•tion
or Kline test

Klip•pel-Feil syn•drome
Klump•ke's pa•ral•y•sis
knee•cap
knee jerk
knee•pan
knee-sprung
Kne•mi•do•kop•tes
knock-knee
knock-kneed
knock•out drops
Knoop hard•ness
knuck•le
knuck•led
knuck•ling
knuck•le•bone
Koch phe•nom•e•non
Koch's ba•cil•lus
or Koch ba•cil•lus

Koch's pos•tu•lates
also Koch's laws

Koch-Weeks ba•cil•lus
koil•onych•ia
koi•lo•ster•nia
ko•jic
ko•la nut
also ko•la
or co•la nut

ko•la tree

Kol•mer
or Kol•mer re•ac•tion
or Kol•mer test
or Kol•mer's test

ko•nim•e•ter
also co•ni•om•e•ter

ko•nio•cor•tex
pl ko•nio•cor•ti•ces

ko•ni•ol•o•gy
also co•ni•ol•o•gy
pl ko•ni•ol•o•gies
also co•ni•ol•o•gies

Kop•lik's spots
also Kop•lik spots

Kor•sa•koff's psy•cho•sis
or Kor•sa•koff's syn•drome
also Kor•sa•kow's psy•cho•sis
or Kor•sa•kow's syn•drome

ko•sin
ko•so
or kos•so
or kous•so

kou•miss
or ku•miss
or ku•mys
or ku•myss

Krab•be's dis•ease
Krae•pe•lin•i•an
krait
kra•me•ria
krau•ro•sis
pl krau•ro•ses

krau•rot•ic
Krau•se's cor•pus•cle

Krau•se's end-bulb
Krau•se's mem•brane
Krebs cy•cle
Kru•ken•berg tu•mor
Kupf•fer cell
also Kupf•fer's cell
ku•ru
Kuss•maul breath•ing
or Kuss•maul res•pi•ra•tion
kwash•i•or•kor
ky•es•te•in
ky•mo•gram
ky•mo•graph
or cy•mo•graph
ky•mo•graph•ic
ky•mog•ra•phy
pl ky•mog•ra•phies
kyn•uren•ic
kyn•uren•ine
ky•pho•sco•li•o•sis
pl ky•pho•sco•li•o•ses
ky•pho•sco•li•ot•ic
ky•pho•sis
pl ky•pho•ses
ky•phot•ic

L

la•bi•al
la•bi•al•ism
la•bi•al•ly
la•bia ma•jo•ra
la•bia mi•no•ra
la•bile
la•bil•i•ty
pl la•bil•i•ties
la•bio•cer•vi•cal
la•bio•den•tal
la•bio•gin•gi•val
la•bio•glos•so•la•ryn•geal
la•bio•men•tal
la•bio•pal•a•tine
la•bio•plas•ty
pl la•bio•plas•ties
la•bi•um
pl la•bia
la•bor
la•brum
lab•y•rinth
lab•y•rin•thec•to•my
pl lab•y•rin•thec•to•mies
lab•y•rin•thine
lab•y•rin•thi•tis
lab•y•rin•thot•o•my
pl lab•y•rin•thot•o•mies
lac•er•ate
lac•er•at•ed
lac•er•at•ing
lac•er•a•tion
la•cer•tus fi•bro•sus
lach•ry•mal
or lac•ri•mal
lac•ri•ma•tion
also lach•ry•ma•tion
lac•ri•ma•tor
or lach•ry•ma•tor
lac•ri•ma•to•ry
or lach•ry•ma•to•ry
lac•ri•mot•o•my
pl lac•ri•mot•o•mies
lac•ta•gogue
lact•al•bu•min
lac•tase
lac•tate
lac•tat•ed
lac•tat•ing
lac•ta•tion
lac•ta•tion•al
lac•ta•tion•al•ly
lac•te•al
lac•tes•cent
lac•tic
lac•tif•er•ous
lac•ti•fuge
lac•tig•e•nous
lac•tim
Lac•to•bac•il•la•ce•ae
lac•to•ba•cil•lus
pl lac•to•ba•cil•li
Lac•to•ba•cil•lus ca•sei fac•tor
lac•to•cele
lac•to•fla•vin
lac•to•gen
lac•to•gen•e•sis
pl lac•to•gen•e•ses
lac•to•gen•ic
lac•to•glob•u•lin
lac•tom•e•ter

lac·tone
lac·to·per·ox·i·dase
lac·to·pro·tein
lac·tor·rhea
lac·tose
lac·tos·uria
lac·to·veg·e·tar·i·an
la·cu·na
pl la·cu·nae
or la·cu·nas
la·cu·nal
or la·cu·nar
la·cu·nule
Laen·nec's cir·rho·sis
la·ge·na
pl la·ge·nae
lag·neia
lag·oph·thal·mos
or lag·oph·thal·mus
lake
laked
lak·ing
laky
lak·i·er
lak·i·est
lal·la·tion
lal·og·no·sis
la·lop·a·thy
pl la·lop·a·thies
lal·o·ple·gia
lal·or·rhea
La·marck·ian
La·marck·ism
lamb·da
lamb·da·cism
lamb·doid
or lamb·doi·dal
lam·bert
Lam·blia
lam·bli·a·sis
lame
la·mel·la
pl la·mel·lae
also la·mel·las
la·mel·lar
lam·i·na
pl lam·i·nae
or lam·i·nas
lam·i·na cri·bro·sa
pl lam·i·nae cri·bro·sae
lam·i·na·gram
or lam·i·no·gram
lam·i·na·graph
or lam·i·no·graph
lam·i·na pro·pria
pl lam·i·nae pro·pri·ae
lam·i·nar
lam·i·nate
lam·i·nat·ed
lam·i·nat·ing
lam·i·na·tion
lam·i·nec·to·my
pl lam·i·nec·to·mies
lam·i·ni·tis
lam·i·not·o·my
pl lam·i·not·o·mies
la·nat·o·side
lance
lanced
lanc·ing
Lance·field group
also Lance·field's group
or Lance·field group·ing
lan·cet
lan·ci·nate
lan·ci·nat·ed
lan·ci·nat·ing
land·mark
Lan·dry's pa·ral·y·sis
lani·ary
lan·o·lin
also lan·o·line
la·nos·ter·ol
lan·tha·num
la·nu·go
pl la·nu·gos
la·pac·tic
lap·a·ror·rha·phy
pl lap·a·ror·rha·phies
lap·a·ro·scope
lap·a·rot·o·my
pl lap·a·rot·o·mies
lap·in·ized
also lap·in·ised
la·pis
lap·pa
large intestine
lar·va
pl lar·vae
also lar·vas
lar·val
lar·va mi·grans
pl lar·vae mi·gran·tes

lar•vate
or lar•vat•ed

lar•vi•cide
also lar•va•cide

la•ryn•ge•al

la•ryn•ge•al•ly

lar•yn•gec•to•mee

lar•yn•gec•to•mize
lar•yn•gec•to•mized
lar•yn•gec•to•miz•ing

lar•yn•gec•to•my
pl lar•yn•gec•to•mies

lar•yn•gis•mus
pl lar•yn•gis•mi

lar•yn•gis•mus stri•du•lus
pl lar•yn•gis•mi stri•du•li

lar•yn•git•ic

lar•yn•gi•tis
pl lar•yn•git•i•des

la•ryn•go•cele

la•ryn•go•fis•sure

la•ryn•go•graph

lar•yn•gol•o•gy
pl lar•yn•gol•o•gies

la•ryn•go•pa•ral•y•sis
pl la•ryn•go•pa•ral•y•ses

lar•yn•gop•a•thy
pl lar•yn•gop•a•thies

la•ryn•go•phan•tom

la•ryn•go•pha•ryn•geal

la•ryn•go•phar•yn•gec•to•my
pl la•ryn•go•phar•yn•gec•to•mies

la•ryn•go•phar•yn•gi•tis
pl la•ryn•go•phar•yn•git•i•des

la•ryn•go•phar•ynx
pl la•ryn•go•pha•ryn•ges
also la•ryn•go•phar•ynx•es

la•ryn•go•plas•ty
pl la•ryn•go•plas•ties

la•ryn•go•ple•gia

la•ryn•go•rhi•nol•o•gy
pl la•ryn•go•rhi•nol•o•gies

la•ryn•go•scle•ro•ma
pl la•ryn•go•scle•ro•mas
or la•ryn•go•scle•ro•ma•ta

la•ryn•go•scope

la•ryn•go•scop•ic

lar•yn•gos•co•py
pl lar•yn•gos•co•pies

la•ryn•go•spasm

la•ryn•go•ste•no•sis
pl la•ryn•go•ste•no•ses

lar•yn•gos•to•my
pl lar•yn•gos•to•mies

lar•yn•got•o•my
pl lar•yn•got•o•mies

la•ryn•go•tra•che•al

la•ryn•go•tra•che•itis

la•ryn•go•tra•cheo•bron•chi•tis
pl la•ryn•go•tra•cheo•bron•chit•i•des

la•ryn•go•tra•che•ot•o•my
pl la•ryn•go•tra•che•ot•o•mies

la•ryn•go•xe•ro•sis
pl la•ryn•go•xe•ro•ses

lar•ynx
pl la•ryn•ges
also lar•ynx•es
part of the trachea
(*see* pharynx)

la•ser

L-as•par•a•gi•nase

la•tah

la•ten•cy
pl la•ten•cies

la•tent

lat•er•ad

lat•er•al

lat•er•al•i•ty
pl lat•er•al•i•ties

lat•ero•ab•dom•i•nal

lat•ero•duc•tion

lat•ero•flex•ion

lat•ero•pul•sion

lat•ero•tor•sion

lat·ero·ver·sion
lath·y·rism
lath·y·rit·ic
la·tis·si·mus dor·si
pl la·tis·si·mi dor·si
Lat·ro·dec·tus
lat·tice
lat·ticed
lat·tic·ing
la·tus
laud·able
lau·dan·o·sine
lau·da·num
laugh·ing gas
lau·ric
la·vage
la·va·tion
la·va·tion·al
lav·en·der
Lav·er·a·nia
lax·a·tion
lax·a·tive
lax·a·tive·ly
lay·er
lay·er of Lang·hans
la·zar
laz·a·ret·to
pl laz·a·ret·tos
L-do·pa
leach
lec·i·thal
also lec·i·thic
lec·i·thin
lec·i·thin·ase
lec·i·tho·blast
lec·i·tho·pro·tein
lec·tin
leech
left-hand·ed
leg·ged
le·gu·min
leio·der·mia
leio·myo·fi·bro·ma
pl leio·myo·fi·bro·mas
also leio·myo·fi·bro·ma·ta
leio·my·o·ma
pl leio my·o·mas
or leio·my·o·ma·ta
leio·myo·sar·co·ma
pl leio·myo·sar·co·mas
or leio·myo·sar·co·ma·ta
lei·ot·ri·chous
leish·man·ia
leish·man·i·a·sis
also leish·man·i·o·sis
pl leish·man·i·a·ses
or leish·man·i·o·ses
le·ma
lem·mo·cyte
lem·nis·cus
pl lem·nis·ci
lens·om·e·ter
len·ti·co·nus
len·tic·u·la
pl len·tic·u·las
or len·tic·u·lae
len·tic·u·lar
len·tic·u·lo·stri·ate
len·tic·u·lo·tha·lam·ic
len·ti·form
len·ti·glo·bus
len·ti·go
pl len·tig·i·nes
le·on·ti·a·sis
pl le·on·ti·a·ses
le·on·ti·a·sis os·sea
lep·er
lep·i·dine
Lep·i·dop·tera
lep·i·dop·ter·an
lep·i·do·sis
pl lep·i·do·ses
lep·o·thrix
pl lep·o·thrix·es
also le·pot·ri·ches
lep·ra
lep·rid
lep·rol·o·gist
lep·rol·o·gy
pl lep·rol·o·gies
lep·ro·ma
pl lep·ro·mas
or lep·ro·ma·ta
lep·ro·ma·tous
lep·ro·min
lep·ro·sar·i·um
pl lep·ro·sar·i·ums
or lep·ro·sar·ia
lep·ro·stat·ic
lep·ro·sy
pl lep·ro·sies

lep·rot·ic
lep·rous
lep·to·ceph·a·lous
also lep·to·ce·phal·ic

lep·to·ceph·a·lus
pl lep·to·ceph·a·li

lep·to·cyte
lep·to·cy·to·sis
lep·to·dac·ty·lous
lep·to·men·in·ge·al
lep·to·men·in·gi·tis
pl lep·to·men·in·git·i·des

lep·to·men·in·gop·a·thy
pl lep·to·men·in·gop·a·thies

lep·to·me·ninx
pl lep·to·me·nin·ges

lep·to·mo·nad
lep·to·mo·nas
lep·to·pel·lic
lep·to·pho·nia
lep·to·pro·so·pia
lep·to·pro·so·pic
also lep·to·pro·so·pous

lep·tor·rhine
lep·to·scope
lep·to·spi·ra
pl lep·to·spi·ra
also lep·to·spi·ras
or lep·to·spi·rae

lep·to·spir·al
lep·to·spire
lep·to·spi·ro·sis
pl lep·to·spi·ro·ses

lep·to·tene
Lep·to·trich·ia
le·re·sis
les·bi·an
les·bi·an·ism
le·sion
le·thal
le·thal·i·ty
pl le·thal·i·ties

le·thal·ly
leth·ar·gy
pl leth·ar·gies

Let·ter·er-Siwe dis·ease
leu·cae·mia, leu·ce·mia
vars of leukemia

leu·cine
leu·cin·uria
leu·co·blast
var of leukoblast

leu·co·ci·din
leu·co·cyte
var of leukocyte

leu·co·cy·the·mia
also leu·co·cy·thae·mia

leu·co·cy·the·mic
also leu·co·cy·thae·mic

leu·co·cyt·ic
var of leukocytic

leu·co·cy·to·blast
var of leukocytoblast

leu·co·cy·to·poi·e·sis
var of leukocytopoiesis

leu·co·cy·to·sis
var of leukocytosis

leu·co·cy·tot·ic
var of leukocytotic

leu·co·der·ma
var of leukoderma

leu·co·en·ceph·a·li·tis
var of leukoencephalitis

leu·co·ma
var of leukoma

leu·co·nos·toc
leu·co·pe·nia
var of leukopenia

leu·co·poi·e·sis
var of leukopoiesis

leu·co·poi·et·ic
var of leukopoietic

leu·co·pro·te·ase
leu·cor·rhea, leu·cor·rhoea
vars of leukorrhea

leu·cor·rhe·al, leu·cor·rhoe·al
vars of leukorrheal

leu·co·sis
var of leukosis

leu·cov·o·rin
leu·ke·mia
also leu·kae·mia
or leu·ce·mia
or leu·cae·mia

leu·ke·mic
also leu·kae·mic

leu·ke·mid
leu·ke·mo·gen

leu•ke•mo•gen•e•sis
pl leu•ke•mo•gen•e•ses

leu•ke•mo•gen•ic

leu•ke•moid

leu•ko•blast
also leu•co•blast

leu•ko•blas•to•sis
pl leu•ko•blas•to•ses

leu•ko•ci•din

leu•ko•cyte
also leu•co•cyte

leu•ko•cy•the•mia

leu•ko•cyt•ic
also leu•co•cyt•ic

leu•ko•cy•to•blast
also leu•co•cy•to•blast

leu•ko•cy•to•gen•e•sis
pl leu•ko•cy•to•gen•e•ses

leu•ko•cy•to•ly•sin

leu•ko•cy•tol•y•sis
pl leu•ko•cy•tol•y•ses

leu•ko•cy•to•lyt•ic

leu•ko•cy•to•ma
pl leu•ko•cy•to•mas
or leu•ko•cy•to•ma•ta

leu•ko•cy•to•pe•nia

leu•ko•cy•to•poi•e•sis
also leu•co•cy•to•poi•e•sis
pl leu•ko•cy•to•poi•e•ses
also leu•co•cy•to•poi•e•ses

leu•ko•cy•to•sis
or leu•co•cy•to•sis
pl leu•ko•cy•to•ses
or leu•co•cy•to•ses

leu•ko•cy•tot•ic
or leu•co•cy•tot•ic

leu•ko•der•ma
also leu•co•der•ma

leu•ko•dys•tro•phy
pl leu•ko•dys•tro•phies

leu•ko•en•ceph•a•li•tis
also leu•co•en•ceph•a•li•tis
pl leu•ko•en•ceph•a•lit•i•des
also leu•co•en•ceph•a•lit•i•des

leu•ko•en•ceph•a•lop•a•thy
pl leu•ko•en•ceph•a•lop•a•thies

leu•ko•ma
also leu•co•ma

leu•kom•a•tous

leu•kon

leuk•onych•ia

leu•kop•a•thy
pl leu•kop•a•thies

leu•ko•pe•de•sis
pl leu•ko•pe•de•ses

leu•ko•pe•nia
or leu•co•pe•nia

leu•ko•pe•nic

leu•ko•phleg•ma•sia

leu•ko•plakia

leu•ko•poi•e•sis
or leu•co•poi•e•sis
pl leu•ko•poi•e•ses
or leu•co•poi•e•ses

leu•ko•poi•et•ic
or leu•co•poi•et•ic

leu•kop•sin

leu•kor•rha•gia

leu•kor•rhea
also leu•kor•rhoea
or leu•cor•rhea
or leu•cor•rhoea

leu•kor•rhe•al
also leu•kor•rhoe•al
or leu•cor•rhe•al
or leu•cor•rhoe•al

leu•ko•sar•co•ma
pl leu•ko•sar•co•mas
or leu•ko•sar•co•ma•ta

leu•ko•sar•co•ma•to•sis
pl leu•ko•sar•co•ma•to•ses

leu•ko•sis
or leu•co•sis
pl leu•ko•ses
or leu•co•ses

leu•ko•tome

leu•kot•o•my
pl leu•kot•o•mies

leu•ko•tox•in

leu•ko•trich•ia

leu•kot•rich•ous

lev•al•lor•phan

lev•ar•te•re•nol

le•va•tor
pl lev•a•to•res
or lev•a•tors

Le•vin tube
also Le•vine tube

lev·i·ta·tion
le·vo·car·dia
le·vo·car·dio·gram
le·vo·duc·tion
le·vo·gy·rate
or le·vo·gyre
le·vo·ro·ta·tion
le·vo·ro·ta·to·ry
or le·vo·ro·ta·ry
le·vo·ver·sion
lev·u·lose
lev·u·los·uria
lew·is·ite
Ley·dig cell
also Ley·dig's cell
li·bid·i·nal
li·bid·i·nal·ly
li·bid·i·ni·za·tion
li·bid·i·nize
li·bid·i·nized
li·bid·i·niz·ing
li·bid·i·nous
li·bid·i·nous·ly
li·bi·do
pl li·bi·dos
lice
pl of louse
li·censed prac·ti·cal nurse
li·censed vo·ca·tion·al nurse
li·chen
li·chen·i·fi·ca·tion
li·chen·in
li·chen·oid
li·chen pla·nus
lic·o·rice
also li·quo·rice
li·do·caine
Lie·ber·kühn's gland
also Lie·ber·kühn's crypt
Lie·ber·mann-Bur·chard re·ac·tion
li·en
li·en·al
li·en·cu·lus
pl li·en·cu·li
li·en·itis
li·en·og·ra·phy
pl li·en·og·ra·phies
li·enop·a·thy
pl li·enop·a·thies
li·eno·re·nal
li·eno·tox·in
li·en·ter·ic
li·en·tery
pl li·en·ter·ies
li·en·un·cu·lus
pl li·en·un·cu·li
Lie·se·gang ring
life
pl lives
life-sup·port sys·tem
lig·a·ment
lig·a·men·ta·ry
lig·a·ment of Coo·per
lig·a·ment of Treitz
lig·a·ment of Wins·low
lig·a·ment of Zinn
lig·a·men·to·pexy
pl lig·a·men·to·pex·ies
lig·a·men·tous
lig·a·men·tum
pl lig·a·men·ta
lig·a·men·tum fla·vum
pl lig·a·men·ta fla·va
lig·a·men·tum nu·chae
pl lig·a·men·ta nu·chae
li·gand
li·gase
li·gate
li·gat·ed
li·gat·ing
li·ga·tion
lig·a·ture
light-adapt·ed
light chain
lig·nin
lig·no·caine
lig·no·cel·lu·lose
lig·no·cel·lu·los·ic
lig·num
pl lig·nums
also lig·na
lig·u·la
pl lig·u·lae
also lig·u·las

lig·ule
lim·bic
lim·bus
li·men
lime·wa·ter
lim·in·al
lim·it
li·mon
li·moph·thi·sis
pl li·moph·thi·ses

li·nar·ia
lin·co·my·cin
linc·tus
lin·dane
lin·ea
pl lin·e·ae

lin·ea al·ba
pl lin·e·ae al·bae

lin·e·ae al·bi·can·tes
lin·ear
lin·gua
pl lin·guae

lin·gual
lin·gual·ly
Lin·guat·u·la
lin·guat·u·lo·sis
pl lin·guat·u·lo·ses

lin·gui·form
lin·gu·la
pl lin·gu·lae

lin·guo·dis·tal
lin·guo·gin·gi·val
lin·guo·ver·sion
lin·i·ment
li·nin
li·ni·tis
link·age
linked
Li·nog·na·thus
lin·ole·ic
lin·o·le·nic
lin·seed
li·pase
li·pec·to·my
pl li·pec·to·mies

li·pe·mia
also li·pae·mia

lip·id
also lip·ide

li·pid·ic
lip·i·do·sis
pl lip·i·do·ses

li·po·blast
li·po·ca·ic
li·po·chon·dro·dys·tro·phy
pl li·po·chon·dro·dys·tro·phies

li·po·chrome
li·po·cyte
li·po·dys·tro·phy
pl li·po·dys·tro·phies

li·po·fi·bro·ma
pl li·po·fi·bro·mas
also li·po·fi·bro·ma·ta

li·po·fus·cin
li·po·gen·e·sis
pl li·po·gen·e·ses

li·pog·e·nous
also lip·o·gen·ic

li·po·gran·u·lo·ma
pl li·po·gran·u·lo·mas
or li·po·gran·u·lo·ma·ta

li·po·ic
li·poid
or lip·oi·dal

li·poi·do·sis
pl li·poi·do·ses

li·pol·y·sis
pl li·pol·y·ses

li·po·lyt·ic
li·po·ma
pl li·po·mas
or li·po·ma·ta

li·pom·a·toid
li·po·ma·to·sis
pl li·po·ma·to·ses

li·po·ma·tous
li·po·me·tab·o·lism
li·po·pe·nia
li·po·phage
li·po·pha·gia
li·po·pha·gic
li·po·phan·er·o·sis
pl li·po·phan·er·o·ses

li·po·phil
li·po·phil·ic
also li·po·phile

li·po·phore
li·po·phre·nia
li·po·poly·sac·cha·ride
li·po·pro·tein
li·po·sar·co·ma
pl li·po·sar·co·mas
or li·po·sar·co·ma·ta

li·po·sis
pl li·po·ses

li·po·sol·u·ble
li·po·thym·ia
or li·poth·y·my
pl li·po·thym·ias
or li·poth·y·mies

li·po·thym·i·al
li·po·trop·ic
also li·po·tro·phic

li·pot·ro·pism
li·po·vac·cine
li·pox·e·nous
li·pox·e·ny
pl li·pox·e·nies

Lip·pes loop
li·pu·ria
liq·ue·fa·cient
liq·ue·fac·tion
liq·ue·fac·tive
li·ques·cent
liq·uid
li·quor
li·quor am·nii
li·quo·rice
var of licorice

Lis·sau·er's tract
Lis·sen·ceph·a·la
lis·sen·ce·phal·ic
or lis·sen·ceph·a·lous

lis·sen·ceph·a·ly
also lis·sen·ce·pha·lia
pl lis·sen·ceph·a·lies
also lis·sen·ce·pha·lias

lis·ter·el·la
lis·te·ria
lis·te·ri·o·sis
also lis·ter·el·losis
pl lis·te·ri·o·ses
also lis·ter·el·lo·ses

lis·ter·ism
lis·ter·ize
lis·ter·ized
lis·ter·iz·ing
li·ter
or li·tre

lith·a·gogue
li·tharge
li·thec·to·my
pl li·thec·to·mies

li·the·mia
also li·thae·mia

li·the·mic
also li·thae·mic

li·thi·a·sis
pl li·thi·a·ses

lith·ic
lith·i·co·sis
lith·i·um
lith·o·cho·lic
litho·di·al·y·sis
pl litho·di·al·y·ses

lith·o·gen·e·sis
pl lith·o·gen·e·ses

li·thog·e·nous
lith·oid
also li·thoi·dal

li·thol·a·paxy
pl li·thol·a·pax·ies

li·thol·o·gy
pl li·thol·o·gies

litho·ne·phri·tis
pl litho·ne·phrit·i·des
litho·ne·phrot·o·my
pl litho·ne·phrot·o·mies

lith·on·trip·tic
also lith·o·trip·tic

lith·o·pe·di·on
litho·phone
litho·scope
li·tho·sis
lith·o·tome
li·thot·o·mist
li·thot·o·mize
li·thot·o·mized
li·thot·o·miz·ing
li·thot·o·my
li·thot·o·mies
litho·trip·sy
pl litho·trip·sies

lith·o·trite
li·thot·ri·tist
lith·o·tri·tor
li·thot·ri·ty
pl li·thot·ri·ties

lith·ure·sis
li·thu·ria
lit·mus
li·tre
var of liter

lit·ter
Lit·tle's dis·ease
Lit·tre's gland
live-born
li·ve·do
liv·er

lives
pl of life

liv•id

li•vid•i•ty
pl li•vid•i•ties

loa

loa•ia•sis
or lo•ia•sis
pl loa•ia•ses
or lo•ia•ses

lo•bar

lo•bate
also lo•bat•ed

lo•bec•to•my
pl lo•bec•to•mies

lo•be•lia

lo•be•line

lo•bot•o•mize
lo•bot•o•mized
lo•bot•o•miz•ing

lo•bot•o•my
pl lo•bot•o•mies

lob•ster claw

lob•u•lar

lob•u•late
also lob•u•lat•ed

lob•u•la•tion

lob•ule

lob•u•lose

lob•u•lus
pl lob•u•li

lo•bus
pl lo•bi

lo•cal

lo•cal•iza•tion

lo•cal•ize
lo•cal•ized
lo•cal•iz•ing

lo•cal•iz•er

lo•cal•ly

lo•chia
pl lo•chia

lo•chia al•ba

lo•chi•al

lo•chio•me•tra

lo•chio•me•tri•tis

lo•chi•or•rhea

lo•chi•os•che•sis
pl lo•chi•os•che•ses

lo•ci
pl of locus

Locke's so•lu•tion
or Locke so•lu•tion

lock•jaw

lo•co
pl lo•cos
or lo•coes

lo•coed

lo•co•ism

lo•co•mo•tive

lo•co•mo•tor
also lo•co•mo•to•ry

lo•co•weed

loc•u•lar

loc•u•late
or loc•u•lat•ed

loc•u•la•tion

loc•u•lus
pl loc•u•li

lo•cum-te•nen•cy
pl lo•cum-te•nen•cies

lo•cum te•nens
pl lo•cum te•nen•tes

lo•cus
pl lo•ci

log•ag•no•sia

log•am•ne•sia

log•apha•sia

log•op•a•thy
pl log•op•a•thies

log•o•pe•dia

log•o•pe•dics

logo•ple•gia

log•or•rhea

log•or•rhe•ic

logo•spasm

lo•ia•sis
var of loaiasis

long bone

lon•gis•si•mus dor•si

lon•gi•tu•di•nal

lon•gi•tu•di•na•lis

lon•gus

loop of Hen•le

loph•o•dont

lo•phoph•o•rine

lo•phot•ri•chous
or lo•phot•ri•chate

lor•do•sis
pl lor•do•ses

lor•dot•ic

lo•tio
pl lo•tios

lo•tion

louse
pl lice

lous•i•ness

lousy
lous•i•er
lous•i•est

lox·ia
Lox·os·ce·les
lox·os·ce·lism
loz·enge
lu·cent
lu·cid·i·ty
pl lu·cid·i·ties
Lud·wig's an·gi·na
Lu·er sy·ringe
lu·es
pl lu·es
lu·et·ic
lu·e·tin
Lu·gol's so·lu·tion
lum·ba·go
pl lum·ba·gos
lum·bar
lum·bar·i·za·tion
lum·bo·co·los·to·my
pl lum·bo·co·los·to·mies
lum·bo·cos·tal
lum·bo·in·gui·nal
lum·bo·sa·cral
lum·bri·cal
lum·bri·ca·lis
pl lum·bri·ca·les
lum·bri·coid
lum·bri·cus
lu·men
pl lu·mi·na
also lu·mens
lu·mi·chrome
lu·mi·nal
also lu·me·nal
lu·mi·nesce
lu·mi·nesced
lu·mi·nesc·ing
lu·mi·nes·cence
lu·mi·nes·cent
lu·mi·nif·er·ous
lu·mis·ter·ol
lumpy jaw
lu·na·cy
pl lu·na·cies
lu·nar
lu·nare
pl lu·nar·ia
lu·na·tic
lu·na·to·ma·la·cia
lu·na·tum
pl lu·na·ta
lung·worm
lu·nule
lu·pi·form
lu·pine
or lu·pin
lu·pi·no·sis
lu·poid
lu·pus
lu·pus er·y·the·ma·to·sus
lu·pus per·nio
lu·pus vul·gar·is
lu·sus
lu·sus na·tu·rae
lu·te·al
lu·tein
lu·tein·iza·tion
lu·tein·ize
lu·tein·ized
lu·tein·iz·ing
lu·te·o·ma
pl lu·te·o·mas
or lu·te·o·ma·ta
lu·teo·tro·phic
or lu·teo·trop·ic
lu·teo·tro·phin
or lu·teo·tro·pin
lu·te·tium
also lu·te·cium
lux·ate
lux·at·ed
lux·at·ing
lux·a·tion
lux·us
ly·ase
ly·can·thrope
ly·can·thro·py
pl ly·can·thro·pies
Ly·co·per·don
ly·co·per·don·o·sis
pl ly·co·per·don·o·ses
or ly·co·per·don·o·sis·es
ly·co·po·di·um
ly·co·rex·ia
ly·go·phil·ia
ly·ing-in
pl ly·ings-in
or ly·ing-ins
Lym·naea
lymph
pl lymphs
lymph·ad·e·nec·to·my
pl lymph·ad·e·nec·to·mies
lymph·ad·e·ni·tis
lymph·ad·e·noid

lymph·ad·e·no·ma
pl lymph·ad·e·no·mas
or lymph·ad·e·no·ma·ta

lymph·ad·e·no·ma·to·sis
pl lymph·ad·e·no·ma·to·ses

lymph·ad·e·nop·a·thy
pl lymph·ad·e·nop·a·thies

lymph·ad·e·no·sis
pl lymph·ad·e·no·ses

lymph·a·gogue

lym·phan·gi·al

lym·phan·gi·ec·ta·sia

lym·phan·gi·ec·ta·sis

lym·phan·gi·ec·tat·ic

lym·phan·gi·ec·to·my
pl lymph·an·gi·ec·to·mies

lym·phan·gio·en·do·the·li·o·ma
pl lym·phan·gio·en·do·the·li·o·mas
or lym·phan·gio·en·do·the·li·o·ma·ta

lym·phan·gi·og·ra·phy
pl lym·phan·gi·og·ra·phies

lymph·an·gi·o·ma
pl lymph·an·gi·o·mas
or lymph·an·gi·o·ma·ta

lymph·an·gi·oma·tous

lym·phan·gio·plas·ty
pl lym·phan·gio·plas·ties

lym·phan·gio·sar·co·ma
pl lym·phan·gio·sar·co·mas
or lym·phan·gio·sar·co·ma·ta

lym·phan·gi·ot·o·my
pl lym·phan·gi·ot·o·mies

lym·phan·gi·tis
pl lym·phan·git·i·des

lym·phat·ic

lym·pha·tism

lymph·ede·ma
also lymph·oe·de·ma

lym·pho·blast

lym·pho·blas·tic

lym·pho·blas·to·ma
pl lym·pho·blas·to·mas
or lym·pho·blas·to·ma·ta

lym·pho·blas·to·sis

lym·pho·cyte

lym·pho·cyt·ic

lym·pho·cy·to·ma
pl lym·pho·cy·to·mas
or lym·pho·cy·to·ma·ta

lym·pho·cy·to·pe·nia

lym·pho·cy·to·poi·e·sis
pl lym·pho·cy·to·poi·e·ses

lym·pho·cy·to·sis
pl lym·pho·cy·to·ses

lym·pho·cy·tot·ic

lym·pho·der·mia

lym·pho·ep·i·the·li·o·ma
pl lym·pho·ep·i·the·li·o·mas
or lym·pho·ep·i·the·li·o·ma·ta

lym·phog·e·nous
also lym·pho·gen·ic

lym·pho·gram

lym·pho·gran·u·lo·ma
pl lym·pho·gran·u·lo·mas
or lym·pho·gran·u·lo·ma·ta

lym·pho·gran·u·lo·ma in·gui·na·le

lym·pho·gran·u·lo·ma·to·sis
pl lym·pho·gran·u·lo·ma·to·ses

lym·pho·gran·u·lo·ma·tous

lym•pho•gran•u•
lo•ma ve•ne•re
um
lym•pho•graph•ic
lym•phog•ra•phy
pl lym•phog•ra•phies
lym•phoid
lym•phoid•o•cyte
lym•pho•ma
pl lym•pho•mas
or lym•pho•ma•ta
lym•pho•ma•toid
lym•pho•ma•to•sis
pl lym•pho•ma•to•ses
lym•pho•ma•tous
lym•pho•path•ia
ve•ne•re•um
lym•pho•pe•nia
lym•pho•poi•e•sis
pl lym•pho•poi•e•ses
lym•pho•poi•et•ic
lym•pho•re•tic•u•
lo•sis
pl lym•pho•re•tic•u•
lo•ses
lym•phor•rhea
lym•pho•sar•co•
ma
pl lym•pho•sar•co•
mas
or lym•pho•sar•co•
ma•ta
lym•pho•sar•co•
ma•to•sis
pl lym•pho•sar•co•
ma•to•ses
lym•pho•sar•co•
ma•tous
lym•phu•ria

lyo•phile
also lyo•phil
lyo•philed
lyo•phil•ic
ly•oph•i•li•za•tion
ly•oph•i•lize
ly•oph•i•lized
ly•oph•i•liz•ing
ly•oph•i•liz•er
lyo•pho•bic
also lyo•phobe
lyo•sorp•tion
lyo•trop•ic
ly•ra
also lyre
ly•sate
lyse
lysed
lys•ing
ly•ser•gic ac•id
di•eth•yl•am•ide
ly•sin
ly•sine
ly•sis
pl ly•ses
ly•so•gen
ly•so•gen•e•sis
pl ly•so•gen•e•ses
ly•so•gen•ic
ly•so•ge•nic•i•ty
pl ly•so•ge•nic•i•ties
ly•sog•e•ni•za•tion
ly•sog•e•nize
ly•sog•e•nized
ly•sog•e•niz•ing
ly•sog•e•ny
pl ly•sog•e•nies

ly•so•ki•nase
ly•so•lec•i•thin
ly•so•som•al
ly•so•som•al•ly
ly•so•some
ly•so•staph•in
ly•so•zyme
lys•sa
lyt•ic

M

Mc•Bur•ney's
point
mac•er•ate
mac•er•at•ed
mac•er•at•ing
mac•er•a•tion
Mach num•ber
*Mac•ra•can•tho•
rhyn•chus*
mac•ren•ce•phal•
ic
also mac•ren•ceph•a•
lous
mac•ren•ceph•a•
ly
pl mac•ren•ceph•a•
lies
mac•ro•bi•ot•ics
mac•ro•blast
mac•ro•ble•phar•
ia
mac•ro•bra•chia
mac•ro•car•di•us
mac•ro•ceph•a•
lous
or mac•ro•ce•phal•ic

mac·ro·ceph·a·lus
pl mac·ro·ceph·a·li

mac·ro·ceph·a·ly
pl mac·ro·ceph·a·lies

mac·ro·chei·lia
mac·ro·chei·ria
mac·ro·cyst
mac·ro·cyte
mac·ro·cyt·ic
mac·ro·cy·to·sis
pl mac·ro·cy·to·ses

mac·ro·dac·ty·ly
pl mac·ro·dac·ty·lies

mac·ro·dont
mac·ro·don·tia
or mac·ro·don·tism

mac·ro·ga·mete
mac·ro·ga·me·to·cyte
mac·ro·gen·i·to·so·mia
mac·rog·lia
mac·rog·li·al
mac·ro·glob·u·lin
mac·ro·glob·u·lin·emia
mac·ro·glob·u·lin·emic
mac·ro·glos·sia
mac·ro·gna·thia
mac·ro·gy·ria
mac·ro·lide
mac·ro·mas·tia
mac·ro·me·lia
ma·crom·e·lus
pl ma·crom·e·li

mac·ro·mere
mac·ro·meth·od
mac·ro·mo·lec·u·lar
mac·ro·mol·e·cule
mac·ro·mono·cyte
mac·ro·my·elo·blast
mac·ro·nor·mo·blast
mac·ro·nu·cle·us
pl mac·ro·nu·clei
also mac·ro·nu·cle·us·es

mac·ro·nych·ia
mac·ro·phage
mac·ro·phag·ic
mac·ro·po·dia
mac·ro·poly·cyte
mac·rop·sia
also mac·rop·sy
pl mac·rop·sias
also mac·rop·sies

mac·ro·scop·ic
also mac·ro·scop·i·cal

mac·ro·scop·i·cal·ly
mac·ros·mat·ic
mac·ro·so·mia
mac·ro·sto·mia
mac·ro·tia
mac·u·la
pl mac·u·lae
also mac·u·las

mac·u·la acu·sti·ca
pl mac·u·lae acu·sti·cae

mac·u·la lu·tea
pl mac·u·lae lu·te·ae

mac·u·lar
mac·u·late
or mac·u·lat·ed

mac·u·la·tion
mac·ule
mac·u·lo·pap·u·lar
mac·u·lo·pap·ule
mad·a·ro·sis
pl mad·a·ro·ses

Mad·dox rod
mad·i·dans
mad·ness
Mad·u·ra foot
mad·u·ro·my·co·sis
pl mad·u·ro·my·co·ses

ma·gen·stras·se
ma·gen·ta
mag·got
mag·is·tery
pl mag·is·ter·ies

ma·gis·tral
mag·ma
mag·ne·sia
mag·ne·sium
mag·ne·to·car·dio·gram
mag·ne·to·car·dio·graph

mag·ne·to·car·dio·graph·ic
mag·ne·to·car·di·og·ra·phy
pl mag·ne·to·car·di·og·ra·phies
mag·ni·fi·ca·tion
mag·ni·fy
mag·ni·fied
mag·ni·fy·ing
mag·num
ma·huang
maid·en·head
ma·ieu·sio·pho·bia
Mai·mon·i·de·an
ma·jor-med·i·cal
Make·ham's law
mal
ma·la
pl of malum
mal·ab·sorp·tion
mal·a·chite
ma·la·cia
mal·a·co·pla·kia
or mal·a·ko·pla·kia
mal·a·cot·ic
mal·ad·ap·ta·tion
mal·adap·tive
mal·ad·just·ed
mal·ad·jus·tive
mal·ad·just·ment
mal·a·dy
pl mal·a·dies
mal·aise
or mal·ease

mal·an·ders
or mal·len·ders
ma·lar
ma·lar·ia
ma·lar·i·ae ma·lar·ia
ma·lar·i·al
also ma·lar·i·an
ma·lar·i·ol·o·gist
ma·lar·i·ol·o·gy
pl ma·lar·i·ol·o·gies
ma·lar·io·ther·a·py
pl ma·lar·io·ther·a·pies
ma·lar·i·ous
mal·as·sim·i·la·tion
ma·late
mal·a·thi·on
ma·lax·ate
ma·lax·at·ed
ma·lax·at·ing
ma·lax·a·tion
mal de ca·de·ras
mal del pin·to
mal de mer
mal·de·vel·op·ment
male
ma·le·ate
ma·le·ic
male-ster·ile
mal·for·ma·tion
mal·formed
mal·func·tion
ma·lic

ma·lig·nan·cy
pl ma·lig·nan·cies
ma·lig·nant
ma·lig·nant·ly
ma·lig·ni·ty
pl ma·lig·ni·ties
ma·lin·ger
ma·lin·ger·er
mal·le·a·tion
mal·le·in
mal·le·in·i·za·tion
mal·leo·in·cu·dal
mal·le·o·lar
mal·le·o·lus
pl mal·le·o·li
Mal·leo·my·ces
mal·le·ot·o·my
pl mal·le·ot·o·mies
mal·let
mal·le·us
pl mal·lei
Mal·loph·a·ga
mal·nour·ished
mal·nour·ish·ment
mal·nu·tri·tion
mal·oc·clu·sion
ma·lo·lac·tic
mal·o·nate
ma·lo·nic
mal·o·nyl
mal·o·nyl·urea
Mal·pi·ghi·an pyr·a·mid
mal·po·si·tion
mal·prac·tice

mal·prac·ti·tion·er
mal·prax·is
pl mal·prax·es

mal·pre·sen·ta·tion
mal·ro·ta·tion
Mal·ta fe·ver
malt·ase
Mal·thu·sian
Mal·thu·sian·ism
malt·ose
ma·lum
pl ma·la

mal·union
mal·unit·ed
mam·ba
mam·e·lon
mam·ma
pl mam·mae

mam·mal
mam·mal·gia
Mam·ma·lia
mam·ma·li·an
mam·ma·plas·ty
pl mam·ma·plas·ties

mam·ma·ry
mam·mec·to·my
pl mam·mec·to·mies

mam·mi·form
mam·mil·la
also ma·mil·la
pl mam·mil·lae
also ma·mil·lae

mam·mil·lar·ia
mam·mil·la·ry
mam·mil·lat·ed
or mam·mil·late
also mam·il·lat·ed
or mam·il·late

mam·mil·la·tion
mam·mil·li·form
mam·mil·li·plas·ty
pl mam·mil·li·plas·ties

mam·mil·li·tis
mam·mi·tis
pl mam·mit·i·des

mam·mo·gen
mam·mo·gen·ic
mam·mo·gen·i·cal·ly
mam·mo·gram
mam·mo·graph·ic
mam·mog·ra·phy
pl mam·mog·ra·phies

mam·mo·plas·ty
pl mam·mo·plas·ties

mam·mose
mam·mot·o·my
pl mam·mot·o·mies

man·ci·nism
man·del·ate
man·del·ic
man·di·ble
man·dib·u·lar
man·dib·u·late
man·drel
also man·dril
shaft holding a dental tool (*see* mandrill)
man·drill
baboon (*see* mandrel)
man·drin
ma·neu·ver
man·ga·nese
man·gan·ic
man·ga·nous
mange
mangy
mang·i·er
mang·i·est
ma·nia
ma·ni·ac
ma·ni·a·cal
ma·ni·a·cal·ly
man·ic
man·i·cal·ly
man·ic-de·pres·sive
man·i·kin
or man·ni·kin

ma·nip·u·la·ble
ma·nip·u·late
ma·nip·u·lat·ed
ma·nip·u·lat·ing
ma·nip·u·la·tion
ma·nip·u·la·tive
ma·nip·u·la·tive·ly
ma·nip·u·la·tor
ma·nip·u·la·to·ry
man·na
man·ner·ism
man·ni·tol
ma·nom·e·ter

mano·met·ric
also mano·met·ri·cal
mano·met·ri·cal·ly
ma·nom·e·try
pl ma·nom·e·tries
Man·son·el·la
man·so·nia
Man·son's disease
man·tle
Man·toux test
ma·nu·bri·al
ma·nu·bri·um
pl ma·nu·bria
also ma·nu·bri·ums
ma·nu·bri·um ster·ni
man·u·duc·tion
ma·nus
pl ma·nus
many·plies
also mani·plies
ma·ran·tic
ma·ras·ma
ma·ras·mic
ma·ras·mus
mar·ble
mar·ble·iza·tion
marc
Mar·ek's disease
Ma·rey's law
Mar·fan's syndrome
Mar·gar·o·pus
mar·gin·ate
mar·gin·at·ed
mar·gin·at·ing
mar·gin·ation
mar·gino·plas·ty
pl mar·gino·plas·ties
mar·i·jua·na
or mar·i·hua·na
mark·er
mar·mo·rate
or mar·mo·rat·ed
mar·mo·ra·tion
mar·row
mar·row·bone
marsh·mal·low
Marsh test
mar·su·pi·al
mar·su·pi·al·iza·tion
mar·su·pi·al·ize
mar·su·pi·al·ized
mar·su·pi·al·iz·ing
mar·su·pi·um
pl mar·su·pia
mas·cu·line
mas·cu·line·ly
mas·cu·line·ness
mas·cu·lin·i·ty
pl mas·cu·lin·i·ties
mas·cu·lin·i·za·tion
mas·cu·lin·ize
mas·cu·lin·ized
mas·cu·lin·iz·ing
mas·cu·lin·ovo·blas·to·ma
ma·ser
mas·och·ism
mas·och·ist
mas·och·is·tic
mas·och·is·ti·cal·ly
mas·sage
mas·se·ter
mas·se·ter·ic
mas·seur
mas·seuse
mas·so·ther·a·pist
mas·so·ther·a·py
pl mas·so·ther·a·pies
mast·ad·e·ni·tis
mas·tal·gia
mas·tec·to·my
pl mas·tec·to·mies
mas·tic
also mas·tich
or mas·ti·che
mas·ti·cate
mas·ti·cat·ed
mas·ti·cat·ing
mas·ti·ca·tion
mas·ti·ca·tor
mas·ti·ca·to·ry
Mas·ti·goph·o·ra
mas·ti·goph·o·ran
mas·ti·goph·o·rous
mas·ti·gote
mas·tit·ic
mas·ti·tis
pl mas·tit·i·des

mas·to·cyte
mas·to·cy·to·ma
pl mas·to·cy·to·mas
or mas·to·cy·to·ma·ta
mas·to·cy·to·sis
mas·to·dyn·ia
mas·toid
mas·toi·dal
also mas·toi·de·al
or mas·toi·de·an
mas·toid·ec·to·my
pl mas·toid·ec·to·mies
mas·toid·i·tis
pl mas·toid·it·i·des
mas·toid·ot·o·my
pl mas·toid·ot·o·mies
mas·ton·cus
mas·to·pa·ri·etal
mas·top·a·thy
pl mas·top·a·thies
mas·to·pexy
pl mas·to·pex·ies
mas·to·pla·sia
mas·to·plas·ty
pl mas·to·plas·ties
mas·tor·rha·gia
mas·to·scir·rhus
pl mas·to·scir·rhi
mas·tot·o·my
pl mas·tot·o·mies
mas·tur·bate
mas·tur·bat·ed
mas·tur·bat·ing
mas·tur·ba·tion
mas·tur·ba·tor
mas·tur·ba·tory
ma·té
or ma·te
ma·te·ria al·ba
ma·te·ri·al
ma·te·ria med·i·ca
ma·ter·nal
ma·ter·ni·ty
pl ma·ter·ni·ties
ma·ti·co
pl ma·ti·cos
ma·tri·cal
mat·ri·car·ia
pl mat·ri·car·ia
or mat·ri·car·ias
ma·tri·cid·al
ma·tri·cide
ma·trix
pl ma·tri·ces
or ma·trix·es
matte
mat·ter
mat·tery
mat·toid
mat·u·rate
mat·u·rat·ed
mat·u·rat·ing
mat·u·ra·tion
mat·u·ra·tion·al
ma·tur·a·tive
ma·ture
ma·tur·er
ma·tur·est
ma·ture
ma·tured
ma·tur·ing
ma·tu·ri·ty
pl ma·tu·ri·ties
ma·tu·ti·nal
ma·tu·ti·nal·ly
Mau·me·né test
Mau·rer's dot
max·il·la
pl max·il·lae
or max·il·las
max·il·lary
max·il·lo·fa·cial
max·il·lo·pal·a·tal
or max·il·lo·pal·a·tine
max·il·lo·tur·bi·nal
max·i·mal
max·i·mal·ly
max·i·mum
pl max·i·ma
or max·i·mums
may·hem
ma·zic
mazo·pla·sia
mea·sled
mea·sles
mea·sly
mea·sli·er
mea·sli·est
me·atal
me·a·tot·o·my
pl me·a·tot·o·mies
me·atus
pl me·atus·es
or me·atus
mec·a·myl·a·mine
me·chan·i·cal

me•chan•i•cal•ly
me•chan•ics
mech•a•nism
mech•a•no•chem•i•cal
mech•a•no•chem•is•try
pl mech•a•no•chem•is•tries
mech•a•no•re•cep•tion
mech•a•no•re•cep•tive
mech•a•no•re•cep•tor
mech•a•no•ther•a•pist
mech•a•no•ther•a•py
pl mech•a•no•ther•a•pies
mech•lor•eth•a•mine
me•cism
Me•cis•to•cir•rus
Meck•el's car•ti•lage
Meck•el's cave
Meck•el's di•ver•tic•u•lum
Meck•el's gan•gli•on
me•com•e•ter
mec•on•ate
me•con•ic
me•co•ni•or•rhea
me•co•ni•um

me•dia
pl of medium
me•dia
pl me•di•ae
me•di•ad
me•di•al
me•di•a•lis
me•di•al•ly
me•di•an
me•di•as•ti•nal
me•di•as•ti•ni•tis
pl me•di•as•ti•nit•i•des
me•di•as•ti•no•peri•car•di•tis
pl me•di•as•ti•no•peri•car•dit•i•des
me•di•as•ti•no•scope
me•di•as•ti•nos•co•py
pl me•di•as•ti•nos•co•pies
me•di•as•ti•not•o•my
pl me•di•as•ti•not•o•mies
me•di•as•ti•num
pl me•di•as•ti•na
me•di•ate
me•di•at•ed
me•di•at•ing
me•di•a•tion
me•di•a•tion•al
me•di•a•tor
med•ic
med•i•ca•ble
med•ic•aid
med•i•cal

me•di•ca•ment
med•i•ca•men•to•sus
me•di•ca•men•tous
med•i•cant
medi•care
med•i•cate
med•i•cat•ed
med•i•cat•ing
med•i•ca•tion
med•i•ca•tive
med•i•ca•tor
me•dic•i•na•ble
me•dic•i•nal
me•dic•i•nal•ly
med•i•cine
med•i•co•le•gal
med•i•co•psy•chol•o•gy
pl med•i•co•psy•chol•o•gies
Me•di•na worm
me•dio•car•pal
me•dio•dor•sal
me•dio•ne•cro•sis
pl me•dio•ne•cro•ses
me•dio•tar•sal
Med•i•ter•ra•nean ane•mia
me•di•um
pl me•di•ums
or me•dia
me•di•us
pl me•dii
me•dul•la
pl me•dul•las
or me•dul•lae

me•dul•la ob•lon•ga•ta
pl me•dul•la ob•lon•ga•tas
or me•dul•lae ob•lon•ga•tae

med•ul•lary
also me•dul•lar

med•ul•lat•ed
med•ul•la•tion
me•dul•lin
me•dul•li•spi•nal
me•dul•li•za•tion
me•dul•lo•blas•to•ma
pl me•dul•lo•blas•to•mas
or me•dul•lo•blas•to•ma•ta

mef•e•nam•ic
mega•ce•phal•ic
also mega•ceph•a•lous

mega•ceph•a•ly
pl mega•ceph•a•lies

mega•co•lon
mega•cy•cle
mega•death
mega•dont
mega•dont•ism
mega•don•ty
pl mega•don•ties

mega•esoph•a•gus
pl mega•esoph•a•gi

mega•ga•mete
mega•ga•me•to•phyte
mega•karyo•blast
mega•karyo•cyte
also mega•caryo•cyte

mega•karyo•cyt•ic
mega•lec•i•thal
meg•a•lo•blast
meg•a•lo•blas•tic
meg•a•lo•car•dia
meg•a•lo•ce•phal•ic
or meg•a•lo•ceph•a•lous

meg•a•lo•ceph•a•ly
pl meg•a•lo•ceph•a•lies

meg•a•lo•cyte
meg•a•lo•cyt•ic
meg•a•lo•ma•nia
meg•a•lo•ma•ni•ac
meg•a•lo•ma•ni•a•cal
or meg•a•lo•man•ic

meg•a•lo•ma•ni•a•cal•ly
meg•al•on•y•cho•sis
meg•a•loph•thal•mos
or meg•a•loph•thal•mus

meg•a•lo•ure•ter
mega•pros•o•pous
mega•spore
mega•spor•ic
mega•spo•ro•gen•e•sis
pl mega•spo•ro•gen•e•ses

mega•vi•ta•min
me•grim
Meh•lis' gland
Mei•bo•mian gland
mei•o•sis
pl mei•o•ses

mei•ot•ic
mei•ot•i•cal•ly
Meiss•ner's cor•pus•cle
me•lae•na
var of melena

me•lal•gia
mel•a•mine
mel•an•cho•lia
pl mel•an•cho•lias
also mel•an•cho•li•ae

mel•an•cho•li•ac
mel•an•chol•ic
mel•an•chol•i•cal•ly
mel•an•choly
pl mel•an•chol•ies

mel•ane•mia
me•lan•geur
Me•la•nia
me•lan•ic
mel•a•nif•er•ous
mel•a•nin
mel•a•nism
mel•a•nis•tic
mel•a•ni•za•tion

mel·a·nize
mel·a·nized
mel·a·niz·ing
me·la·no·blast
me·la·no·blas·tic
me·la·no·blas·to·ma
pl me·la·no·blas·to·mas
or me·la·no·blas·to·ma·ta
mel·a·no·car·ci·no·ma
pl me·la·no·car·ci·no·mas
or me·la·no·car·ci·no·ma·ta
mel·a·noch·roi
me·la·no·chro·ic
mel·a·noch·ro·ous
mel·a·noc·o·mous
me·la·no·cyte
me·la·no·cyte-stim·u·lat·ing hor·mone
me·la·no·derm
me·la·no·der·ma
mel·a·no·der·ma·ti·tis
me·la·no·der·mic
me·la·no·gen
me·la·no·gen·e·sis
pl me·la·no·gen·e·ses
me·la·no·ge·net·ic
me·la·no·gen·ic
mel·a·no·glos·sia
mel·a·noid
mel·a·no·ma
pl mel·a·no·mas
or mel·a·no·ma·ta
mel·a·no·ma·to·sis
pl mel·a·no·ma·to·ses
mel·a·no·nych·ia
mel·a·no·phage
me·la·no·phore
me·la·no·phor·ic
mel·a·no·pla·kia
mel·a·no·sis
pl mel·a·no·ses
mel·a·not·ic
mel·a·not·ri·chous
mel·a·nous
mel·an·uria
mel·an·uric
me·las·ma
me·las·mic
mel·a·to·nin
me·le·na
or me·lae·na
me·lez·i·tose
mel·i·bi·ose
mel·i·oi·do·sis
pl mel·i·oi·do·ses
me·lis·sa
me·lis·sic
mel·i·ten·sis
me·li·tis
mel·i·tu·ria
or mel·li·tu·ria
melo·ma·nia
Me·loph·a·gus
mel·o·plas·ty
pl mel·o·plas·ties
mem·ber
mem·bra·na
pl mem·bra·nae
mem·bra·na·ceous
mem·bran·al
mem·bra·nate
mem·brane
mem·bra·noid
mem·bra·nous
mem·bra·nous·ly
mem·brum
pl mem·bra
mem·o·ry
pl mem·o·ries
men·ac·me
men·a·di·one
me·naph·thone
men·ar·che
men·ar·che·al
also men·ar·chi·al
men·a·zon
Men·de·lian
Men·de·lian·ism
Men·de·lian·ist
Men·del·ism
Men·del·ist
men·del·ize
men·del·ized
men·del·iz·ing
Men·del's law
Mé·nière's dis·ease
or Mé·nière's syn·drome

men·in·ge·al
me·nin·ges
pl of me·ninx
me·nin·gi·o·ma
pl me·nin·gi·o·mas
or me·nin·gi·o·ma·ta
men·in·gis·mus
also me·nin·gism
pl men·in·gis·mi
also me·nin·gisms
men·in·git·ic
men·in·gi·tis
pl men·in·git·i·des
me·nin·go·cele
or me·nin·go·coele
me·nin·go·coc·cal
also me·nin·go·coc·cic
me·nin·go·coc·ce·mia
also me·nin·go·coc·cae·mia
me·nin·go·coc·cus
pl me·nin·go·coc·ci
me·nin·go·en·ceph·a·lit·ic
me·nin·go·en·ceph·a·li·tis
pl me·nin·go·en·ceph·a·lit·i·des
me·nin·go·en·ceph·a·lo·cele
me·nin·go·en·ceph·a·lo·my·eli·tis
pl me·nin·go·en·ceph·a·lo·my·elit·i·des
me·nin·go·my·eli·tis
pl me·nin·go·my·elit·i·des
me·nin·go·my·elo·cele
men·in·gop·a·thy
pl men·in·gop·a·thies
me·ninx
pl me·nin·ges
men·is·cec·to·my
pl men·is·cec·to·mies
men·is·ci·tis
me·nis·co·cyte
me·nis·co·cy·to·sis
pl me·nis·co·cy·to·ses
me·nis·cus
pl me·nis·ci
also me·nis·cus·es
meno·me·tror·rha·gia
meno·paus·al
meno·pause
Men·o·pon
men·or·rha·gia
men·or·rhag·ic
men·or·rhal·gia
men·or·rhea
meno·tax·is
pl meno·tax·es
men·ses
men·stru·al
men·stru·ant
men·stru·ate
men·stru·at·ed
men·stru·at·ing
men·stru·a·tion
men·stru·ous
men·stru·um
pl men·stru·ums
or men·strua
men·su·al
men·tal
men·tal·is
pl men·tal·es
men·tal·i·ty
pl men·tal·i·ties
men·tal·ly
men·ta·tion
Men·tha
men·thane
men·thol
men·tho·lat·ed
men·thyl
men·ti·cide
men·ton
men·tum
pl men·ta
mep·a·crine
me·per·i·dine
me·phen·e·sin
me·phit·ic
also me·phit·i·cal
me·pho·bar·bi·tal
mep·ro·bam·ate
me·ral·gia
mer·al·lu·ride
mer·bro·min
mer·cap·tal
mer·cap·tan

mer•cap•tide
mer•cap•to•ace•tic
mer•cap•tole
mer•cap•tom•er•in
mer•cap•to•pu•rine
mer•cap•tu•ric
mer•cu•ri•al
mer•cu•ri•al•ism
mer•cu•ri•al•iza•tion
mer•cu•ri•al•ize
  mer•cu•ri•al•ized
  mer•cu•ri•al•iz•ing
mer•cu•ric
mer•cu•ro•phyl•line
mer•cu•rous
mer•cu•ry
  pl mer•cu•ries
me•rid•i•an
me•rid•ic
me•rid•i•o•nal
me•ris•tic
me•ris•ti•cal•ly
Mer•kel-Ran•vier cor•pus•cle
Mer•kel's cor•pus•cle
  or Mer•kel's disc
mero•blas•tic
mero•blas•ti•cal•ly
mero•crine
mero•gen•e•sis
  pl mero•gen•e•ses
mero•ge•net•ic
  or mero•gen•ic
mer•o•gon
  also mer•o•gone
mer•o•gon•ic
  or me•rog•o•nous
me•rog•o•ny
  pl me•rog•o•nies
mero•my•o•sin
me•ro•pia
me•ros•mia
me•rot•o•my
  pl me•rot•o•mies
mer•o•zo•ite
mer•sal•yl
mes•ad
  also mesi•ad
me•sal
  var of mesial
me•sal•ly
  var of mesially
mes•aor•ti•tis
mes•a•ra•ic
mes•ar•ter•i•tis
me•sati•ce•phal•ic
  also me•sati•ceph•a•lous
me•sati•pel•lic
me•sati•pel•ly
  pl me•sati•pel•lies
mes•cal
mes•ca•line
mes•cal•ism
mes•ec•to•derm
mes•ec•to•der•mal
  or mes•ec•to•der•mic
mes•en•ce•phal•ic
mes•en•ceph•a•lon
mes•en•chy•ma
mes•en•chy•mal
mes•en•chy•ma•tous
mes•en•chyme
me•sen•na
  var of musenna
mes•en•ter•ic
mes•en•ter•i•tis
mes•en•ter•on
  pl mes•en•tera
mes•en•tery
  pl mes•en•ter•ies
mesh•work
mesi•ad
  var of mesad
me•si•al
  also me•sal
me•si•al•ly
  also me•sal•ly
me•sio•buc•cal
me•sio•clu•sion
  also me•sio•oc•clu•sion
me•sio•dis•tal
mes•mer•ism
mes•mer•ist
mes•mer•iza•tion
mes•mer•ize
  mes•mer•ized
  mes•mer•iz•ing
mes•mer•iz•er

me•so•ap•pen•di•ceal
me•so•ap•pen•dix
pl me•so•ap•pen•dix•es
or me•so•ap•pen•di•ces

me•so•blast
me•so•blas•te•ma
pl me•so•blas•te•mas
or me•so•blas•te•ma•ta

me•so•blas•te•mic
me•so•blas•tic
me•so•car•dia
me•so•car•di•um
me•so•ce•cum
pl me•so•ce•ca

me•so•ce•phal•ic
me•so•ceph•a•ly
pl me•so•ceph•a•lies

me•so•cne•mic
me•so•co•lon
me•so•conch
also me•so•conch•ic

me•so•derm
me•so•der•mal
or me•so•der•mic

me•so•dont
me•so•don•ty
pl me•so•don•ties

me•so•du•o•de•num
pl me•so•du•o•de•na
or me•so•du•o•de•nums

me•so•esoph•a•gus
pl me•so•esoph•a•gi

me•so•gas•ter
me•so•gas•tric
me•so•gas•tri•um
pl me•so•gas•tria

me•so•gna•thi•on
me•sog•na•thous
also me•sog•nath•ic

me•sog•na•thy
pl me•sog•na•thies

me•so•lec•i•thal
me•so•mere
me•so•mer•ic
me•som•er•ism
me•so•me•tri•al
or me•so•me•tric

me•so•me•tri•um
pl me•so•me•tria

me•so•morph
me•so•mor•phic
me•so•mor•phism
me•so•mor•phy
pl me•so•mor•phies

me•son
me•so•neph•ric
me•so•neph•ros
also me•so•neph•ron
pl me•so•neph•roi
also me•so•neph•ra

me•so-on•to•morph
me•so•phile
me•so•phil•ic
also me•soph•i•lous

me•so•phrag•ma
me•so•phrag•mal
me•soph•ry•on
pl me•soph•rya

me•so•pic
me•so•pro•sop•ic
me•so•pro•so•py
pl me•so•pro•so•pies

me•sor•chi•um
pl me•sor•chia

me•so•rec•tum
me•sor•rhi•nal
or me•so•rhi•nal

me•sor•rhine
also me•sor•rhin•ic
or me•so•rhine

me•so•sal•pinx
pl me•so•sal•pin•ges

me•so•seme
me•so•sig•moid
me•so•ster•num
pl me•so•ster•na

me•so•the•li•al
me•so•the•li•o•ma
pl me•so•the•li•o•mas
or me•so•the•li•o•ma•ta

me•so•the•li•um
pl me•so•the•lia

me•so•tron
mes•ovar•i•um
pl mes•ovar•ia

Me•so•zoa
me•so•zo•an
mes•sen•ger RNA
mes•tra•nol
me•tab•a•sis
pl me•tab•a•ses

meta•bi•o•sis
pl meta•bi•o•ses

meta•bi•ot•ic
meta•bi•ot•i•cal•ly

met·a·bol·ic
also met·a·bol·i·cal

met·a·bol·i·cal·ly
me·tab·o·lism
me·tab·o·lite
me·tab·o·liz·abil·i·ty
pl me·tab·o·liz·abil·i·ties

me·tab·o·liz·able
me·tab·o·lize
me·tab·o·lized
me·tab·o·liz·ing
meta·car·pal
meta·car·po·pha·lan·ge·al
meta·car·pus
meta·cer·car·ia
meta·cer·car·i·al
meta·chro·ma·sia
or meta·chro·ma·sy
pl meta·chro·ma·sias
or meta·chro·ma·sies

meta·chro·mat·ic
meta·chro·ma·tism
meta·chro·sis
pl meta·chro·ses

meta·cone
meta·co·nid
meta·co·nule
meta·cre·sol
meta·gen·e·sis
pl meta·gen·e·ses

meta·ge·net·ic
meta·ge·net·i·cal·ly
meta·gen·ic
Meta·gon·i·mus
me·tal·lo·en·zyme
met·al·loid
also met·al·loi·dal

me·tal·lo·pho·bia
me·tal·lo·por·phy·rin
meta·mere
meta·mer·ic
meta·mer·i·cal·ly
me·tam·er·ism
meta·mor·phic
meta·mor·phop·sia
meta·mor·phose
meta·mor·phosed
meta·mor·phos·ing
meta·mor·pho·sis
pl meta·mor·pho·ses

meta·my·elo·cyte
meta·neph·ric
also meta·ne·phrit·ic

meta·neph·ro·gen·ic
meta·neph·ros
also meta·neph·ron
pl meta·neph·roi
also meta·neph·ra

meta·phase
me·taph·y·se·al
me·taph·y·sis
pl me·taph·y·ses

me·taph·y·si·tis
meta·pla·sia
meta·plas·tic
meta·pneu·mon·ic
meta·poph·y·sis
pl meta·poph·y·ses

meta·pro·tein
meta·ram·i·nol
me·tas·ta·sis
pl me·tas·ta·ses

me·tas·ta·size
me·tas·ta·sized
me·tas·ta·siz·ing
met·a·stat·ic
met·a·stat·i·cal·ly
meta·ster·num
Meta·stron·gy·lus
meta·tar·sal
meta·tar·sal·gia
meta·tar·sal·ly
meta·tar·so·pha·lan·ge·al
meta·tar·sus
meta·thal·a·mus
meta·tro·phic
me·tat·ro·phy
pl me·tat·ro·phies

Meta·zoa
met·en·ce·phal·ic
met·en·ceph·a·lon
me·te·or·ism
me·ter
met·es·trous
or met·oes·trous

met·es·trus
or met·oes·trus
also met·es·trum
or met·oes·trum

metha·cho·line
meth·ac·ry·late
meth·a·done
or meth·a·don

meth·am·phet·amine
meth·a·nal
meth·ane
meth·a·nol
meth·an·the·line
met·hem·al·bu·min
met·he·mo·glo·bin
met·he·mo·glo·bin·emia
met·he·mo·glo·bin·uria
me·the·na·mine
meth·ene
meth·i·cil·lin
me·thim·a·zole
meth·io·dal
me·thi·o·nine
meth·od
meth·o·trex·ate
meth·ox·amine
me·thoxy·chlor
me·thoxy·flu·rane
meth·yl
me·thyl·amine
meth·yl·ase
meth·yl·ate
meth·yl·at·ed
meth·yl·at·ing
meth·yl·a·tion
meth·yl·do·pa
meth·y·lene
meth·yl·mor·phine
meth·yl·para·ben
meth·yl·phe·ni·date
meth·yl·pred·nis·o·lone
meth·yl·ros·an·i·line
me·thyl·tes·tos·ter·one
me·thyl·thio·ura·cil
met·oes·trous
var of metestrous

met·oes·trum, met·oes·trus
vars of metestrus

me·top·ic
me·to·pi·on
met·o·pism
met·o·pon
me·tra
pl me·trae

met·ra·pec·tic
met·ra·to·nia
met·rec·ta·sia
met·reu·ryn·ter
met·reu·ry·sis
me·tria
met·ric
or met·ri·cal
met·ri·cal·ly
me·tri·tis
me·tro·cele
me·tro·clyst
me·tro·col·po·cele
me·tro·cys·to·sis
pl me·tro·cys·to·ses
or me·tro·cys·to·sis·es

me·tro·cyte
me·tro·dy·na·mom·e·ter
me·trog·ra·phy
pl me·trog·ra·phies

me·tro·ma·la·cia
met·ro·ni·da·zole
me·tro·pa·ral·y·sis
pl me·tro·pa·ral·y·ses

me·trop·a·thy
pl me·trop·a·thies

me·tro·phle·bi·tis
me·trop·to·sis
pl me·trop·to·ses

me·tror·rha·gia
me·tror·rhag·ic
me·tror·rhea
me·tror·rhex·is
pl me·tror·rhex·es

me·tro·sal·pin·gi·tis
me·tro·sal·pin·gog·ra·phy
pl me·tro·sal·pin·gog·ra·phies

me·tro·scope

me•tro•stax•is
me•tro•ste•no•sis
pl me•tro•ste•no•ses
me•tro•tome
me•tyr•a•pone
mev•a•lon•ic
mho
pl mhos
mi•as•ma
also mi•asm
pl mi•as•mas
or mi•as•ma•ta
also mi•asms
mi•as•mal
mi•as•mat•ic
mi•as•mic
mi•ca
mi•ca•ceous
mice
pl of mouse
mi•cel•lar
mi•celle
also mi•cel•la
pl mi•celles
also mi•cel•lae
Mi•chae•lis con•stant
mi•cra
pl of micron
mi•cracous•tic
mi•cren•ceph•a•lon
pl mi•cren•ceph•a•la
mi•cren•ceph•a•lous
mi•cren•ceph•a•ly
pl mi•cren•ceph•a•lies
mi•cro•ab•scess
mi•cro•aero•phile
mi•cro•aero•phil•ic
also mi•cro•aero•phile
or mi•cro•aer•oph•i•lous
mi•cro•anal•y•sis
pl mi•cro•anal•y•ses
mi•cro•an•a•lyst
mi•cro•an•a•lyt•ic
or mi•cro•an•a•lyt•i•cal
mi•cro•an•a•tom•i•cal
mi•cro•anat•o•mist
mi•cro•anat•o•my
pl mi•cro•anat•o•mies
mi•cro•an•eu•rysm
mi•cro•bac•te•ri•um
pl mi•cro•bac•te•ria
mi•cro•bal•ance
mi•crobe
mi•cro•bi•al
also mi•cro•bic
mi•cro•bi•an
or mi•cro•bic
mi•cro•bi•ci•dal
mi•cro•bi•cide
mi•cro•bi•o•log•i•cal
also mi•cro•bi•o•log•ic
mi•cro•bi•o•log•i•cal•ly
mi•cro•bi•ol•o•gist
mi•cro•bi•ol•o•gy
pl mi•cro•bi•ol•o•gies
mi•cro•bi•on
pl mi•cro•bia
mi•cro•bi•o•sis
pl mi•cro•bi•o•ses
mi•cro•bi•ot•ic
mi•cro•bism
mi•cro•blast
mi•cro•bleph•a•ron
mi•cro•body
pl mi•cro•bod•ies
mi•cro•bra•chia
mi•cro•bu•rette
or mir•cro•bu•ret
mi•cro•cap•sule
mi•cro•car•dia
mi•cro•cen•trum
pl mi•cro•cen•trums
or mi•cro•cen•tra
mi•cro•ce•phal•ic
also mi•cro•ceph•a•lous
mi•cro•ceph•a•lism
mi•cro•ceph•a•lus
pl mi•cro•ceph•a•li
mi•cro•ceph•a•ly
pl mi•cro•ceph•a•lies
mi•cro•chei•lia
mi•cro•chem•i•cal
mi•cro•chem•is•try
pl mi•cro•chem•is•tries

mi•cro•chi•ria
mi•cro•cin•e•mat•o•graph•ic
mi•cro•cin•e•ma•tog•ra•phy
also mi•cro•kin•e•ma•tog•ra•phy
pl mi•cro•cin•e•ma•tog•ra•phies
also mi•cro•kin•e•ma•tog•ra•phies
mi•cro•cir•cu•la•tion
mi•cro•cir•cu•la•to•ry
Mi•cro•coc•ca•ce•ae
mi•cro•coc•cal
mi•cro•coc•cin
mi•cro•coc•cus
pl mi•cro•coc•ci
mi•cro•co•lon
mi•cro•co•nid•i•um
pl mi•cro•co•nid•ia
mi•cro•cor•nea
mi•cro•cou•lomb
mi•cro•crys•tal•line
mi•cro•crys•tal•lin•i•ty
pl mi•cro•crys•tal•lin•i•ties
mi•cro•cul•tur•al
mi•cro•cul•ture
mi•cro•cu•rie
mi•cro•cyst
mi•cro•cyte
mi•cro•cy•the•mia
also mi•cro•cy•te•mia
mi•cro•cy•the•mic
mi•cro•cyt•ic
mi•cro•cy•to•sis
pl mi•cro•cy•to•ses
mi•cro•dac•ty•ly
or mi•cro•dac•tyl•ia
pl mi•cro•dac•ty•lies
or mi•cro•dac•tyl•i•as
mi•cro•de•ter•mi•na•tion
mi•cro•dis•sec•tion
mi•cro•dont
mi•cro•dont•ism
mi•cro•drep•a•no•cy•to•sis
pl mi•cro•drep•a•no•cy•to•ses
mi•cro•elec•tro•pho•re•sis
mi•cro•elec•tro•pho•ret•ic
or mi•cro•elec•tro•pho•ret•i•cal
mi•cro•elec•tro•pho•ret•i•cal•ly
mi•cro•en•cap•su•late
mi•cro•en•cap•su•lat•ed
mi•cro•en•cap•su•lat•ing
mi•cro•en•cap•su•la•tion
mi•cro•en•ceph•a•ly
pl mi•cro•en•ceph•a•lies
mi•cro•eryth•ro•cyte
mi•cro•far•ad
mi•cro•fi•bril
mi•cro•fi•bril•lar
mi•cro•fil•a•re•mia
also mi•cro•fil•a•rae•mia
mi•cro•fi•lar•ia
mi•cro•fi•lar•ial
mi•cro•ga•mete
mi•cro•gas•tria
mi•cro•ge•nia
mi•cro•gen•i•tal•ism
mi•crog•lia
mi•crog•li•al
mi•cro•glos•sia
mi•cro•gna•thia
mi•cro•go•nio•scope
mi•cro•gram
mi•cro•graph
mi•cro•graph•ic
mi•crog•ra•phy
pl mi•crog•ra•phies
mi•cro•gy•ria
mi•crohm
mi•cro•in•cin•er•a•tion
mi•cro•in•va•sion

mi•cro•kin•e•ma•tog•ra•phy
var of microcinematography

mi•cro•li•ter

mi•cro•lith

mi•cro•li•thi•a•sis
pl mi•cro•li•thi•a•ses

mi•cro•log•i•cal
or mi•cro•log•ic

mi•crol•o•gist

mi•crol•o•gy
pl mi•crol•o•gies

mi•cro•ma•nia

mi•cro•ma•nip•u•la•tion

mi•cro•ma•nip•u•la•tor

mi•cro•mas•tia

mi•cro•me•lia

mi•cro•mel•ic

mi•crom•e•lus
pl mi•crom•e•li

mi•crom•e•ter
measuring instrument

mi•cro•me•ter
unit of length

mi•cro•meth•od

mi•cro•mi•cron

mi•cro•mil•li•me•ter

mi•cro•mor•pho•log•ic
or mi•cro•mor•pho•log•i•cal

mi•cro•mor•pho•log•i•cal•ly

mi•cro•mor•phol•o•gy
pl mi•cro•mor•phol•o•gies

mi•cro•mo•to•scope

mi•cro•my•elia

mi•cro•my•elo•blast

mi•cron
pl mi•crons
also mi•cra

mi•cro•nu•cle•us
pl mi•cro•nu•clei
also mi•cro•nu•cle•us•es

mi•cro•nu•tri•ent

mi•cro•nych•ia

mi•cro•or•gan•ic

mi•cro•or•gan•ism

mi•cro•pe•nis
pl mi•cro•pe•nes
or mi•cro•pe•nis•es

mi•cro•phage

mi•cro•pha•kia

mi•cro•phal•lus
pl mi•cro•phal•li
or mi•cro•phal•lus•es

mi•cro•pho•bia

mi•cro•phone

mi•cro•pho•nia

mi•cro•pho•to•graph

mi•cro•pho•tog•ra•pher

mi•cro•pho•to•graph•ic

mi•cro•pho•tog•ra•phy
pl mi•cro•pho•tog•ra•phies

mi•croph•thal•mia

mi•croph•thal•mic

mi•croph•thal•mus
or mi•croph•thal•mos
pl mi•croph•thal•mi
or mi•croph•thal•moi

mi•cro•phys•i•cal

mi•cro•phys•i•cal•ly

mi•cro•phys•ics

mi•cro•pi•pette
or mi•cro•pi•pet

mi•cro•po•dia

mi•cro•probe

mi•crop•sia
also mi•crop•sy
pl mi•crop•sias
or mi•crop•sies

mi•crop•tic

mi•cro•punc•ture

mi•cro•py•lar

mi•cro•pyle

mi•cro•ra•dio•graph

mi•cro•ra•dio•graph•ic

mi•cro•ra•di•og•ra•phy
pl mi•cro•ra•di•og•ra•phies

mi•cro•scope

mi•cro•scop•ic
or mi•cro•scop•i•cal

mi•cro•scop•i•cal•ly

mi•cros•co•pist

mi•cros•co•py
pl mi•cros•co•pies

mi•cros•mat•ic

mi•cro•som•al

mi•cro•some

mi•cro•so•mia

mi•cro•spec•tro•pho•tom•e•ter

mi•cro•spec•tro•pho•to•met•ric
also mi•cro•spec•tro•pho•to•met•ri•cal

mi•cro•spec•tro•pho•to•met•ri•cal•ly

mi•cro•spec•tro•pho•tom•e•try
pl mi•cro•spec•tro•pho•tom•e•tries

mi•cro•sphero•cy•to•sis

Mi•cros•po•ron

mi•cro•spo•ro•sis
pl mi•cro•spo•ro•ses

Mi•cros•po•rum

mi•cro•sto•mia
also mi•cros•to•mus
pl mi•cro•sto•mi•as
also mi•cros•to•mi

mi•cro•struc•tur•al

mi•cro•struc•ture

mi•cro•sur•gery
pl mi•cro•sur•ger•ies

mi•cro•sur•gi•cal

mi•cro•tia

mi•cro•tome

mi•cro•tom•ic
also mi•cro•tom•i•cal

mi•crot•o•my
pl mi•crot•o•mies

mi•cro•tu•bu•lar

mi•cro•tu•bule

Mi•cro•tus

mi•cro•vas•cu•lar

mi•cro•vas•cu•la•ture

mi•cro•vil•lar

mi•cro•vil•lous

mi•cro•vil•lus
pl mi•cro•vil•li

mi•cro•volt

mi•cro•wave

mi•cro•zo•on
pl mi•cro•zoa

mi•crur•gi•cal
or mi•crur•gic

mi•crur•gist

mi•crur•gy
pl mi•crur•gies

Mi•cru•rus

mic•tion

mic•tu•rate
mic•tu•rat•ed
mic•tu•rat•ing

mic•tu•ri•tion

mid•body

mid•brain

mid•car•pal

mid•dor•sal

mid•fron•tal

midge

midg•et

mid•gut

mid•line

mid•pain

mid•plane

mid•riff

mid•sec•tion

mid•tar•sal

mid•wife
pl mid•wives

mid•wife
mid•wifed
or mid•wived
mid•wif•ing
or mid•wiv•ing

mid•wife•ry
pl mid•wife•ries

mi•graine

mi•grain•oid

mi•grain•ous

mi•grate
mi•grat•ed
mi•grat•ing

mi•gra•tion

mi•gra•tion•al

mi•grat•or

mi•gra•to•ry

Miles' op•er•a•tion

mil•i•ar•ia

mil•i•ary

mi•lieu
pl mi•lieus
also mi•lieux

mil·i·um
pl mil·ia
Milk·man's syn·drome
Mil·ler-Ab·bott tube
mil·li·am·me·ter
mil·li·am·pere
mil·li·bar
mil·li·cu·rie
mil·li·equiv·a·lent
mil·li·gram
mil·li·li·ter
mil·li·me·ter
mil·li·met·ric
mil·li·mi·cron
mil·li·mol·ar
mil·li·mo·lar·i·ty
pl mil·li·mo·lar·i·ties
mil·li·mole
mil·li·nor·mal
mil·li·pede
or mil·le·pede
mil·li·roent·gen
mil·li·volt
Mil·lon's re·agent
or Mil·lon re·agent
mil·pho·sis
Mil·roy's dis·ease
mi·me·sis
pl mi·me·ses
mi·met·ic
mim·ic
mim·icked
mim·ick·ing
mim·ic·ry
pl mim·ic·ries
mim·ma·tion
mind-blow·ing
mind-ex·pand·ing
min·er·al
min·er·al·iza·tion
min·er·alo·cor·ti·coid
min·im
mini·pig
min·is·ter
min·is·tered
min·is·ter·ing
Min·ne·so·ta Mul·ti·pha·sic Per·son·al·i·ty In·ven·to·ry
mi·nom·e·ter
mi·nor
mio·car·dia
mio·did·y·mus
mi·o·pus
mi·o·sis
also my·o·sis
pl mi·o·ses
also my·o·ses
mi·ot·ic
or my·ot·ic
mi·ra·cid·i·um
pl mi·ra·cid·ia
mi·rage
mir·ror
mis·an·dry
pl mis·an·dries
mis·an·thrope
mis·an·throp·ic
also mis·an·throp·i·cal
mis·an·throp·i·cal·ly
mis·an·thro·py
pl mis·an·thro·pies
mis·car·riage
mis·car·ry
mis·car·ried
mis·car·ry·ing
mis·ce·ge·na·tion
mis·ci·bil·i·ty
pl mis·ci·bil·i·ties
mis·ci·ble
mis·di·ag·nose
mis·di·ag·nosed
mis·di·ag·nos·ing
mis·di·ag·no·sis
pl mis·di·ag·no·ses
miso·cai·nea
mi·sog·a·mist
mi·sog·a·my
pl mi·sog·a·mies
miso·gy·nic
also mi·sog·y·nous
mi·sog·y·nist
mi·sog·y·nis·tic
mi·sog·y·ny
pl mi·sog·y·nies
mi·sol·o·gy
pl mi·sol·o·gies
miso·ne·ism
miso·ne·ist
miso·ne·is·tic
miso·pe·dia
miso·pe·dist
mis·sense
mith·ri·date

mith·ri·da·tism
mi·ti·cid·al
mi·ti·cide
mit·i·gate
mit·i·gat·ed
mit·i·gat·ing
mit·i·ga·tion
mit·i·ga·tive
mi·tis
mi·to·chon·dri·al
mi·to·chon·dri·on
pl mi·to·chon·dria
mi·to·gen
mi·to·gen·e·sis
pl mi·to·gen·e·ses
mi·to·ge·net·ic
mi·to·gen·ic
mi·to·ge·nic·i·ty
pl mi·to·ge·nic·i·ties
mi·tome
mi·to·my·cin
mi·to·sis
pl mi·to·ses
mi·to·some
mi·to·spore
mi·tot·ic
mi·tot·i·cal·ly
mi·tral
mi·tral·iza·tion
mit·tel·schmerz
Mi·ya·ga·wa·nel·la
mne·mic
mne·mon·ic
also mne·mon·i·cal
mne·mon·i·cal·ly
mne·mon·ics
mo·bile
mo·bil·i·ty
pl mo·bil·i·ties
mo·bi·li·za·tion
mo·bi·lize
mo·bi·lized
mo·bi·liz·ing
moc·ca·sin
mo·dal·i·ty
pl mo·dal·i·ties
mod·er·a·tor
mod·i·fi·er
mo·di·o·lus
pl mo·di·o·li
mod·u·la·tion
mod·u·la·tor
mo·gi·graph·ia
mo·gi·la·lia
Mohs' scale
moi·ety
pl moi·eties
mol·al
mo·lal·i·ty
pl mo·lal·i·ties
mo·lar
mo·lar·i·form
mo·lar·i·ty
pl mo·lar·i·ties
mold
or mould
moldy
or mouldy
mold·i·er
or mould·i·er
mold·i·est
or mould·i·est
mole
bodily spot or *an abnormal growth*
mole
also mol
weight
mo·lec·u·lar
mo·lec·u·lar·ly
mol·e·cule
mo·li·men
pl mo·lim·i·na
Mo·lisch re·ac·tion
or Mo·lisch test
mol·li·ti·es
Mol·lus·ca
mol·lus·can
also mol·lus·kan
mol·lus·coid
mol·lus·cous
mol·lus·cum
pl mol·lus·ca
mol·lus·cum con·ta·gi·o·sum
pl mol·lus·ca con·ta·gi·o·sa
mol·lusk
or mol·lusc
molt
or moult
mo·lyb·date
mo·lyb·de·num
mo·lyb·dic
mo·lyb·dous
mo·lys·mo·pho·bia

mo•men•tum
pl mo•men•ta
or mo•men•tums

mo•nad
Mo•nad•i•dae
mon•amine
var of monoamine

mon•ar•thric
mon•ar•thri•tis
pl mon•ar•thrit•i•des

mon•ar•tic•u•lar
mo•nas
pl mon•a•des

mon•as•ter
mon•ath•e•to•sis
pl mon•ath•e•to•ses

mon•atom•ic
mon•au•ral
mon•au•ral•ly
mon•ax•on•ic
Möncke•berg's ar•te•rio•scle•ro•sis
Mon•dor's dis•ease
Mo•ne•ra
mon•e•tite
mon•gol
mon•go•lian
mon•gol•ism
or mon•go•lian•ism

mon•gol•oid
Mo•nie•zia
mo•nil•e•thrix
or mo•nil•i•thrix
pl mon•i•let•ri•ches
or mon•i•lit•ri•ches

mo•nil•ia
pl mo•nil•ias
or mo•nil•ia

mo•nil•i•al
mon•i•li•a•sis
pl mon•i•li•a•ses

mo•nil•i•form
Mo•nil•i•for•mis
mo•nil•i•form•ly
mo•nil•iid
mo•nism
mo•nis•tic
mon•i•tor
mono
mono•amine
also mon•amine

mono•am•i•ner•gic
mono•ba•sic
mono•blast
mono•blep•sia
mono•bra•chi•us
mono•car•di•an
mono•cel•lu•lar
mon•o•ceph•a•lus
pl mon•o•ceph•a•li

mono•chord
mono•cho•rea
mono•cho•ri•on•ic
mono•chro•ma•sy
pl mono•chro•ma•sies

mono•chro•mat
mono•chro•mat•ic
mono•chro•mat•i•cal•ly

mono•chro•ma•tism
also mono•chro•ma•sy
pl mono•chro•ma•tisms
or mono•chro•ma•sies

mon•o•cle
mon•o•cled
mono•clin•ic
mono•con•tam•i•nate
mono•con•tam•i•nat•ed
mono•con•tam•i•nat•ing
mono•con•tam•i•na•tion
mono•crot•ic
mon•oc•u•lar
mon•oc•u•lar•ly
mon•oc•u•lus
pl mon•oc•u•li

mono•cys•tic
mono•cyte
mono•cyt•ic
mono•cyt•oid
mono•cy•to•pe•nia
mono•cy•to•sis
pl mono•cy•to•ses

mono•dac•tyl•ism
or mono•dac•ty•ly
pl mono•dac•tyl•isms
or mono•dac•ty•lies

mono•dip•lo•pia
mono•es•ter
mono•fac•to•ri•al

mono·fil·a·ment
mono·func·tion·al
mo·nog·a·my
pl mo·nog·a·mies
mono·gas·tric
mono·gen·e·sis
pl mono·gen·e·ses
mono·ge·net·ic
mono·gen·ic
mono·gen·i·cal·ly
mo·nog·e·nous
mono·ger·mi·nal
mono·graph
mono·graph·ic
mono·hy·brid
mono·hy·drate
mono·hy·drat·ed
mono·hy·dric
mono·ide·ism
mono·ide·is·tic
mono·lay·er
mono·loc·u·lar
mono·ma·nia
mono·ma·ni·ac
mono·mas·ti·gote
mono·mel·ic
mono·mer
mo·no·mer·ic
mono·me·tal·lic
mono·mo·lec·u·lar
mono·mo·lec·u·lar·ly
mono·mor·phic
or mono·mor·phous
mono·mor·phism
mo·nom·pha·lus
pl mo·nom·pha·li
mono·neu·ral
mono·neu·ri·tis
pl mono·neu·rit·i·des
or mono·neu·ri·tis·es
mono·nu·cle·ar
mono·nu·cle·o·sis
pl mono·nu·cle·o·ses
mono·nu·cle·o·tide
mono·pa·re·sis
pl mono·pa·re·ses
mono·pha·sia
mono·pha·sic
mono·pho·bia
mon·oph·thal·mic
mon·oph·thal·mus
mono·phy·let·ic
mono·phy·le·tism
or mono·phy·le·ty
pl mono·phy·le·tisms
or mono·phy·le·ties
mono·phy·odont
mono·ple·gia
mono·ple·gic
mono·ploid
mono·po·dia
mon·o·pus
mon·or·chid
mon·or·chi·dism
also mon·or·chism
mon·or·chis
pl mon·or·chi·des
mono·sac·cha·ride
mono·sex·u·al
mono·sex·u·al·i·ty
pl mono·sex·u·al·i·ties
mono·so·di·um glu·ta·mate
mono·some
mono·so·mic
mono·stot·ic
mono·stra·tal
mono·sub·sti·tut·ed
mono·sub·sti·tu·tion
mono·symp·tom·at·ic
mono·syn·ap·tic
mono·syn·ap·ti·cal·ly
mono·ther·mia
mo·not·o·cous
Mono·trema·ta
mono·treme
mo·not·ri·chous
also mono·trich·ic
or mo·not·ri·chate
mono·va·lent
mon·ovu·lar
mon·ox·ide
mono·zy·got·ic
mons
pl mon·tes
mons pu·bis
mon·ster
mon·stros·i·ty
pl mon·stros·i·ties
mon·strous
mons ve·ner·is

Mon•teg•gia's frac•ture
Mon•te•zu•ma's re•venge
Mont•gom•ery's glands
month•lies
mon•tic•u•lus
moon-blind
moon blind•ness
mo•rale
Mo•rax-Ax•en•feld con•junc•ti•vi•tis
mor•bid
mor•bid•i•ty
pl mor•bid•i•ties

mor•bid•ly
mor•bif•ic
mor•bil•li
mor•bil•li•form
mor•bus
pl mor•bi

mor•cel•la•tion
mor•dant
Mor•ga•gni's crypt
morgue
mo•ria
mor•i•bund
mor•i•bun•di•ty
pl mor•i•bun•di•ties

morn•ing-af•ter pill
mo•ron
mo•ron•ic
mo•ron•ism
mo•ron•i•ty
pl mo•ron•i•ties

Mo•ro re•flex
mor•phal•lax•is
pl mor•phal•lax•es

mor•phea
also mor•phoea
pl mor•phe•ae
or mor•phoe•ae

mor•pheme
mor•phe•mic
mor•phe•mi•cal•ly
mor•phia
mor•phine
mor•phin•ic
mor•phin•ism
mor•phin•ize
mor•phin•ized
mor•phin•iz•ing
mor•phi•no•ma•nia
also mor•phi•o•ma•nia

mor•phi•no•ma•ni•ac
also mor•phi•o•ma•ni•ac

mor•pho•gen•e•sis
pl mor•pho•gen•e•ses

mor•pho•ge•net•ic
mor•pho•ge•net•i•cal•ly
mor•pho•gen•ic
mor•pho•graph•ic
mor•phog•ra•phy
pl mor•phog•ra•phies
mor•pho•log•i•cal
also mor•pho•log•ic

mor•pho•log•i•cal•ly
mor•phol•o•gist
mor•phol•o•gy
pl mor•phol•o•gies

mor•phom•e•try
pl mor•phom•e•tries

mor•pho•phys•i•o•log•i•cal
mor•pho•phys•i•ol•o•gy
pl mor•pho•phys•i•ol•o•gies

mor•pho•sis
pl mor•pho•ses

mor•phot•ic
mor•sal
mor•sus
mor•tal
mor•tal•i•ty
pl mor•tal•i•ties

mor•tal•ly
mor•tar
mor•ti•fi•ca•tion
mor•ti•fy
mor•ti•fied
mor•ti•fy•ing
Mor•ton's toe
also Mor•ton's dis•ease

mor•tu•ary
pl mor•tu•ar•ies

mor•u•la
pl mor•u•lae

mor•u•lar

mor·u·la·tion
mo·sa·ic
mo·sa·icism
mos·qui·to
pl mos·qui·toes
also mos·qui·tos
Moss·man fe·ver
moth·er
mo·tile
mo·til·i·ty
pl mo·til·i·ties
mo·tion
mo·ti·vate
mo·ti·vat·ed
mo·ti·vat·ing
mo·ti·va·tion
mo·ti·va·tion·al
mo·ti·va·tion·al·ly
mo·tive
mo·to·neu·ron
also mo·to·neu·rone
mo·tor
mo·to·ri·al
mo·to·ri·um
pl mo·to·ria
mot·tled
mot·tling
mou·lage
mould
var of mold
mouldy
var of moldy
moult
var of molt
mound·ing
moun·te·bank
moun·te·bank·ery
pl moun·te·bank·er·ies
mount·ing
mouse
pl mice
mouse·pox
mous·sena
var of musenna
mouth·piece
mouth-to-mouth
mouth·wash
moxa
mox·i·bus·tion
mu·cic
mu·ci·car·mine
mu·cif·er·ous
mu·cif·ic
mu·ci·fi·ca·tion
mu·ci·fy
mu·ci·fied
mu·ci·fy·ing
mu·ci·gen
mu·ci·lage
mu·ci·lag·i·nous
mu·ci·lag·i·nous·ly
mu·cin
mu·cin·o·gen
mu·cin·oid
mu·ci·no·lyt·ic
mu·ci·no·sis
pl mu·ci·no·ses
mu·ci·nous
mu·cip·a·rous
mu·co·cele
also mu·co·coele
mu·co·col·pos
mu·co·cu·ta·ne·ous
mu·co·en·ter·i·tis
pl mu·co·en·ter·it·i·des
or mu·co·en·ter·i·tis·es
mu·co·epi·der·moid
mu·coid
mu·coi·tin
mu·coi·tin·sul·fu·ric
mu·co·lyt·ic
mu·co·peri·os·te·al
mu·co·peri·os·te·um
pl mu·co·peri·os·tea
mu·co·poly·sac·cha·ride
mu·co·pro·tein
mu·co·pu·ru·lent
mu·co·pus
mu·cor
Mu·co·ra·ce·ae
Mu·co·ra·les
mu·cor·my·co·sis
pl mu·cor·my·co·ses
mu·co·sa
pl mu·co·sae
or mu·co·sas
mu·co·sal
mu·co·san·guin·e·ous
mu·co·se·rous
mu·co·sin

mu•co•si•tis
mu•cos•i•ty
pl mu•cos•i•ties
mu•co•stat•ic
mu•cous
adjective (*see* mucus)
mu•co•vis•ci•do sis
pl mu•co•vis•ci•do• ses
mu•cro
pl mu•cro•nes
also mu•cros
mu•cro•nate
also mu•cro•nat•ed
Mu•cu•na
mu•cus
noun (*see* mucous)
Muel•le•ri•us
mu•lat•to
pl mu•lat•toes
or mu•lat•tos
Mules op•er•a• tion
mu•li•ebria
mu•li•eb•ri•ty
pl mu•li•eb•ri•ties
mull•er
Mül•le•ri•an
also Muel•le•ri•an
Mül•le•ri•an duct
Mül•ler's flu•id
Mül•ler's mus•cle
mult•an•gu•lar
mult•an•gu•lum
pl mult•an•gu•la
mul•ti•cel•lu•lar
mul•ti•cel•lu•lar•i• ty
pl mul•ti•cel•lu•lar•i• ties
mul•ti•cen•tric
mul•ti•cen•tri•cal• ly
mul•ti•cen•tric•i• ty
pl mul•ti•cen•tric•i• ties
mul•ti•ceps
mul•ti•cus•pid
mul•ti•fac•to•ri•al
mul•ti•fa•mil•ial
mul•ti•fid
mul•ti•fid•ly
mul•tif•i•dus
pl mul•tif•i•di
mul•ti•glan•du• lar
mul•ti•grav•i•da
pl mul•ti•grav•i•das
also mul•ti•grav•i• dae
mul•ti•in•fec•tion
mul•ti•lay•ered
mul•ti•lob•u•lar
mul•ti•loc•u•lar
mul•ti•mam•mae
mul•ti•nod•u•lar
mul•ti•nu•cle•ate
or mul•ti•nu•cle•ar
also mul•ti•nu•cle•at• ed
mul•tip•a•ra
pl mul•tip•a•ras
or mul•tip•a•rae
mul•ti•par•i•ty
pl mul•ti•par•i•ties
mul•tip•a•rous
mul•ti•po•lar
mul•ti•re•sis• tance
mul•ti•re•sis•tant
mul•ti•sen•so•ry
mul•tiv•a•lence
mul•ti•va•lent
mul•ti•vi•ta•min
mum•mi•fi•ca• tion
mum•mi•fy
mum•mi•fied
mum•mi•fy•ing
Mun•chau•sen syn•drome
mu•ral
mu•ram•ic
mu•rein
mu•rex•ide
mu•ri•ate
mu•ri•at•ic
mu•rine
mur•mur
mur•rain
mur•ri•na
Mus
Mus•ca
mus•cae vo•li• tan•tes
mus•ca•rine
mus•ca•rin•ic
mus•ca•rin•ism
Mus•ci•dae
mus•cle

mus·cle-bound
mus·cled
mus·cu·lar
mus·cu·la·ris
mus·cu·lar·i·ty
pl mus·cu·lar·i·ties

mus·cu·lar·ly
mus·cu·la·tion
mus·cu·la·ture
mus·cu·lo·apo·neu·rot·ic
mus·cu·lo·cu·ta·ne·ous
mus·cu·lo·mem·bra·nous
mus·cu·lo·phren·ic
mus·cu·lo·skel·e·tal
mus·cu·lo·spi·ral
mus·cu·lo·ten·di·nous
mus·cu·lo·trop·ic
mus·cu·lus
pl mus·cu·li

mu·sen·na
also me·sen·na
or mous·sena

mush·room
mu·si·co·ther·a·py
pl mu·si·co·ther·a·pies

mus·si·ta·tion
mus·tard
mu·ta·fa·cient
mu·ta·gen
mu·ta·gen·e·sis
pl mu·ta·gen·e·ses

mu·ta·gen·ic
mu·ta·gen·i·cal·ly
mu·ta·ge·nic·ity
pl mu·ta·ge·nic·ities

mu·tant
mu·ta·ro·tase
mu·ta·ro·ta·tion
mu·tase
mu·tate
mu·tat·ed
mu·tat·ing
mu·ta·tion
mu·ta·tion·al
mu·ta·tion·al·ly
mu·ta·tor
mu·ti·late
mu·ti·lat·ed
mu·ti·lat·ing
mu·ti·la·tion
mu·ti·la·tor
mu·tism
mu·tu·al·ism
mu·tu·al·ist
muz·zle
muz·zled
muz·zling
my·al·gia
my·al·gic
my·as·the·nia
my·as·the·nia grav·is
my·as·then·ic
my·a·to·nia
muscular flabbiness
(*see* myotonia)
my·ce·li·al
my·ce·li·oid
my·ce·li·um
pl my·ce·lia

my·ce·tism
my·ce·tis·mus
pl my·ce·tis·mi

my·ce·to·gen·ic
my·ce·toid
my·ce·to·ma
pl my·ce·to·mas
or my·ce·to·ma·ta

My·ce·to·zoa
my·ce·to·zo·an
My·co·bac·te·ri·a·ce·ae
my·co·bac·te·ri·al
my·co·bac·te·ri·o·sis
pl my·co·bac·te·ri·o·ses

my·co·bac·te·ri·um
pl my·co·bac·te·ria

my·co·cide
My·co·der·ma
my·co·der·ma·toid
or my·co·der·ma·tous

my·col·ic
my·co·log·i·cal
also my·co·log·ic

my·co·log·i·cal·ly
my·col·o·gist
my·col·o·gy
pl my·col·o·gies

my·co·my·cin
my·coph·a·gous
my·co·plas·ma
pl my·co·plas·mas
or my·co·plas·ma·ta
my·co·plas·mal
my·co·sis
pl my·co·ses
my·co·sis fun·goid·es
my·co·stat·ic
my·cos·ter·ol
my·cot·ic
my·co·tox·ic
my·co·tox·ic·i·ty
pl my·co·tox·ic·i·ties
my·co·tox·i·co·sis
pl my·co·tox·i·co·ses
my·co·tox·in
my·dri·a·sis
pl my·dri·a·ses
myd·ri·at·ic
my·ec·to·my
pl my·ec·to·mies
my·el·at·ro·phy
pl my·el·at·ro·phies
my·el·en·ce·phal·ic
my·el·en·ceph·a·lon
pl my·el·en·ceph·a·la
my·el·ic
my·elin
my·elin·at·ed
my·elin·a·tion
or my·elin·iza·tion
my·elin·ic
my·eli·noc·la·sis
pl my·eli·noc·la·ses
my·eli·no·gen·e·sis
pl my·eli·no·gen·e·ses
my·elin·ol·y·sis
pl my·elin·ol·y·ses
my·eli·no·sis
pl my·eli·no·ses
or my·eli·no·sis·es
my·elit·ic
my·eli·tis
pl my·elit·i·des
my·elo·blast
my·elo·blas·te·mia
my·elo·blas·tic
my·elo·blas·to·ma
pl my·elo·blas·to·mas
or my·elo·blas·to·ma·ta
my·elo·blas·to·sis
pl my·elo·blas·to·ses
my·elo·cele
also my·elo·coele
my·elo·cys·to·cele
my·elo·cyte
my·elo·cyt·ic
my·elo·cy·to·ma
pl my·elo·cy·to·mas
or my·elo·cy·to·ma·ta
my·elo·cy·to·sis
pl my·elo·cy·to·ses
my·elo·dys·pla·sia
my·elo·en·ceph·a·li·tis
pl my·elo·en·ceph·a·lit·i·des
my·elo·fi·bro·sis
pl my·elo·fi·bro·ses
my·elo·fi·brot·ic
my·elo·gen·e·sis
pl my·elo·gen·e·ses
my·elo·gen·ic
my·elog·e·nous
also my·elo·gen·ic
my·elo·gram
my·elo·graph·ic
my·elo·graph·i·cal·ly
my·elog·ra·phy
pl my·elog·ra·phies
my·eloid
my·elo·li·po·ma
pl my·elo·li·po·mas
or my·elo·li·po·ma·ta
my·elo·lym·pho·cyte
my·elo·ma
pl my·elo·mas
or my·elo·ma·ta
my·elo·ma·la·cia
my·elo·ma·to·sis
pl my·elo·ma·to·ses
my·elo·ma·tous
my·elo·men·in·gi·tis
pl my·elo·men·in·git·i·des
my·elo·me·nin·go·cele
my·elo·mere

my•elo•mono•cyte
my•elo•neu•ri•tis
pl my•elo•neu•rit•i•des
or my•elo•neu•ri•tis•es

my•elon•ic
my•elo•pa•ral•y•sis
pl my•elo•pa•ral•y•ses

my•elo•path•ic
my•elop•a•thy
pl my•elop•a•thies

my•elop•e•tal
my•elo•phthis•ic
my•elo•phthi•sis
pl my•elo•phthi•ses

my•elo•plast
my•elo•plax
pl my•elo•plax•es
or my•e•lop•la•ces

my•elo•ple•gia
my•elo•poi•e•sis
pl my•elo•poi•e•ses

my•elo•poi•et•ic
my•elo•pro•lif•er•a•tive
my•elo•ra•dic•u•li•tis
my•elo•ra•dic•u•lo•dys•pla•sia
my•elo•ra•dic•u•lop•a•thy
pl my•elo•ra•dic•u•lop•a•thies

my•elo•rrha•gia
my•elo•sar•co•ma
pl my•elo•sar•co•mas
or my•elo•sar•co•ma•ta

my•elos•chi•sis
pl my•elos•chi•ses
or my•elos•chi•sis•es

my•elo•scle•ro•sis
my•elo•sis
pl my•elo•ses

my•elo•spon•gi•um
pl my•elo•spon•gia

my•elo•tox•ic
my•en•ter•ic
my•en•ter•on
my•es•the•sia
my•ia•sis
pl my•ia•ses

my•lo•hy•oid
my•lo•hy•oi•de•an
my•lo•hy•oi•de•us
pl my•lo•hy•oi•dei

myo•ar•chi•tec•ton•ic
myo•blast
myo•blas•tic
myo•car•di•al
myo•car•dio•graph
myo•car•di•op•a•thy
pl myo•car•di•op•a•thies

myo•car•di•tis
myo•car•di•um
pl myo•car•dia
myo•car•do•sis
pl myo•car•do•ses

myo•clo•nia
myo•clon•ic
my•oc•lo•nus
myo•coel
also myo•coele

myo•com•ma
pl myo•com•ma•ta
also myo•com•mas

myo•cyte
myo•dy•nam•ics
myo•dys•to•nia
or myo•dys•to•ny
pl myo•dys•to•ni•as
or myo•dys•to•nies

myo•dys•tro•phy
pl myo•dys•tro•phies

myo•ede•ma
pl myo•ede•mas
or myo•ede•ma•ta

myo•elas•tic
myo•elec•tric
also myo•elec•tri•cal

myo•elec•tri•cal•ly
myo•ep•i•the•li•al
myo•ep•i•the•li•o•ma
pl myo•ep•i•the•li•o•mas
or myo•ep•i•the•li•o•ma•ta

myo•fas•ci•tis
myo•fi•bril
also myo•fi•bril•la

myo•fi•bro•ma
pl myo•fi•bro•mas
also myo•fi•bro•ma•ta

myo·fi·bro·sis
pl myo·fi·bro·ses

myo·fi·bro·si·tis
myo·fil·a·ment
myo·gen
myo·gen·ic
myo·ge·nic·i·ty
pl myo·ge·nic·i·ties

my·og·e·nous
myo·glo·bin
myo·glo·bin·uria
myo·gram
myo·graph
myo·graph·ic
myo·graph·i·cal·ly
my·og·ra·phy
pl my·og·ra·phies

myo·he·mo·glo·bin
my·oid
myo·ki·nase
myo·ky·mia
myo·lem·ma
pl myo·lem·mas
or myo·lem·ma·ta

myo·li·po·ma
pl myo·li·po·mas
or myo·li·po·ma·ta

my·o·log·ic
or my·o·log·i·cal

my·ol·o·gy
pl my·ol·o·gies

my·o·ma
pl my·o·mas
or my·o·ma·ta

myo·ma·la·cia
my·o·ma·tous
myo·mec·to·my
pl myo·mec·to·mies

myo·mere
myo·mer·ic
myo·me·tri·al
myo·me·tri·tis
myo·me·tri·um
myo·neme
also myo·ne·ma

myo·neu·ral
myo·pal·mus
myo·pa·ral·y·sis
pl myo·pa·ral·y·ses

myo·pa·re·sis
pl myo·pa·re·ses

myo·path·ic
my·op·a·thy
pl my·op·a·thies

my·ope
myo·peri·car·di·tis
pl myo·peri·car·dit·i·des

my·o·pia
my·o·pic
my·o·pi·cal·ly
myo·plas·ty
pl myo·plas·ties

myo·psy·cho·sis
pl myo·psy·cho·ses

my·or·rha·phy
pl my·or·rha·phies

myo·sar·co·ma
pl myo·sar·co·mas
or myo·sar·co·ma·ta

myo·scle·ro·sis
pl myo·scle·ro·ses

myo·sep·tum
pl myo·sep·ta

my·o·sin
my·o·sis
var of miosis

myo·si·tis
myo·tac·tic
my·ot·a·sis
myo·tat·ic
myo·ten·o·si·tis
myo·te·not·o·my
pl myo·te·not·o·mies

my·ot·ic
var of miotic

myo·tome
my·ot·o·my
pl my·ot·o·mies

myo·to·nia
tonic muscular spasm (*see* myatonia)

myo·ton·ic
my·ot·o·nus
my·ot·ro·phy
pl my·ot·ro·phies

my·rin·ga
myr·in·gec·to·my
pl myr·in·gec·to·mies

myr·in·gi·tis
my·rin·go·dec·to·my
pl my·rin·go·dec·to·mies

my·rin·go·my·co·sis
pl my·rin·go·my·co·ses

my·rin·go·plas·ty
pl my·rin·go·plas·ties

my·rin·go·tome
myr·in·got·o·my
pl myr·in·got·o·mies

my·ris·tic
myrrh
my·so·phil·ia
my·so·pho·bia
my·so·pho·bic
my·ta·cism
mytho·ma·nia
mytho·ma·ni·ac
myx·ad·e·ni·tis
myx·ad·e·no·ma
pl myx·ad·e·no·mas
or myx·ad·e·no·ma·ta

myx·as·the·nia
myx·ede·ma
pl myx·ede·mas
or myx·ede·ma·ta

myx·ede·ma·tous
myx·id·i·o·cy
pl myx·id·i·o·cies

myxo·chon·dro·fi·bro·sar·co·ma
pl myxo·chon·dro·fi·bro·sar·co·mas
or myxo·chon·dro·fi·bro·sar·co·ma·ta

myxo·chon·dro·ma
pl myxo·chon·dro·mas
also myxo·chon·dro·ma·ta

myxo·cyte
myxo·fi·bro·ma
pl myxo·fi·bro·mas
or myxo·fi·bro·ma·ta

myxo·fi·bro·sar·co·ma
pl myxo·fi·bro·sar·co·mas
or myxo·fi·bro·sar·co·ma·ta

myxo·li·po·ma
pl myxo·li·po·mas
or myxo·li·po·ma·ta

myx·o·ma
pl myx·o·mas
or myx·o·ma·ta

myx·o·ma·to·sis
pl myx·o·ma·to·ses

myx·o·ma·tous
myxo·my·cete
Myxo·my·ce·tes
myxo·my·ce·tous
myxo·neu·ro·ma
pl myxo·neu·ro·mas
or myxo·neu·ro·ma·ta

myx·or·rhea
myxo·sar·co·ma
pl myxo·sar·co·mas
or myxo·sar·co·ma·ta

myxo·sar·co·ma·tous
myxo·spore
Myxo·spo·rid·ia
myxo·vi·ral
myxo·vi·rus

N

na·bo·thi·an
na·cre·ous
also na·crous

nae·void
var of nevoid

nae·vus
var of nevus

na·ga·na
or n'ga·na

na·ive
or na·ïve

na·iv·er
or na·ïv·er

na·iv·est
or na·ïv·est

Na·ja
na·li·dix·ic
na·lor·phine
nal·ox·one
na·nism
na·nit·ic
nano·gram
na·noid
na·no·so·mia
na·no·so·mus
naph·tha
naph·tha·lene
naph·thi·on·ic
naph·thol
naph·tho·qui·none
also naph·tha·qui·none

naph·thyl
na·pi·form

nap·ra·path
na·prap·a·thy
pl na·prap·a·thies

nar·ce·ine
nar·cism
nar·cis·sine
nar·cis·sism
nar·cis·sist
nar·cis·sis·tic
nar·cis·sis·ti·cal·ly
nar·co·anal·y·sis
pl nar·co·anal·y·ses

nar·co·an·es·the·sia
also nar·co·an·aes·the·sia

nar·co·di·ag·no·sis
pl nar·co·di·ag·no·ses

nar·co·hyp·nia
nar·co·hyp·no·sis
pl nar·co·hyp·no·ses

nar·co·lep·sy
pl nar·co·lep·sies

nar·co·lep·tic
nar·co·ma
pl nar·co·mas
also nar·co·ma·ta

nar·co·ma·nia
nar·cose
also nar·cous

nar·co·sis
pl nar·co·ses

nar·co·syn·the·sis
pl nar·co·syn·the·ses

nar·co·ther·a·py
pl nar·co·ther·a·pies

nar·cot·ic
nar·cot·i·cal·ly
nar·cot·i·cism
nar·co·tine
nar·co·tism
nar·co·ti·za·tion
nar·co·tize
nar·co·tized
nar·co·tiz·ing
na·ris
pl na·res

na·sal
na·sa·lis
na·scent
na·si·on
Nas·myth's mem·brane
na·so·cil·i·ary
na·so·la·bi·al
na·so·lac·ri·mal
also na·so·lach·ry·mal

na·so·pal·a·tine
also na·so·pal·a·tal

na·so·pha·ryn·geal
na·so·phar·yn·gi·tis
pl na·so·phar·yn·git·i·des

na·so·pha·ryn·go·scope
na·so·pha·ryn·go·scop·ic
na·so·phar·ynx
pl na·so·pha·ryn·ges
also na·so·phar·ynx·es

na·so·scope
na·so·si·nus·itis
also na·so·si·nu·itis

na·so·spi·na·le
na·so·tur·bi·nal
na·sus
pl na·si

na·tal
na·tal·i·ty
pl na·tal·i·ties

na·tes
na·tive
na·tri·um
na·tri·ure·sis
also na·tru·re·sis

na·tri·uret·ic
na·tu·ro·path
na·tu·ro·path·ic
na·tu·rop·a·thy
also na·ture·op·a·thy

nau·sea
nau·se·ant
nau·se·ate
nau·se·at·ed
nau·se·at·ing
nau·seous
nau·seous·ly
na·vel
na·vic·u·la
na·vic·u·lar
na·vic·u·la·re
near·sight·ed
near·sight·ed·ly

near·sight·ed·ness
ne·ar·thro·sis
pl ne·ar·thro·ses
ne·ben·kern
neb·u·la
pl neb·u·las
or neb·u·lae
neb·u·lar
neb·u·li·za·tion
neb·u·lize
neb·u·lized
neb·u·liz·ing
neb·u·liz·er
ne·ca·tor
neck·lace
nec·ro·bac·il·lary
nec·ro·bac·il·lo·sis
pl nec·ro·bac·il·lo·ses
nec·ro·bi·o·sis
pl nec·ro·bi·o·ses
nec·ro·bi·ot·ic
nec·ro·gen·ic
or ne·crog·e·nous
nec·ro·log·i·cal
also nec·ro·log·ic
ne·crol·o·gist
ne·crol·o·gy
pl ne·crol·o·gies
nec·ro·pha·gia
or ne·croph·a·gy
pl nec·ro·pha·gias
or ne·croph·a·gies
ne·croph·a·gous
nec·ro·phile
nec·ro·phil·ia
nec·ro·phil·ic
ne·croph·i·lism
ne·croph·i·lous
nec·ro·pho·bia
nec·ro·pho·bic
nec·rop·sy
pl nec·rop·sies
nec·rop·sy
nec·rop·sied
nec·rop·sy·ing
ne·crose
nec·ro·sin
ne·cro·sis
pl ne·cro·ses
nec·ro·sper·mia
ne·crot·ic
nec·ro·tize
nec·ro·tized
nec·ro·tiz·ing
ne·crot·o·my
pl ne·crot·o·mies
nee·dle
ne·en·ceph·a·lon
pl ne·en·ceph·a·la
neg·a·tive
neg·a·tiv·ist·ic
Ne·gri body
Ne·groid
Neis·se·ria
ne·ma·thel·minth
Ne·ma·thel·min·thes
ne·ma·to·cid·al
also ne·ma·ti·cid·al
ne·ma·to·cide
also ne·ma·ti·cide
Nem·a·to·da
nem·a·tode
ne·ma·to·di·a·sis
pl ne·ma·to·di·a·ses
Nem·a·to·di·rus
nem·a·toid
or nem·a·toi·de·an
nem·a·to·log·i·cal
nem·a·tol·o·gist
nem·a·tol·o·gy
pl nem·a·tol·o·gies
neo·ars·phen·a·mine
neo·blas·tic
neo·cer·e·bel·lar
neo·cer·e·bel·lum
pl neo·cer·e·bel·lums
or neo·cer·e·bel·la
neo·cor·tex
pl neo·cor·ti·ces
or neo·cor·tex·es
neo·cor·ti·cal
neo·dym·i·um
neo·fe·tus
neo·for·ma·tion
neo-Freud·ian
neo·gen·e·sis
pl neo·gen·e·ses
neo·ge·net·ic
or neo·gen·ic
neo·la·lia
ne·ol·o·gism
neo·morph
neo·mor·phic
neo·mor·phism
neo·my·cin
ne·on

neo·na·tal
neo·na·tal·ly
ne·o·nate
neo·pal·li·um
pl neo·pal·lia
or neo·pal·li·ums

neo·pho·bia
neo·pho·bic
neo·pine
neo·pla·sia
neo·plasm
neo·plas·tic
neo·stig·mine
neo·stri·a·tum
pl neo·stri·a·tums
or neo·stria·ta

ne·o·ten·ic
ne·o·te·ny
also ne·o·tei·nia
pl ne·o·te·nies
also ne·o·tei·nias

neo·thal·a·mus
pl neo·thal·a·mi

neph·a·lism
neph·a·list
neph·a·lis·tic
neph·e·lom·e·ter
neph·e·lo·met·ric
neph·e·lo·met·ri·cal·ly
neph·e·lom·e·try
pl neph·e·lom·e·tries

ne·phrec·to·mize
ne·phrec·to·mized
ne·phrec·to·miz·ing

ne·phrec·to·my
pl ne·phrec·to·mies

neph·ric
ne·phrid·i·al
ne·phrid·i·um
pl ne·phrid·ia

ne·phrit·ic
ne·phri·tis
pl ne·phrit·i·des
or ne·phri·tis·es

neph·ro·cal·ci·no·sis
pl neph·ro·cal·ci·no·ses

neph·ro·cele
neph·ro·cyte
neph·ro·gen·ic
also ne·phrog·e·nous

neph·roid
neph·ro·lith
neph·ro·li·thi·a·sis
pl neph·ro·li·thi·a·ses

neph·ro·lith·ic
neph·ro·li·thot·o·my
pl neph·ro·li·thot·o·mies

ne·phrol·o·gist
ne·phrol·o·gy
pl ne·phrol·o·gies

ne·phro·ma
pl ne·phro·mas
also ne·phro·ma·ta

neph·ro·mere
neph·ron
also neph·rone

ne·phrop·a·thy
pl ne·phrop·a·thies

neph·ro·pexy
pl neph·ro·pex·ies

neph·rop·to·sis
pl neph·rop·to·ses

ne·phror·rha·phy
pl ne·phror·rha·phies

neph·ro·scler·o·sis
pl neph·ro·scler·o·ses

ne·phro·sis
pl ne·phro·ses

neph·ro·stome
also neph·ro·stom
or ne·phros·to·ma
pl neph·ro·stomes
also neph·ro·stoms
or neph·ro·sto·ma·ta

neph·ro·sto·mic
ne·phrot·ic
neph·ro·tome
ne·phrot·o·my
pl ne·phrot·o·mies

neph·ro·tox·ic
neph·ro·tox·ic·i·ty
pl neph·ro·tox·ic·i·ties

nep·tu·ni·um
ner·o·li oil
ner·va·tion
nerve of Lan·ci·si
nerve of Wris·berg
ner·vos·i·ty
pl ner·vos·i·ties

ner·vous
ner·vous·ly

ner•vous•ness
ner•vus
pl ner•vi

ner•vus ter•mi•
nal•is
ness•ler•iza•tion
ness•ler•ize
ness•ler•ized
ness•ler•iz•ing
Ness•ler's re•
agent
or Ness•ler's so•lu•
tion

net•work
neu•rad
neu•ral
neu•ral•gia
neu•ral•gic
neu•ral•gi•form
neu•ral•ly
neur•amin•ic
neur•amin•i•dase
neur•apoph•y•sis
pl neur•apoph•y•ses

neur•as•the•nia
neur•as•then•ic
neur•as•then•i•
cal•ly
neur•ax•is
pl neur•ax•es

neur•ax•on
also neur•ax•one

neu•rec•to•my
pl neu•rec•to•mies

neur•en•ter•ic
neu•rer•gic

neu•ri•lem•ma
also neu•ri•lema
or neu•ro•lem•ma

neu•ri•lem•mal
or neu•ri•lem•mat•ic
or neu•ri•lem•ma•
tous

neu•ri•lem•mo•
ma
or neu•ri•le•mo•ma
pl neu•ri•lem•mo•
mas
or neu•ri•lem•mo•
ma•ta
or neu•ri•le•mo•mas
or neu•ri•le•mo•ma•
ta

neu•ril•i•ty
pl neu•ril•i•ties

neu•rine
also neu•rin

neu•ri•no•ma
pl neu•ri•no•mas
or neu•ri•no•ma•ta

neu•rite
neu•rit•ic
neu•ri•tis
pl neu•rit•i•des
or neu•ri•tis•es

neu•ro•ac•tive
neu•ro•anat•o•
mist
neu•ro•anat•o•my
pl neu•ro•anat•o•
mies

neu•ro•bi•o•log•i•
cal
neu•ro•bi•ol•o•gist
neu•ro•bi•ol•o•gy
pl neu•ro•bi•ol•o•gies

neu•ro•bio•tax•is
pl neu•ro•bio•tax•es

neu•ro•blast
neu•ro•blas•tic
neu•ro•blas•to•ma
pl neu•ro•blas•to•mas
or neu•ro•blas•to•ma•
ta

neu•ro•ca•nal
neu•ro•cen•trum
pl neu•ro•cen•trums
or neu•ro•cen•tra

neu•ro•chem•i•cal
neu•ro•chem•ist
neu•ro•chem•is•
try
pl neu•ro•chem•is•
tries

neu•ro•chord
neu•ro•cir•cu•la•
to•ry
neu•ro•coele
or neu•ro•coel
also neu•ro•cele

neu•ro•cra•ni•um
pl neu•ro•cra•ni•ums
or neu•ro•cra•nia

neu•ro•crine
neu•ro•crin•ism
neu•ro•cu•ta•ne•
ous
neu•ro•cyte
neu•ro•cy•to•ma
pl neu•ro•cy•to•mas
or neu•ro•cy•to•ma•ta

neu•ro•den•drite
or neu•ro•den•dron

neu•ro•der•ma•
tit•ic

neu·ro·der·ma·ti·tis
pl neu·ro·der·ma·ti·ti·ses
or neu·ro·der·ma·tit·i·des

neu·ro·ec·to·derm
neu·ro·ec·to·der·mal
neu·ro·en·do·crine
neu·ro·en·do·cri·nol·o·gy
pl neu·ro·en·do·cri·nol·o·gies

neu·ro·epi·der·mal
neu·ro·ep·i·the·li·al
neu·ro·ep·i·the·li·um
pl neu·ro·ep·i·the·lia

neu·ro·fi·bril
neu·ro·fi·bril·la
pl neu·ro·fi·bril·lae

neu·ro·fi·bril·lary
neu·ro·fi·bro·ma
pl neu·ro·fi·bro·mas
also neu·ro·fi·bro·ma·ta

neu·ro·fi·bro·ma·to·sis
pl neu·ro·fi·bro·ma·to·ses

neu·ro·gen
neu·ro·gen·ic
neu·ro·gen·i·cal·ly
neu·rog·e·nous
neu·ro·glia
neu·ro·gli·al
neu·ro·gli·ar
neu·ro·gli·o·ma
pl neu·ro·gli·o·mas
or neu·ro·gli·o·ma·ta

neu·ro·gli·o·sis
pl neu·ro·gli·o·ses

neu·ro·gram
neu·ro·gram·mic
neu·ro·graph·ic
neu·rog·ra·phy
pl neu·rog·ra·phies

neu·ro·hor·mon·al
neu·ro·hor·mone
neu·ro·hu·mor
neu·ro·hu·mor·al
neu·ro·hy·poph·y·se·al
or neu·ro·hy·po·phys·i·al

neu·ro·hy·poph·y·sis
pl neu·ro·hy·poph·y·ses

neu·roid
neu·ro·ker·a·tin
neu·ro·ki·nin
neu·ro·kyme
neu·ro·lem·ma
var of neurilemma

neu·ro·lept·an·al·ge·sia
or neu·ro·lep·to·an·al·ge·sia

neu·ro·lept·an·al·ge·sic
neu·ro·lep·tic
neu·ro·log·i·cal
or neu·ro·log·ic

neu·ro·log·i·cal·ly
neu·rol·o·gist
neu·rol·o·gize
neu·rol·o·gized
neu·rol·o·giz·ing
neu·rol·o·gy
pl neu·rol·o·gies

neu·ro·lym·pho·ma·to·sis
pl neu·ro·lym·pho·ma·to·ses

neu·rol·y·sis
pl neu·rol·y·ses

neu·ro·lyt·ic
neu·ro·ma
pl neu·ro·mas
or neu·ro·ma·ta

neu·ro·mere
neu·rom·er·ism
neu·ro·mo·tor
neu·ro·mus·cu·lar
neu·ro·my·al
neu·ro·my·e·li·tis
pl neu·ro·my·e·lit·i·des

neu·ron
also neu·rone

neu·ro·nal
also neu·ron·ic

neu·ron·ism
neu·ron·i·tis

neu·ro·no·pha·gia
also neu·ro·noph·a·gy
pl neu·ro·no·pha·gias
also neu·ro·noph·a·gies

neu·ro·path

neu·ro·path·ic

neu·ro·path·i·cal·ly

neu·ro·patho·log·ic
or neu·ro·patho·log·i·cal

neu·ro·pa·thol·o·gist

neu·ro·pa·thol·o·gy
pl neu·ro·pa·thol·o·gies

neu·rop·a·thy
pl neu·rop·a·thies

neu·ro·phar·ma·co·log·ic
or neu·ro·phar·ma·co·log·i·cal

neu·ro·phar·ma·col·o·gist

neu·ro·phar·ma·col·o·gy
pl neu·ro·phar·ma·col·o·gies

neu·ro·phile
or neu·ro·phil·ic

neu·ro·phys·i·o·log·i·cal
also neu·ro·phys·i·o·log·ic

neu·ro·phys·i·ol·o·gist

neu·ro·phys·i·ol·o·gy
pl neu·ro·phys·i·ol·o·gies

neu·ro·pil
also neu·ro·pile

neu·ro·pi·lar

neu·ro·plasm

neu·ro·plas·mat·ic
or neu·ro·plas·mic

neu·ro·po·di·um
pl neu·ro·po·dia

neu·ro·pore

neu·ro·psy·chi·at·ric

neu·ro·psy·chi·at·ri·cal·ly

neu·ro·psy·chi·a·trist

neu·ro·psy·chi·a·try
pl neu·ro·psy·chi·a·tries

neu·ro·psy·chic
also neu·ro·psy·chi·cal

neu·ro·psy·cho·log·i·cal

neu·ro·psy·chol·o·gist

neu·ro·psy·chol·o·gy
pl neu·ro·psy·chol·o·gies

neu·ro·ret·i·ni·tis
pl neu·ro·ret·i·nit·i·des

neu·ro·sci·ence

neu·ro·sci·en·tist

neu·ro·se·cre·tion

neu·ro·se·cre·to·ry

neu·ro·sen·so·ry

neu·ro·sis
pl neu·ro·ses

neu·ro·some

neu·ro·spon·gi·um
pl neu·ro·spon·gia

neu·ros·po·ra

neu·ro·sur·geon

neu·ro·sur·gery
pl neu·ro·sur·ger·ies

neu·ro·sur·gi·cal

neu·ro·syph·i·lis

neu·rot·ic

neu·rot·i·cal·ly

neu·rot·i·cism

neu·roto·gen·ic

neu·ro·tome

neu·rot·o·my
pl neu·rot·o·mies

neu·ro·tox·ic

neu·ro·tox·ic·i·ty
pl neu·ro·tox·ic·i·ties

neu·ro·tox·in

neu·ro·trans·mit·ter

neu·ro·troph·ic

neu·ro·trop·ic

neu·rot·ro·pism

neu•ro•tu•bule
neu•ro•vas•cu•lar
neu•ro•veg•e•ta•tive
neu•ru•la
pl neu•ru•las
or neu•ru•lae
neu•ru•lar
neu•ru•la•tion
neu•tral
neu•tral•iza•tion
neu•tral•ize
neu•tral•ized
neu•tral•iz•ing
neu•tri•no
pl neu•tri•nos
neu•tro•clu•sion
neu•tro•cyte
neu•tro•cyt•ic
neu•tron
neu•tro•pe•nia
neu•tro•pe•nic
neu•tro•phil
neu•tro•phile
neu•tro•phil•ia
neu•tro•phil•ic
neu•tro•phil•ine
also neu•tro•phil•in
ne•void
also nae•void
ne•vus
also nae•vus
pl ne•vi
also nae•vi
new•born
New•cas•tle dis•ease
new•ton
New•ton's disk
nex•us
pl nex•uses
or nex•us
n'ga•na
var of nagana
ni•a•cin
ni•a•cin•a•mide
ni•al•amide
nick•el
nic•o•tin•amide
nic•o•tin•amide-ad•e•nine di•nu•cle•o•tide
nic•o•tin•amide-ad•e•nine di•nu•cle•o•tide phos•phate
nic•o•tin•ate
nic•o•tine
nic•o•tin•ic
nic•o•tin•ism
nic•o•tin•ize
nic•o•tin•ized
nic•o•tin•iz•ing
nic•o•tin•uric
nic•tate
nic•tat•ed
nic•tat•ing
nic•ta•tion
nic•ti•tate
nic•ti•tat•ed
nic•ti•tat•ing
nic•ti•ta•tion
ni•dal
ni•da•tion
ni•dus
pl ni•di
or ni•dus•es
Niel•sen meth•od
Nie•mann-Pick Dis•ease
night-blind
night blind•ness
night•mare
night•shade
nig•ra
ni•gro•sine
also ni•gro•sin
ni•hi•lism
nik•eth•amide
nin•hy•drin
ni•o•bi•um
nip•per
nip•ple
ni•sin
Nissl bod•ies
or Nissl gran•ules
Nissl sub•stance
ni•sus
pl ni•sus
ni•ter
also ni•tre
ni•trate
ni•tric
ni•trid•a•tion
ni•tride
ni•tri•fi•ca•tion
ni•tri•fy
ni•tri•fied
ni•tri•fy•ing
ni•trile
ni•trite

ni·tri·toid
ni·tro·ben·zene
ni·tro·cel·lu·lose
ni·tro·cel·lu·los·ic
ni·tro·fu·ran
ni·tro·fu·ran·to·in
ni·tro·fu·ra·zone
ni·tro·gen
ni·tro·ge·nase
ni·tro·gen·iza·tion
ni·tro·ge·nize
ni·tro·ge·nized
ni·tro·ge·niz·ing
ni·tro·gen nar·co·sis
ni·trog·e·nous
ni·tro·glyc·er·in
or ni·tro·glyc·er·ine
ni·tro·mer·sol
ni·trom·e·ter
ni·tro·met·ric
ni·tro·prus·side
ni·tro·sa·mine
also ni·tro·so·amine
ni·tro·syl
ni·trous
ni·trox·yl
ni·tryl
no·bel·i·um
no·car·dia
no·car·di·o·sis
pl no·car·di·o·ses
no·ci·cep·tive
no·ci·cep·tor
no·ci·fen·sor
no·ci·per·cep·tion
no·ci·per·cep·tive
noct·am·bu·la·tion
noct·am·bule
noct·am·bu·lic
also noct·am·bu·lis·tic
noct·am·bu·lism
noct·am·bu·list
noc·tu·ria
noc·tur·nal
noc·tur·nal·ly
noc·u·ous
noc·u·ous·ly
nod·al
nod·al·ly
node of Ran·vier
no·dose
also no·dous
no·dos·i·ty
pl no·dos·i·ties
nod·u·lar
nod·u·late
nod·u·lat·ed
nod·u·lat·ing
nod·u·la·tion
nod·ule
nod·u·lose
also nod·u·lous
nod·u·lus
pl nod·u·li
no·dus
pl no·di
no·e·ma·tach·o·graph
no·e·ma·ta·chom·e·ter
no·e·mat·ic
no·e·sis
no·et·ic
no·ma
no·mad·ic
no·men·cla·ture
nom·o·gram
nom·o·graph
nom·o·thet·ic
non·ac·cess
non·ad·di·tive
non·ad·di·tiv·i·ty
pl non·ad·di·tiv·i·ties
non·al·le·lic
non·aque·ous
non·chro·mo·som·al
non com·pos men·tis
non·con·duc·tor
non·con·trac·tile
non·con·trib·u·to·ry
non·cross·over
Non·de·cid·u·a·ta
non·di·a·bet·ic
non·di·rec·tive
non·dis·junc·tion
non·dis·junc·tion·al
non·di·vid·ing
non·elec·tro·lyte
non·en·zy·mat·ic
or non·en·zy·mic
also non·en·zyme
non·en·zy·mat·i·cal·ly

non·fat
non·func·tion·al
non·hi·ber·nat·ing
non·his·tone
non·iden·ti·cal
non·in·fect·ed
non·in·fec·tious
non·in·flam·ma·to·ry
non·in·sec·ti·cid·al
non·ma·lig·nant
non·med·u·lat·ed
non·mo·tile
non·mus·cu·lar
non·neo·plas·tic
non·nu·cle·at·ed
non·opaque
non·par·a·sit·ic
non·par·a·sit·i·cal·ly
non·patho·gen·ic
non·per·sis·tent
non·pig·ment·ed
non·preg·nant
non·pre·scrip·tion
non·pro·pri·etary
non·pro·tein
non·pro·tein·aceous
non·re·com·bi·nant
non·re·pro·duc·tive
non·re·straint
non·se·cre·tor
non·sed·i·ment·able
non·sex·u·al
non·spe·cif·ic
non·ste·roid
non·ste·roi·dal
non·sur·gi·cal
non·tar·get
non·tox·ic
non·union
non·vec·tor
non·vi·a·ble
no·olog·i·cal
no·ol·o·gy
pl no·ol·o·gies
nor·adren·a·line
also nor·adren·a·lin
nor·ephed·rine
nor·epi·neph·rine
nor·eth·in·drone
nor·ethyn·o·drel
nor·leu·cine
nor·ma
pl nor·mae
nor·mal·cy
pl nor·mal·cies
nor·mal·i·ty
pl nor·mal·i·ties
nor·mal·iza·tion
nor·mal·ize
nor·mal·ized
nor·mal·iz·ing
nor·mal·iz·er
nor·mer·gy
pl nor·mer·gies
nor·mo·blast
nor·mo·blas·tic
nor·mo·chro·mia
nor·mo·chro·mic
nor·mo·cyte
nor·mo·cyt·ic
nor·mo·ten·sion
nor·mo·ten·sive
nor·mo·ther·mia
nor·mo·ther·mic
nor·trip·ty·line
nor·va·line
nose·bleed
No·se·ma
nose·piece
nos·o·co·mi·al
noso·geo·graph·ic
or noso·geo·graph·i·cal
noso·ge·og·ra·phy
pl noso·ge·og·ra·phies
nos·o·graph·ic
no·sog·ra·phy
pl no·sog·ra·phies
no·so·log·i·cal
or no·so·log·ic
no·so·log·i·cal·ly
no·sol·o·gist
no·sol·o·gy
no·sol·o·gies
Nos·o·psyl·lus
nos·tal·gia
nos·tal·gic
nos·tal·gi·cal·ly
nos·tril
nos·trum
no·tal

no·ti·fi·able
no·to·chord
no·to·chord·al
No·to·ed·res
no·to·ed·ric
no·vo·bi·o·cin
no·vo·caine
noxa
pl nox·ae

nox·ious
nox·ious·ness
nu·bile
nu·bil·i·ty
pl nu·bil·i·ties

nu·cha
pl nu·chae

nu·chal
nu·cle·ar
nu·cle·ase
nu·cle·at·ed
or nu·cle·ate

nu·cle·ation
nu·cle·ic
nu·cle·in
nu·cleo·cap·sid
nu·cleo·cy·to·plas·mic
nu·cleo·his·tone
nu·cle·oid
nu·cle·o·lar
nu·cle·o·lo·ne·ma
nu·cle·o·lus
pl nu·cle·o·li

nu·cle·on
nu·cle·on·ic
nu·cle·on·ics
nu·cleo·phil·ic
nu·cleo·phil·i·cal·ly
nu·cleo·plasm
nu·cleo·plas·mat·ic
or nu·cleo·plas·mic

nu·cleo·pro·tein
nu·cle·o·sid·ase
nu·cle·o·side
nu·cle·o·tid·ase
nu·cle·o·tide
nu·cleo·tox·ic
nu·cle·us
pl nu·clei
also nu·cle·us·es

nu·cle·us dor·sa·lis
pl nu·clei dor·sa·les

nu·cle·us of Pan·der
nu·cle·us pul·po·sus
pl nu·clei pul·po·si

nu·clide
nu·clid·ic
nul·li·grav·i·da
pl nul·li·grav·i·das
or nul·li·grav·i·dae

nul·lip·a·ra
pl nul·lip·a·ras
also nul·lip·a·rae

nul·lip·a·rous
nul·li·some
nul·li·so·mic
num·mi·form
num·mu·lar
nun·na·tion
nurs·ery
pl nurs·er·ies

nurse's aide
nurs·ling
also nurse·ling

nu·ta·tion
nu·ta·tion·al
nut·gall
nu·tri·ent
nu·tri·ment
nu·tri·tion
nu·tri·tion·al
nu·tri·tion·al·ly
nu·tri·tion·ist
nu·tri·tious
nu·tri·tious·ly
nu·tri·tive
nu·tri·tive·ly
nu·tri·to·ry
nu·tri·ture
Nut·tal·lia
nut·tal·li·a·sis
or nut·tal·li·o·sis
pl nut·tal·li·a·ses
or nut·tal·li·o·ses

nux vom·i·ca
pl nux vom·i·ca

nyc·ta·lope
nyc·ta·lo·pia
nyc·ta·lop·ic
nyc·tu·ria
ny·lon
nym·pha
pl nym·phae

nym·pho·lep·sy
pl nym·pho·lep·sies

nym·pho·lept

nym·pho·lep·tic
nym·pho·ma·nia
nym·pho·ma·ni·ac
nym·pho·ma·ni·a·cal
nys·tag·mic
nys·tag·moid
nys·tag·mus
ny·stat·in
nyx·is
pl nyx·es

O

ob·ce·ca·tion
ob·dor·mi·tion
ob·duc·tion
obe·li·al
also obe·li·ac
obe·li·on
pl obe·lia
obe·si·ty
pl obe·si·ties
obex
ob·fus·cate
ob·fus·cat·ed
ob·fus·cat·ing
ob·fus·ca·tion
ob·fus·ca·to·ry
ob·ject
ob·jec·tive
ob·jec·tive·ly
ob·li·gate
oblig·a·to·ri·ly
oblig·a·to·ry
oblique
obliq·ui·ty
pl obliq·ui·ties
oblit·er·ate
oblit·er·at·ed
oblit·er·at·ing
oblit·er·a·tion
oblit·er·a·tive
ob·li·ves·cence
ob·lon·ga·ta
pl ob·lon·ga·tas
or ob·lon·ga·tae
ob·lon·gat·al
ob·mu·tes·cence
ob·nu·bi·la·tion
ob·ses·sion
ob·ses·sion·al
ob·ses·sive
ob·ses·sive·ly
ob·ses·sive·ness
ob·stet·ric
or ob·stet·ri·cal
ob·stet·ri·cal·ly
ob·ste·tri·cian
ob·stet·rics
ob·sti·na·cy
pl ob·sti·na·cies
ob·sti·pate
ob·sti·pat·ed
ob·sti·pat·ing
ob·sti·pa·tion
ob·struc·tion
ob·struc·tive
ob·struc·tive·ness
ob·stru·ent
ob·tund
ob·tun·dent
ob·tu·rate
ob·tu·rat·ed
ob·tu·rat·ing
ob·tu·ra·tion
ob·tu·ra·tor
ob·tu·sion
oc·cip·i·tal
oc·cip·i·ta·lis
oc·cip·i·tal·ly
oc·cip·i·to·fron·tal
oc·cip·i·to·fron·ta·lis
oc·cip·i·to·mas·toid
oc·cip·i·to·pa·ri·etal
oc·ci·put
pl oc·ci·puts
or oc·cip·i·ta
oc·clude
oc·clud·ed
oc·clud·ing
oc·clu·sal
oc·clu·sion
oc·clu·sive
oc·clu·som·e·ter
oc·cult
oc·cu·pa·tion
oc·cu·pa·tion·al
oc·cu·pa·tion·al·ly
ocel·lar
ocel·lus
pl ocel·li
och·lo·pho·bia
och·ra·tox·in

ochro·no·sis
pl ochro·no·ses

ochro·not·ic
oc·tad
oc·ta·deca·di·e·no·ic
oc·ta·dec·a·no·ic
oc·ta·dec·e·no·ic
oc·ta·meth·yl·py·ro·phos·phor·amide
oc·ta·no·ic
oc·ta·pep·tide
oc·ta·va·lent
oc·to·ge·nar·i·an
oc·to·roon
oc·tose
oc·u·lar
oc·u·list
oc·u·lo·gy·ric
also oc·u·lo·gy·ral

oc·u·lo·mo·tor
oc·u·lo·my·co·sis
pl oc·u·lo·my·co·ses

oc·u·lus
pl oc·u·li

OD
OD'd
OD'ing
OD's
odax·es·mus
Od·di's sphinc·ter
odon·tal·gia
odon·tal·gic
odon·tec·to·my
pl odon·tec·to·mies

odon·ti·a·sis
pl odon·ti·a·ses

odon·ti·tis
pl odon·tit·i·des

odon·to·blast
odon·to·blas·tic
odon·to·cele
odon·to·clast
odon·to·gen·ic
odon·to·graph
odon·tog·ra·phy
pl odon·tog·ra·phies

odon·toid
odont·o·log·i·cal
odon·tol·o·gist
odon·tol·o·gy
pl odon·tol·o·gies

odon·to·lox·ia
odon·to·ma
pl odon·to·mas
also odon·to·ma·ta

odon·to·pri·sis
odon·to·sis
pl odon·to·ses

odon·tot·o·my
pl odon·tot·o·mies

odor·ant
odor·if·er·ous
odor·if·er·ous·ly
odor·if·er·ous·ness
odor·im·e·ter
odor·im·e·try
pl odor·im·e·tries

odor·i·phore
oe·coid
var of ecoid

oe·de·ma
var of edema

oe·di·pal
Oed·i·pe·an
Oe·di·pus
pl Oe·di·pus·es

oe·nol·o·gy
var of enology

oe·soph·a·ge·al
var of esophageal

Oe·soph·a·gos·to·mum
oe·soph·a·gus
var of esophagus

oes·tra·di·ol
var of estradiol

oes·tral
var of estral

oes·trid
oes·trin
var of estrin

oes·tri·ol
var of estriol

oes·tro·gen
var of estrogen

oes·tro·gen·ic
var of estrogenic

oes·trone
var of estrone

oes·trous
var of estrous

oes·tru·al
var of estrual

Oes·trus
oes·trus, oes·trum
vars of estrus

of•fal
of•fi•cial
of•fi•ci•nal
of•fi•ci•nal•ly
ohm-am•me•ter
ohm•me•ter
oid•io•my•co•sis
pl oid•io•my•co•ses
oid•i•um
pl oid•ia
oint•ment
ole•ag•i•nous
ole•an•der
ole•an•do•my•cin
ole•ate
olec•ra•nal
olec•ran•ar•thri•tis
olec•ra•non
ole•fin
also ole•fine
ole•fin•ic
ole•ic
ole•in
oleo•mar•ga•rine
also oleo•mar•ga•rin
ole•om•e•ter
oleo•res•in
oleo•sac•cha•rum
pl oleo•sac•cha•ra
oleo•tho•rax
pl oleo•tho•rax•es
or oleo•tho•ra•ces
oleo•vi•ta•min
ole•um
pl olea
ole•yl
ol•fac•tion
ol•fac•tol•o•gy
pl ol•fac•tol•o•gies
ol•fac•tom•e•ter
ol•fac•to•met•ric
ol•fac•to•met•ri•cal•ly
ol•fac•tom•e•try
pl ol•fac•tom•e•tries
ol•fac•to•ry
ol•fac•tron•ics
olib•a•num
ol•i•ge•mia
ol•i•ge•mic
ol•i•gid•ic
ol•i•go•chro•me•mia
ol•i•go•cy•the•mia
ol•i•go•cy•the•mic
ol•i•go•dac•tyl•ia
ol•i•go•dac•tyl•ism
also ol•i•go•dac•tyly
pl ol•i•go•dac•tyl•isms
also ol•i•go•dac•tyl•ies
ol•i•go•den•dro•cyte
ol•i•go•den•drog•lia
ol•i•go•den•dro•gli•o•ma
pl ol•i•go•den•dro•gli•o•mas
or ol•i•go•den•dro•gli•o•ma•ta
ol•i•go•don•tia
ol•i•go•dy•nam•ic
ol•i•go•gen•ic
ol•i•go•hy•dram•ni•os
ol•i•go•lec•i•thal
ol•i•go•men•or•rhea
oligo•mer
oligo•mer•ic
oligo•mer•iza•tion
oli•go•my•cin
ol•i•go•nu•cle•o•tide
ol•i•go•phre•nia
ol•i•go•phren•ic
ol•i•go•py•rene
oli•go•sac•cha•ride
ol•i•go•sper•mat•ic
ol•i•go•sper•mia
ol•i•go•trich•ia
ol•i•go•zoo•sper•mia
ol•i•gu•ria
ol•i•vary
ol•ive
olo•li•u•qui
oma•si•tis
oma•sum
pl oma•sa
omen•tal
omen•tec•to•my
pl omen•tec•to•mies
omen•to•pexy
pl omen•to•pex•ies
omen•tu•lum
pl omen•tu•la

omen·tum
pl omen·ta
or omen·tums

om·ma·tid·i·um
pl om·ma·tid·ia

om·ni·fo·cal
om·odyn·ia
omo·hy·oid
omo·hy·oi·de·us
pl omo·hy·oi·dei

om·phal·ic
om·pha·li·tis
pl om·pha·lit·i·des

om·pha·lo·mes·en·ter·ic
om·pha·lo·phle·bi·tis
pl om·pha·lo·phle·bit·i·des

om·pha·los
pl om·pha·li

onan·ism
onan·ist
onan·is·tic
On·cho·cer·ca
on·cho·cer·cal
on·cho·cer·ci·a·sis
pl on·cho·cer·ci·a·ses

on·cho·cer·co·ma
on·cho·cer·co·sis
pl on·cho·cer·co·ses

on·cho·sphere
also on·co·sphere

on·co·cyte
on·co·cy·to·ma
on·co·gen·e·sis
pl on·co·gen·e·ses

on·co·gen·ic
also on·cog·e·nous

on·co·ge·nic·i·ty
pl on·co·ge·nic·i·ties

on·cog·e·ny
pl on·cog·e·nies

on·co·graph
on·cog·ra·phy
pl on·cog·ra·phies

on·co·log·i·cal
also on·co·log·ic

on·col·o·gist
on·col·o·gy
pl on·col·o·gies

on·col·y·sis
pl on·col·y·ses

on·co·lyt·ic
On·co·me·la·nia
on·com·e·ter
on·cot·o·my
pl on·cot·o·mies

onei·ric
onio·ma·nia
onio·ma·ni·ac
oni·um
on·o·ma·tol·o·gy
pl on·o·ma·tol·o·gies

on·o·mato·ma·nia
on·o·mato·poi·e·sis
pl on·o·mato·poi·e·ses

on·to·gen·e·sis
pl on·to·gen·e·ses

on·to·ge·net·ic
on·to·ge·net·i·cal·ly
on·to·gen·ic
on·to·gen·i·cal·ly
on·tog·e·ny
pl on·tog·e·nies

on·ych·aux·is
pl on·ych·aux·es

onych·ia
on·y·chi·tis
pl on·y·chit·i·des

on·y·cho·gry·po·sis
pl on·y·cho·gry·po·ses

on·y·choid
on·y·chol·y·sis
pl on·y·chol·y·ses

on·y·cho·ma·de·sis
on·y·cho·ma·la·cia
on·y·cho·my·co·sis
pl on·y·cho·my·co·ses

on·y·cho·pha·gia
on·y·choph·a·gy
pl on·y·choph·a·gies

on·y·chor·rhex·is
pl on·y·chor·rhex·es

on·y·cho·schiz·ia
on·y·cho·sis
pl on·y·cho·ses

on·yx
onyx·is
oo·blast

oo•cy•e•sis
pl oo•cy•e•ses

oo•cyst
oo•cyte
oo•gen•e•sis
pl oo•gen•e•ses

oo•ge•net•ic
oo•go•ni•al
oo•go•ni•um
oo•ki•ne•sis
pl oo•ki•ne•ses

oo•ki•nete
oo•ki•net•ic
oo•lem•ma
oo•pho•rec•to•mize
oo•pho•rec•to•mized
oo•pho•rec•to•miz•ing
oo•pho•rec•to•my
pl oo•pho•rec•to•mies

oo•pho•ri•tis
oo•phoro•cys•tec•to•my
pl oo•phoro•cys•tec•to•mies

ooph•o•ron
oo•plasm
oo•plas•mic
oo•por•phy•rin
oo•sperm
Oos•po•ra
oo•spore
oo•the•ca
pl oo•the•cae

oo•the•cal
oo•tid
oo•type
opaci•fi•ca•tion
opaci•fy
opaci•fied
opaci•fy•ing
opac•i•ty
pl opac•i•ties

opal•es•cent
opei•do•scope
open-heart
op•er•a•bil•i•ty
pl op•er•a•bil•i•ties

op•er•a•ble
op•er•a•bly
op•er•ant
op•er•ate
op•er•at•ed
op•er•at•ing
op•er•a•tion
op•er•a•tive
op•er•a•tive•ly
op•er•a•tor
oper•cu•lar
oper•cu•late
also oper•cu•lat•ed

oper•cu•lum
pl oper•cu•la
also oper•cu•lums

op•er•on
ophi•a•sis
Ophid•ia
ophry•on
Oph•ryo•sco•lec•i•dae
oph•thal•mec•to•my
pl oph•thal•mec•to•mies

oph•thalm•en•ceph•a•lon
pl oph•thalm•en•ceph•a•la

oph•thal•mia
oph•thal•mia neo•na•to•rum
oph•thal•mic
oph•thal•mo•cen•te•sis
oph•thal•mo•di•a•stim•e•ter
oph•thal•mo•dy•na•mom•e•ter
oph•thal•mo•dyn•ia
oph•thal•mo•graph
oph•thal•mo•leu•ko•scope
also oph•thal•mo•leu•co•scope

oph•thal•mo•log•ic
also oph•thal•mo•log•i•cal

oph•thal•mol•o•gist
oph•thal•mol•o•gy
pl oph•thal•mol•o•gies

oph•thal•mo•ma•la•cia

oph·thal·mom·e·ter
oph·thal·mom·e·try
pl oph·thal·mom·e·tries
oph·thal·mo·my·co·sis
pl oph·thal·mo·my·co·ses
oph·thal·mop·a·thy
pl oph·thal·mop·a·thies
oph·thal·mo·ple·gia
oph·thal·mo·ple·gic
oph·thal·mo·re·ac·tion
oph·thal·mor·rhex·is
oph·thal·mo·scope
oph·thal·mo·scop·ic
or oph·thal·mo·scop·i·cal
oph·thal·mo·scop·i·cal·ly
oph·thal·mos·co·py
pl oph·thal·mos·co·pies
oph·thal·mos·ta·sis
pl oph·thal·mos·ta·ses
oph·thal·mo·trope
oph·thal·mo·tro·pom·e·ter
opi·ate
opis·the·nar
opis·thi·on
pl opis·thia
or opis·thi·ons
opis·tho·cra·ni·on
op·is·thog·na·thism
opis·thor·chi·a·sis
Op·is·thor·chis
op·is·thot·ic
opis·tho·ton·ic
op·is·thot·o·nos
opi·um
op·o·bal·sam
or op·o·bal·sa·mum
op·po·nens
pl op·po·nen·tes
op·por·tun·is·tic
or op·por·tun·ist
op·sin
op·son·ic
op·so·nin
op·so·nize
op·so·nized
op·so·niz·ing
op·so·no·cy·to·phag·ic
op·tic
op·ti·cal
op·ti·cian
op·ti·coel
op·ti·co·pu·pil·lary
op·tics
op·tim·e·ter
op·to·gram
op·to·ki·net·ic
op·tom·e·ter
op·to·met·ric
also op·to·met·ri·cal
op·tom·e·trist
op·tom·e·try
pl op·tom·e·tries
op·to·type
ora
pl of os
orad
oral
of the mouth (*see* aural)
ora·le
oral·i·ty
pl oral·i·ties
oral·ly
oral·o·gy
pl oral·o·gies
ora ser·ra·ta
pl orae ser·ra·tae
or·bic·u·lar
or·bi·cu·lar·is
pl or·bi·cu·la·res
or·bic·u·lar·i·ty
pl or·bic·u·lar·i·ties
or·bic·u·lar·ly
or·bit
or·bit·al
or·bi·to·sphe·noid
also or·bi·to·sphe·noi·dal
or·ce·in
or·chi·dec·to·my
pl or·chi·dec·to·mies

or·chi·do·pexy
or or·chi·o·pexy
pl or·chi·do·pex·ies
or or·chi·o·pex·ies

or·chi·ec·to·my
also or·chec·to·my
pl or·chi·ec·to·mies
also or·chec·to·mies

or·chil
var of archil

or·chio·plas·ty
pl or·chio·plas·ties

or·chit·ic
or·chi·tis
or·cin
or·cin·ol
or·der
or·der·ly
pl or·der·lies

or·di·nate
orec·tic
orex·ia
orex·is
or·gan
or·gan·elle
also or·gan·el·la

or·gan·ic
or·gan·i·cal·ly
or·gan·i·cism
or·gan·i·cist
or·gan·i·cis·tic
or·gan·ism
or·ga·niz·er
or·gan of Cor·ti
or·gan of Ja·cob·son
or·gano·gel
or·gan·o·gen·e·sis
pl or·gan·o·gen·e·ses

or·gan·o·ge·net·ic
or·gan·o·ge·net·i·cal·ly
or·gan·o·gen·ic
or·ga·nog·e·ny
pl or·ga·nog·e·nies

or·gano·graph·ic
or·gan·og·ra·phy
pl or·gan·og·ra·phies

or·gan·oid
or·gan·o·lep·tic
or·gan·o·lep·ti·cal·ly
or·gan·o·log·ic
or or·gan·o·log·i·cal

or·gan·ol·o·gy
pl or·gan·ol·o·gies

or·gano·mer·cu·ri·al
or·gano·me·tal·lic
or·ga·non
or·gano·phos·phate
or·gano·phos·pho·rus
or·ga·nos·co·py
pl or·ga·nos·co·pies

or·gano·sol
or·gan·o·ther·a·peu·tic
or·gan·o·ther·a·py
pl or·gan·o·ther·a·pies

or·gan·o·tro·phic
or·gan·o·trop·ic
or·gan·o·trop·i·cal·ly
or·gan·ot·ro·pism
or·ga·not·ro·py
pl or·ga·not·ro·pies

or·ga·num
or·gasm
or·gas·mic
or or·gas·tic

or·i·fice
or·i·fi·cial
orig·a·num
or·i·gin
or·ni·thine
Or·ni·thod·o·ros
or·ni·tho·sis
pl or·ni·tho·ses

or·nith·uric
oro·pha·ryn·geal
oro·phar·ynx
pl oro·pha·ryn·ges
also oro·phar·ynx·es

orot·ic
Oroya fe·ver
or·tho·ce·phal·ic
or or·tho·ceph·a·lous

or·tho·ceph·a·ly
pl or·tho·ceph·a·lies

or·tho·chro·mat·ic
or·tho·cre·sol
or·tho·di·a·gram
orth·odon·tia
orth·odon·tic
orth·odon·tics

orth·odon·tist
or·tho·drom·ic
or·tho·gen·e·sis
pl or·tho·gen·e·ses
or·tho·ge·net·ic
or·tho·ge·net·i·cal·ly
or·tho·gen·ic
or·tho·grade
or·thom·e·ter
or·tho·mo·lec·u·lar
or·tho·pe·dic
also or·tho·pae·dic
or·tho·pe·dics
also or·tho·pae·dics
or·tho·pe·dist
also or·tho·pae·dist
or·tho·pho·ria
or·tho·phos·phate
or·thop·nea
also or·thop·noea
or·thop·ne·ic
also or·thop·noe·ic
or·tho·praxy
pl or·tho·prax·ies
or·tho·psy·chi·at·ric
also or·tho·psy·chi·at·ri·cal
or·tho·psy·chi·a·trist
or·tho·psy·chi·a·try
pl or·tho·psy·chi·a·tries
or·thop·tic
or·thop·tics
or·thop·tist
or·tho·scope
or·tho·scop·ic
or·tho·sis
pl or·tho·ses
or·tho·stat·ic
or·tho·ste·reo·scope
or·tho·ste·reo·scop·ic
or·thot·ic
or·thot·ics
or·tho·tist
or·thot·o·nus
or·tho·top·ic
os
pl os·sa
bone
os
pl ora
mouth
osa·zone
os cal·cis
pl os·sa cal·cis
os·cil·la·tion
os·cil·la·tor
os·cil·la·to·ry
os·cil·lo·gram
os·cil·lo·graph
os·cil·lo·graph·ic
os·cil·lo·graph·i·cal·ly
os·cil·log·ra·phy
pl os·cil·log·ra·phies
os·cil·lom·e·ter
os·cil·lo·met·ric
os·cil·lom·e·try
pl os·cil·lom·e·tries
os·cil·lo·scope
os·cil·lo·scop·ic
os·cil·lo·scop·i·cal·ly
os·cine
Os·cin·i·dae
os·ci·ta·tion
os cox·ae
pl os·sa cox·ae
os·cu·la·tion
os·cu·lum
pl os·cu·la
os·mate
os·mat·ic
or os·mic
os·me·sis
os·mic
os·mics
os·mi·dro·sis
pl os·mi·dro·ses
os·mio·phil
or os·mio·phil·ic
os·mi·um
os·mol
os·mol·al
os·mo·lal·i·ty
pl os·mo·lal·i·ties
os·mo·lar
os·mo·lar·i·ty
pl os·mo·lar·i·ties
os·mom·e·ter
os·mo·met·ric
os·mom·e·try
pl os·mom·e·tries
os·mo·phore

os·mo·phor·ic
os·mo·re·cep·tor
os·mo·reg·u·la·tion
os·mo·reg·u·la·tor
os·mo·reg·u·la·to·ry
os·mose
 os·mosed
 os·mos·ing
os·mo·sis
 pl os·mo·ses
os·mot·ic
os·mot·i·cal·ly
os·phre·sis
os·phret·ic
os·sa
 pl of os
os·se·in
os·se·let
os·seo·car·ti·lag·i·nous
os·se·ous
os·se·ous·ly
os·si·cle
os·sic·u·lar
os·si·cu·lec·to·my
 pl os·si·cu·lec·to·mies
os·si·cu·lot·o·my
 pl os·si·cu·lot·o·mies
os·sic·u·lum
 pl os·sic·u·la
os·sif·ic
os·si·fi·ca·tion
os·sif·i·ca·to·ry
os·si·fy
 os·si·fied
 os·si·fy·ing
os·tal·gia
os·te·al
os·tec·to·my
 pl os·tec·to·mies
os·te·in
os·te·it·ic
os·te·i·tis
 pl os·te·it·i·des
os·te·i·tis de·for·mans
os·te·i·tis fi·bro·sa
os·teo·ar·thrit·ic
os·teo·ar·thri·tis
 pl os·teo·ar·thrit·i·des
os·teo·ar·throp·a·thy
 pl os·teo·ar·throp·a·thies
os·teo·ar·throt·o·my
 pl os·teo·ar·throt·o·mies
os·teo·blast
os·teo·blas·tic
os·teo·car·ti·lag·i·nous
os·teo·chon·dri·tis
os·teo·chon·dro·ma
 pl os·teo·chon·dro·mas
 also os·teo·chon·dro·ma·ta
os·teo·chon·dro·ma·to·sis
os·teo·chon·drop·a·thy
 pl os·teo·chon·drop·a·thies
os·teo·chon·dro·sar·co·ma
 pl os·teo·chon·dro·sar·co·mas
 or os·teo·chon·dro·sar·co·ma·ta
os·teo·chon·dro·sis
 pl os·teo·chon·dro·ses
os·teo·chon·drot·ic
os·teo·chon·drous
 also os·teo·chon·dral
os·te·oc·la·sis
os·teo·clast
os·teo·clas·tic
os·teo·com·ma
os·teo·cra·ni·um
 pl os·teo·cra·ni·ums
 or os·teo·cra·nia
os·teo·cyte
os·teo·den·tin
 or os·teo·den·tine
os·teo·der·ma·tous
 also os·teo·der·mous
os·teo·dyn·ia
os·teo·dys·tro·phia
os·teo·dys·tro·phic

os·teo·dys·tro·phy
pl os·teo·dys·tro·phies

os·teo·fi·bro·ma
pl os·teo·fi·bro·mas
also os·teo·fi·bro·ma·ta

os·teo·fi·bro·sis
pl os·teo·fi·bro·ses

os·teo·fi·brous

os·teo·gen·e·sis
pl os·teo·gen·e·ses

os·teo·gen·e·sis im·per·fec·ta

os·teo·gen·ic
also os·teo·ge·net·ic

os·te·og·e·nous

os·te·og·ra·phy
pl os·te·og·ra·phies

os·te·oid

os·teo·log·ic
or os·teo·log·i·cal

os·teo·log·i·cal·ly

os·te·ol·o·gist

os·te·ol·o·gy
pl os·te·ol·o·gies

os·te·ol·y·sis
pl os·te·ol·y·ses

os·teo·lyt·ic

os·te·o·ma
pl os·te·o·mas
or os·te·o·ma·ta

os·teo·ma·la·cia

os·te·o·ma·toid

os·te·o·ma·tous

os·teo·met·ric
or os·teo·met·ri·cal

os·te·om·e·try
pl os·te·om·e·tries

os·teo·my·elit·ic

os·teo·my·eli·tis
pl os·teo·my·elit·i·des

os·te·on

os·teo·ne·cro·sis
pl os·teo·ne·cro·ses

os·teo·path

os·teo·path·ic

os·teo·path·i·cal·ly

os·te·op·a·thist

os·te·op·a·thy
pl os·te·op·a·thies

os·teo·peri·os·ti·tis

os·teo·pe·tro·sis
pl os·teo·pe·tro·ses

os·teo·pe·trot·ic

os·teo·phage

os·teo·pha·gia

os·teo·phyte

os·teo·phyt·ic

os·teo·plast

os·teo·plas·tic

os·teo·plas·ty
pl os·teo·plas·ties

os·teo·po·ro·sis
pl os·teo·po·ro·ses

os·teo·po·rot·ic

os·te·op·sath·y·ro·sis
pl os·te·op·sath·y·ro·ses

os·teo·ra·dio·ne·cro·sis
pl os·teo·ra·dio·ne·cro·ses

os·teo·sar·co·ma
pl os·teo·sar·co·mas
or os·teo·sar·co·ma·ta

os·teo·scle·ro·sis
pl os·teo·scle·ro·ses

os·teo·scle·rot·ic

os·teo·syn·the·sis
pl os·teo·syn·the·ses

os·teo·tome

os·te·ot·o·my
pl os·te·ot·o·mies

os·teo·tribe

Os·ter·ta·gia

os·ti·al

os·ti·um
pl os·tia

os·to·my
pl os·to·mies

ot·ac·a·ri·a·sis
pl ot·ac·a·ri·a·ses

ot·acous·tic

otal·gia

otal·gic

ot·he·ma·to·ma

otic

otit·ic

oti·tis
pl otit·i·des

oti·tis ex·ter·na

oti·tis me·dia

Oto·bi·us

oto·ce·phal·ic

oto·ceph·a·ly
pl oto·ceph·a·lies

oto·co·ni·um
pl oto·co·nia

oto·cyst
oto·cys·tic
Oto·dec·tes
oto·dec·tic
otog·e·nous
or oto·gen·ic

oto·lar·yn·go·log·i·cal
oto·lar·yn·gol·o·gist
oto·lar·yn·gol·o·gy
pl oto·lar·yn·gol·o·gies

oto·lith
olo·lith·ic
oto·log·ic
also oto·log·i·cal

oto·log·i·cal·ly
otol·o·gist
otol·o·gy
pl otol·o·gies

oto·my·co·sis
pl oto·my·co·ses

oto·my·cot·ic
oto·plas·ty
pl oto·plas·ties

oto·rhi·no·lar·yn·gol·o·gy
pl oto·rhi·no·lar·yn·gol·o·gies

otor·rhea
also otor·rhoea

oto·sal·pinx
pl oto·sal·pin·ges

oto·scle·ro·sis
pl oto·scle·ro·ses

oto·scle·rot·ic
oto·scope
oto·scop·ic
otos·co·py
pl otos·co·pies

oto·sis
pl oto·ses

ot·os·te·al
otos·te·on
otot·o·my
pl otot·o·mies

oto·tox·ic
oto·tox·ic·i·ty
pl oto·tox·ic·i·ties

oua·bain
out·pa·tient
out·pock·et·ing
ova
pl of ovum

ov·al·bu·min
ovalo·cyte
ovalo·cyt·ic
ovalo·cy·to·sis
pl ovalo·cy·to·ses

ovar·i·al
ovar·i·an
ovari·ec·to·mize
ovari·ec·to·miz·ed
ovari·ec·to·miz·ing
ovari·ec·to·my
pl ovari·ec·to·mies

ovar·io·hys·ter·ec·to·my
pl ovar·io·hys·ter·ec·to·mies

ovar·io·tes·tis
pl ovar·io·tes·tes

ovar·i·ot·o·my
pl ovar·i·ot·o·mies

ova·ri·tis
pl ova·rit·i·des

ova·ry
pl ova·ries

over·achieve
over·achieved
over·achiev·ing
over·achiev·er
over·bite
over·com·pen·sate
over·com·pen·sat·ed
over·com·pen·sat·ing
over·com·pen·sa·tion
over·cor·rec·tion
over·dos·age
over·dose
over·ex·ten·sion
over·growth
over·hang
over·hung
over·hang·ing
over·jet
over·nu·tri·tion
over·ven·ti·la·tion
over·weight

ovi·cid·al
ovi·du·cal
ovi·duct
ovi·duc·tal
ovi·form
ovi·gen·e·sis
pl ovi·gen·e·ses
ovi·ge·net·ic
ovig·er·ous
ovi·na·tion
ovip·a·rous
ovip·a·rous·ly
ovip·a·rous·ness
ovi·pos·it
ovi·po·si·tion
ovi·po·si·tion·al
ovi·pos·i·tor
ovi·sac
ovo·cyte
ovo·fla·vin
ovo·gen·e·sis
pl ovo·gen·e·ses
ovo·mu·cin
ovo·mu·coid
ovo·plasm
ovo·plas·mic
ovo·tes·tic·u·lar
ovo·tes·tis
pl ovo·tes·tes
ovo·vi·tel·lin
ovo·vi·vi·par·i·ty
pl ovo·vi·vi·par·i·ties
ovo·vi·vip·a·rous
ovo·vi·vip·a·rous·ly
ovo·vi·vip·a·rous·ness
ovu·lar
ovu·late
ovu·lat·ed
ovu·lat·ing
ovula·tion
ovu·la·to·ry
ovum
pl ova
ox·a·cil·lin
ox·a·late
ox·al·ic
ox·a·lo·suc·cin·ic
ox·al·uria
ox·al·uric
ox·a·lyl
ox·a·lyl·urea
ox·am·ide
ox·az·e·pam
ox·gall
ox·i·dant
ox·i·dase
ox·i·da·sic
ox·i·da·tion
ox·i·da·tion-re·duc·tion
ox·i·da·tive
ox·i·da·tive·ly
ox·ide
ox·id·ic
ox·i·di·za·tion
ox·i·dize
ox·i·dized
ox·i·diz·ing
ox·i·do·re·duc·tase
ox·ime
ox·im·e·ter
ox·i·met·ric
ox·im·e·try
pl ox·im·e·tries
ox·o·ni·um
oxo·phen·ar·sine
oxo·trem·o·rine
oxy·acan·thine
oxy·ac·id
oxy·bi·o·tin
oxy·blep·sia
oxy·cal·o·rim·e·ter
oxy·ce·phal·ic
or oxy·ceph·a·lous
oxy·ceph·a·ly
pl oxy·ceph·a·lies
oxy·chlo·ride
oxy·chro·mat·ic
or oxy·chro·ma·tin·ic
oxy·chro·ma·tin
ox·y·gen
ox·y·gen·ase
ox·y·gen·ate
ox·y·gen·at·ed
ox·y·gen·at·ing
ox·y·gen·a·tion
ox·y·gen·a·tor
ox·y·gen·ic
ox·y·gen·ic·i·ty
pl ox·y·gen·ic·i·ties
ox·y·gen·ize
ox·y·gen·ized
ox·y·gen·iz·ing
oxy·he·mo·glo·bin
oxy·hy·dro·gen
ox·y·mel

oxy·myo·glo·bin
oxy·neu·rine
ox·yn·tic
oxy·opia
also oxy·opy
pl oxy·opias
also oxy·opies

oxy·phil
oxy·phil·ic
also ox·yph·i·lous

oxy·poly·gel·a·tin
oxy·some
Oxy·spi·ru·ra
oxy·tet·ra·cy·cline
oxy·to·cia
oxy·to·cic
oxy·to·cin
oxy·uri·a·sis
pl oxy·uri·a·ses

oxy·uric
oxy·uri·cide
oxy·urid
Oxy·uris
oze·na
also ozae·na
or ozoe·na

ozon·a·tor
ozone
ozon·ide
ozon·iza·tion
ozon·ize
ozon·ized
ozon·iz·ing
ozon·iz·er
ozon·ol·y·sis
pl ozon·ol·y·ses

ozo·sto·mia

P

Pac·chi·o·ni·an body
or Pac·chi·o·ni·an cor·pus·cle

pace·mak·er
pachy·ac·ria
pachy·ce·pha·lia
or pachy·ceph·a·ly
pl pachy·ce·pha·lias
or pachy·ceph·a·lies

pachy·chei·lia
pachy·der·ma·tous
pachy·der·mia
pachy·der·mi·al
pachy·lep·to·men·in·gi·tis
pl pachy·lep·to·men·in·git·i·des

pachy·men·in·gi·tis
pl pachy·men·in·git·i·des

pachy·me·ninx
pl pachy·me·nin·ges

pachy·o·nych·ia
pachy·peri·to·ni·tis
pachy·tene
Pa·cin·i·an cor·pus·cle
also Pa·ci·ni's cor·pus·cle

pae·di·at·ric
var of pediatric

pae·di·at·rics
var of pediatrics

pae·do·phil·ia
var of pedophilia

pag·et·oid
Pag·et's dis·ease
pain·kill·er
pain·kill·ing
paired-as·so·ci·ate learn·ing
pa·ja·ro·el·lo
also pa·ja·huel·lo

pal·a·tal
pal·ate
pal·a·tine
pal·a·ti·tis
pal·a·to·glos·sal
pal·a·to·glos·sus
pl pal·a·to·glos·si

pal·a·to·gram
pal·a·to·graph·ic
pal·a·tog·ra·phy
pl pal·a·tog·ra·phies

pal·a·to·max·il·lary
pal·a·to·na·sal
pal·a·to·pha·ryn·geal
pal·a·to·pha·ryn·ge·us
pal·a·to·plas·ty
pl pal·a·to·plas·ties

pal·a·to·ple·gia
pal·a·tor·rha·phy
pl pal·a·tor·rha·phies

pal·a·tos·chi·sis
pl pal·a·tos·chi·ses
also pal·a·tos·chi·sis·es

pal·a·tum
pl pal·a·ta

pa·le·en·ceph·a·lon
pl pa·le·en·ceph·a·la

pa·leo·cer·e·bel·lar

pa·leo·cer·e·bel·lum
pl pa·leo·cer·e·bel·lums
or pa·leo·cer·e·bel·la

pa·leo·cor·tex
pl pa·leo·cor·ti·ces

pa·leo·en·ceph·a·lon
pl pa·leo·en·ceph·a·la

pa·leo·pal·li·um
pl pa·leo·pal·lia
or pa·leo·pal·li·ums

pa·leo·stri·a·tal

pa·leo·stri·a·tum
pl pa·leo·stri·a·ta

pa·leo·thal·a·mus
pl pa·leo·thal·a·mi

pali·ki·ne·sia

pali·la·lia

pal·in·dro·mia

pa·lin·drom·ic

pal·in·drom·i·cal·ly

pal·la·di·um

pall·an·es·the·sia

pall·es·the·sia

pal·li·al

pal·li·ate
pal·li·at·ed
pal·li·at·ing

pal·li·a·tion

pal·lia·tive

pal·lia·tive·ly

pal·li·dal

pal·li·um
pl pal·lia
or pal·li·ums

pal·mar

pal·mar·is

pal·ma·ture

pal·mi·tate

pal·mit·ic

pal·mod·ic

pal·mo·spas·mus

pal·mus
pl pal·mi

pal·pa·ble

pal·pate
pal·pat·ed
pal·pat·ing

pal·pa·tion
examination by touch (see palpitation)

pal·pe·bra
pl pal·pe·brae

pal·pe·bral

pal·pe·brate
pal·pe·brat·ed
pal·pe·brat·ing

pal·pe·bra·tion

pal·pi·tate
pal·pi·tat·ed
pal·pi·tat·ing

pal·pi·ta·tion
rapid beating of the heart (see palpation)

pal·sied

pal·sy
pl pal·sies

pa·lu·dal

pal·u·dism

pam·a·quine
also pam·a·quin

pan·ag·glu·ti·na·bil·i·ty
pl pan·ag·glu·ti·na·bil·i·ties

pan·ag·glu·ti·na·ble

pan·ag·glu·ti·na·tion

pan·ar·ter·i·tis

pan·ar·thri·tis
pl pan·ar·thri·ti·des

pan·at·ro·phy
pl pan·at·ro·phies

pan·car·di·tis

pan·col·ec·to·my
pl pan·col·ec·to·mies

pan·cre·as

pan·cre·atec·to·mize
pan·cre·atec·to·mized
pan·cre·atec·to·miz·ing

pan·cre·atec·to·my
pl pan·cre·atec·to·mies

pan·cre·at·ic

pan·cre·at·i·co·du·o·de·nal

pan·cre·at·i·co·en·ter·os·to·my
pl pan·cre·at·i·co·en·ter·os·to·mies

pan·cre·at·i·co·gas·tros·to·my
pl pan·cre·at·i·co·gas·tros·to·mies

pan·cre·at·i·co·je·ju·nos·to·my
pl pan·cre·at·i·co·je·ju·nos·to·mies

pan·cre·atin
pan·cre·a·tism
pan·cre·ati·tis
pl pan·cre·atit·i·des

pan·cre·a·tog·e·nous
pan·cre·ato·lith
pan·cre·ato·li·thot·o·my
pl pan·cre·ato·li·thot·o·mies

pan·cre·a·tot·o·my
pl pan·cre·a·tot·o·mies

pan·cy·to·pe·nia
pan·cy·to·pe·nic
pan·dem·ic
pan·dic·u·la·tion
pan·en·do·scope
pan·en·do·scop·ic
pan·en·dos·co·py
pl pan·en·dos·co·pies

pan·hy·po·pi·tu·ita·rism
pan·hy·po·pi·tu·itary
pan·hys·ter·ec·to·my
pl pan·hys·ter·ec·to·mies

pan·hys·tero·sal·pin·gec·to·my
pl pan·hys·tero·sal·pin·gec·to·mies

pan·hys·tero·sal·pingo-oo·pho·rec·to·my
pl pan·hys·tero·sal·pingo-oo·pho·rec·to·mies

pan·leu·co·pe·nia
also pan·leu·ko·pe·nia

pan·my·elop·a·thy
pl pan·my·elop·a·thies

pan·my·elo·phthi·sis
pl pan·my·elo·phthi·ses

pan·nic·u·li·tis
pan·nic·u·lus
pl pan·nic·u·li

pan·nus
pl pan·ni

pan·oph·thal·mi·tis
pan·op·tic
also pan·op·ti·cal

pan·oti·tis
pl pan·otit·i·des

pan·scle·ro·sis
pl pan·scle·ro·ses

pan·si·nus·itis
pan·sper·mia
also pan·sper·ma·tism

pan·te·the·ine
pan·to·the·nate
pan·to·then·ic
pan·trop·ic
pan·zo·ot·ic
pa·pa·in
Pa·pa·ni·co·laou test
Pa·pa·ver
pa·pav·er·ine
pa·pil·la
pl pa·pil·lae

pa·pil·la of Va·ter
pap·il·lar
pap·il·lary
pa·pil·late
or pa·pil·lat·ed

pap·il·lec·to·my
pl pap·il·lec·to·mies

pap·ill·ede·ma
also pap·ill·oe·de·ma
pl pap·ill·ede·mas
or pap·ill·ede·ma·ta
also pap·ill·oe·de·mas
or pap·ill·oe·de·ma·ta

pap·il·lif·er·ous
pa·pil·li·form
pap·il·li·tis

pap·il·lo·ma
pl pap·il·lo·mas
or pap·il·lo·ma·ta

pap·il·lo·ma·to·sis
pl pap·il·lo·ma·to·ses

pap·il·lo·ma·tous

pap·il·lo·ret·i·ni·tis
pl pap·il·lo·ret·i·nit·i·des

pa·po·va·vi·rus

pap·pose
also pap·pous

pap·pus
pl pap·pi

Pap smear
also Pap test

pap·u·lar

pap·u·la·tion

pap·ule

pap·u·lo·er·y·them·a·tous

pap·u·lo·pus·tu·lar

pap·u·lo·squa·mous

pap·u·lo·ve·sic·u·lar

pap·y·ra·ceous

para
pl par·as
or par·ae

para-ami·no·ben·zo·ic

para-ami·no·hip·pu·ric

para-an·al·ge·sia

para-an·es·the·sia

para·bi·o·sis
pl para·bi·o·ses

para·bi·ot·ic

para·bi·ot·i·cal·ly

para·blep·sia
also para·blep·sis
or para·blep·sy
pl para·blep·sias
or para·blep·ses
or para·blep·sies

para·bu·lia

para·car·mine

Par·a·cel·sian

para·cen·te·sis
pl para·cen·te·ses

para·cen·tral

para·chord·al

para·chro·ma·tism

para·co·li·tis

para·col·pi·tis

par·a·col·pi·um

para·cone

par·acu·sia
or par·acu·sis
pl par·acu·sias
or par·acu·ses

para·cys·tic

para·cys·ti·tis
pl para·cys·tit·i·des

para·cys·ti·um
pl para·cys·tia

para·den·tal

para·den·ti·tis

para·den·tium
pl para·den·tia

para·den·to·sis
pl para·den·to·ses

para·did·y·mis
pl para·did·y·mi·des

par·a·dox·i·cal sleep

par·aes·the·sia
var of paresthesia

par·aes·thet·ic
var of paresthetic

par·af·fin
also par·af·fine

par·af·fin·oma
pl par·af·fin·omas
or par·af·fin·oma·ta

para·gam·ma·cism
also para·gam·ma·cis·mus
pl para·gam·ma·cisms
also para·gam·ma·cis·mus·es

para·gan·gli·o·ma
pl para·gan·gli·o·mas
or para·gan·gli·o·ma·ta

para·gan·gli·on
pl para·gan·glia
also para·gan·gli·ons

para·gan·gli·on·ic

para·geu·sia

par·ag·glu·ti·na·tion

para·glos·sia

pa·rag·na·thus

par·a·gon·i·mi·a·sis
pl par·a·gon·i·mi·a·ses

Par·a·gon·i·mus

para·graph·ia
para·he·mo·phil·ia
para·he·pat·ic
para·hor·mone
or para·hor·mo·nic
para·hy·droxy·ben·zo·ic
para·in·flu·en·za
para·ker·a·to·sis
pl para·ker·a·to·ses
para·ker·a·tot·ic
para·ki·ne·sia
or para·ki·ne·sis
pl para·ki·ne·sias
or para·ki·ne·ses
para·ki·net·ic
para·la·lia
para·lamb·da·cism
par·al·de·hyde
para·lex·ia
para·lex·ic
par·al·ge·sia
par·al·ge·sic
para·lo·gia
pa·ral·o·gism
pa·ral·y·sis
pl pa·ral·y·ses
pa·ral·y·sis ag·i·tans
par·a·lyt·ic
also par·a·lyt·i·cal
par·a·ly·zant
also par·a·ly·sant
par·a·ly·za·tion
par·a·lyze
also par·a·lyse
par·a·lyzed
also par·a·lysed
par·a·lyz·ing
also par·a·lys·ing
par·a·lyz·er
para·mas·ti·tis
pl para·mas·tit·i·des
para·mas·toid
para·me·di·an
para·med·ic
para·med·i·cal
para·me·nia
para·metha·di·one
para·me·tri·al
para·me·tri·tis
para·me·tri·um
pl para·me·tria
para·mim·ia
par·am·ne·sia
Par·am·phis·to·mum
para·mu·sia
par·am·y·lum
para·my·oc·lo·nus mul·ti·plex
para·myo·to·nia
par·a·nee
para·neph·ric
para·ne·phri·tis
pl para·ne·phrit·i·des
para·neu·ral
para·noia
para·noi·ac
para·no·ic
para·noid
para·no·mia
para·nu·cle·ar
para·nu·cle·us
pl para·nu·clei
also para·neu·cle·us·es
para·ox·on
para·pan·cre·at·ic
para·pa·re·sis
pl para·pa·re·ses
par·a·pha·sia
par·a·pha·sic
para·phenyl·ene·di·amine
para·phil·ia
para·phil·i·ac
para·phi·mo·sis
pl para·phi·mo·ses
para·pho·nia
pl para·pho·nias
also para·phon·i·ae
para·phra·sia
para·phre·nia
para·phren·ic
pa·raph·y·se·al
or par·a·phys·i·al
pa·raph·y·sis
pl pa·raph·y·ses
para·ple·gia
para·ple·gic
par·ap·o·plexy
pl par·ap·o·plexies
para·prax·ia
or para·prax·is
pl para·prax·ias
or para·prax·es
para·proc·ti·tis
para·proc·tium
pl para·proc·tia

para·pro·tein
para·pro·tein·emia
para·pso·ri·a·sis
pl para·pso·ri·a·ses
para·psy·cho·log·i·cal
para·psy·chol·o·gist
para·psy·chol·o·gy
pl para·psy·chol·o·gies
para·rec·tal
para·ros·an·i·line
par·ar·thria
para·sa·cral
Par·as·ca·ris
para·se·cre·tion
para·sex·u·al
para·sex·u·al·i·ty
pl para·sex·u·al·i·ties
para·sig·ma·tism
par·a·site
par·a·sit·emia
par·a·sit·ic
also par·a·sit·i·cal
par·a·sit·i·cal·ly
par·a·sit·i·cid·al
also par·a·sit·i·cid·ic
par·a·sit·i·cide
par·a·sit·ism
par·a·sit·iza·tion
par·a·sit·ize
par·a·sit·ized
par·a·sit·iz·ing
para·si·to·gen·ic
par·a·si·to·log·i·cal
also par·a·si·to·log·ic
par·a·si·tol·o·gist
par·a·si·tol·o·gy
pl par·a·si·tol·o·gies
par·a·sit·osis
pl par·a·sit·o·ses
par·a·si·to·trop·ic
para·spa·di·as
para·ster·nal
para·ster·nal·ly
para·sym·pa·thet·ic
para·sym·pa·thet·i·co·mi·met·ic
para·sym·pa·tho·lyt·ic
para·sym·pa·tho·mi·met·ic
para·syph·i·lit·ic
para·thi·on
para·thy·roid
also para·thy·roi·dal
para·thy·roid·ec·to·mized
para·thy·roid·ec·to·my
pl para·thy·roid·ec·to·mies
para·thy·ro·pri·val
also para·thy·ro·priv·ic
para·thy·ro·trop·ic
para·troph·ic
pa·rat·ro·phy
pl pa·rat·ro·phies
para·tu·ber·cu·lo·sis
pl para·tu·ber·cu·lo·ses
para·tu·ber·cu·lous
para·ty·phoid
para·typ·ic
also para·typ·i·cal
para·um·bil·i·cal
para·ure·thral
para·vag·i·nal
para·vag·i·nal·ly
para·vag·i·ni·tis
para·ver·te·bral
para·ver·te·bral·ly
para·ves·i·cal
par·ax·i·al
par·ax·i·al·ly
par·ec·ta·sis
or par·ec·ta·sia
pl par·ec·ta·ses
or par·ec·ta·sias
par·e·go·ric
pa·ren·chy·ma
also par·en·chyme
pa·ren·chy·mal
or pa·ren·chy·mous
par·en·chy·ma·tous
or pa·ren·chy·mat·ic
par·en·chy·ma·tous·ly
par·en·ter·al

par·en·ter·al·ly
par·ep·i·did·y·mis
pl par·ep·i·did·y·mi·des
par·er·ga·sia
pa·re·sis
pl pa·re·ses
par·es·the·sia
also par·aes·the·sia
par·es·thet·ic
also par·aes·thet·ic
pa·ret·ic
pa·ret·i·cal·ly
par·gy·line
par·i·es
pl pa·ri·etes
pa·ri·etal
pa·ri·e·to·fron·tal
pa·ri·e·to-oc·cip·i·tal
par·kin·so·nian
par·kin·son·ism
Par·kin·son's dis·ease
Par·kin·son's syn·drome
par·oc·cip·i·tal
par·odon·tal
par·odon·ti·tis
pl par·odon·tit·i·des
par·o·don·ti·um
par·o·mo·my·cin
par·o·nych·ia
par·ooph·o·ron
par·oph·thal·mia
par·o·rex·ia
par·os·mia
par·os·ti·tis
par·otic
pa·rot·id
pa·rot·i·dec·to·my
pl pa·rot·i·dec·to·mies
pa·rot·i·di·tis
pl pa·rot·i·di·tis·es
par·otit·ic
par·oti·tis
par·ous
par·ovar·ian
par·ovar·i·ot·o·my
pl par·ovar·i·ot·o·mies
par·ovar·i·um
pl par·ovar·ia
par·ox·ysm
par·ox·ys·mal
par·ox·ys·mic
pars ner·vo·sa
par·the·no·gen·e·sis
pl par·the·no·gen·e·ses
par·the·no·ge·net·ic
or par·the·no·gen·ic
par·the·no·ge·net·i·cal·ly
par·tu·ri·ent
par·tu·ri·fa·cient
par·tu·ri·tion
pa·ru·lis
pl pa·ru·li·des
par·um·bil·i·cal
par·vi·cel·lu·lar
Par·vo·bac·te·ri·a·ce·ae
par·vule
pas·tern
Pas·teur ef·fect
pas·teu·rel·la
pl pas·teu·rel·las
or pas·teu·rel·lae
pas·teu·rel·lo·sis
pl pas·teu·rel·lo·ses
pas·teur·iza·tion
pas·teur·ize
pas·teur·ized
pas·teur·iz·ing
pas·teur·iz·er
Pas·teur treat·ment
pas·tille
also pas·til
pa·tel·la
pl pa·tel·lae
or pa·tel·las
pa·tel·lar
pat·el·lec·to·my
pl pat·el·lec·to·mies
pa·tel·li·form
pa·ten·cy
pl pa·ten·cies
pa·tent
pa·tent·ly
pa·ter·ni·ty
pl pa·ter·ni·ties
pa·thet·i·cus
pl pa·thet·i·ci
path·odon·tia
patho·gen
also patho·gene
patho·gen·e·sis
pl patho·gen·e·ses

patho·ge·net·ic
patho·gen·ic
patho·gen·i·cal·ly
patho·ge·nic·i·ty
pl patho·ge·nic·i·ties

pa·thog·e·ny
pl pa·thog·e·nies

pa·tho·gno·mon·ic
also pa·tho·gno·mon·i·cal

pa·tho·gno·mon·i·cal·ly
pa·tho·gno·my
pl pa·tho·gno·mies

patho·log·i·cal
or patho·log·ic

patho·log·i·cal·ly
pa·thol·o·gist
pa·thol·o·gy
pl pa·thol·o·gies

pa·thom·e·ter
patho·mor·pho·log·i·cal
or patho·mor·pho·log·ic

patho·mor·phol·o·gy
pl patho·mor·phol·o·gies

patho·neu·ro·sis
pl patho·neu·ro·ses

patho·phys·i·o·log·i·cal
or patho·phys·i·o·log·ic

patho·phys·i·ol·o·gy
pl patho·phys·i·ol·o·gies

patho·psy·chol·o·gy
pl patho·psy·chol·o·gies

pa·tho·sis
pl pa·tho·ses

pa·tient
pat·ri·lin·eal
pat·u·lin
pat·u·lous
pat·u·lous·ly
Pav·lov·ian
Pav·lov pouch
pa·vor
pec·cant
pec·tase
pec·ten
pl pec·tens
also pec·ti·nes

pec·tic
pec·tin
pec·tin·ase
pec·tin·e·al
pec·tin·es·ter·ase
pec·tin·e·us
pl pec·tin·ei

pec·to·ral
pec·to·ra·lis
pl pec·to·ra·les

pec·to·ril·o·quy
pl pec·to·ril·o·quies

pec·tus
pl pec·to·ra

ped·al

ped·er·ast
ped·er·as·tic
ped·er·as·ti·cal·ly
ped·er·as·ty
pl ped·er·as·ties

pe·des
pl of pes

pe·di·at·ric
also pae·di·at·ric

pe·di·a·tri·cian
also pe·di·a·trist

pe·di·at·rics
also pae·di·at·rics

ped·i·cel
ped·i·cel·late
also ped·i·cel·lat·ed

ped·i·cle
ped·i·cled
pe·dic·u·lar
pe·dic·u·late
pe·dic·u·lat·ed
pe·dic·u·la·tion
pe·dic·u·li·ci·dal
pe·dic·u·li·cide
pe·dic·u·lo·sis
pl pe·dic·u·lo·ses

pe·dic·u·lous
pe·dic·u·lus
pl pe·dic·u·li
or pe·dic·u·lus

ped·i·cure
pe·do·don·tia
pe·do·don·tic
pe·do·don·tics
pe·do·don·tist
pe·do·log·ic
or pe·do·log·i·cal

pe·dol·o·gist
pe·dol·o·gy
pl pe·dol·o·gies
pe·do·phile
pe·do·phil·ia
or pae·do·phil·ia
pe·do·phil·i·ac
or pe·do·phil·ic
pe·dun·cle
pe·dun·cled
pe·dun·cu·lar
pe·dun·cu·late
or pe·dun·cu·lat·ed
pe·dun·cu·la·tion
pe·dun·cu·lus
pl pe·dun·cu·li
pel·la·gra
pel·la·gra·gen·ic
pel·la·gric
pel·la·grin
pel·la·groid
pel·la·grous
pel·li·cle
pel·lic·u·lar
pel·mat·o·gram
pel·oid
pelo·ther·a·py
pl pelo·ther·a·pies
pel·vic
pel·vi·graph
pel·vim·e·ter
pel·vim·e·try
pl pel·vim·e·tries
pel·vis
pl pel·vis·es
or pel·ves
pel·vi·sa·cral
pel·vi·scope
pem·o·line
pem·phi·goid
pem·phi·gus
pl pem·phi·gus·es
or pem·phi·gi
pe·ni·al
pen·i·cil·la·mine
pen·i·cil·lin
pen·i·cil·lin·ase
pen·i·cil·lin·ic
pen·i·cil·li·o·sis
pl pen·i·cil·li·o·ses
pen·i·cil·li·um
pl pen·i·cil·lia
pen·i·cil·lo·ic
pen·i·cil·lus
pl pen·i·cil·li
pe·nile
pe·nis
pl pe·nes
or pe·nis·es
pen·nate
also pen·nat·ed
pen·ny·weight
pen·ta·chlo·ro·phe·nol
pen·ta·dac·tyl
also pen·ta·dac·ty·late
pen·ta·dac·tyl·ism
pen·ta·eryth·ri·tol tet·ra·ni·trate
pen·ta·gas·trin
pen·tal·o·gy
pl pen·tal·o·gies
pent·am·i·dine
pen·tane
pen·taz·o·cine
pen·to·bar·bi·tal
pen·to·bar·bi·tone
pen·to·side
pen·tos·uria
pen·tyl·ene·tet·ra·zol
peo·til·lo·ma·nia
pep·si·gogue
pep·sin
pep·sin·if·er·ous
pep·sin·o·gen
pep·tic
pep·ti·dase
pep·tide
pep·ti·do·gly·can
pep·tone
pep·to·ni·za·tion
pep·to·nize
pep·to·nized
pep·to·niz·ing
pep·to·noid
pep·ton·uria
per·ace·tic
per·acute
per anum
per·cep·tion
per·co·la·tion
per·co·la·tor
per·cuss
per·cus·sion
per·cus·sor
per·cu·ta·ne·ous
per·cu·ta·ne·ous·ly
per·fec·tion·ism

per•fla•tion
per•fo•rans
per•fo•rate
per•fo•rat•ed
per•fo•rat•ing
per•fo•ra•tion
per•fo•ra•tor
per•fri•ca•tion
per•fus•ate
per•fuse
per•fused
per•fus•ing
per•fu•sion
peri•ac•i•nal
also peri•ac•i•nous
peri•ad•e•ni•tis
peri•anal
peri•an•gi•i•tis
pl peri•an•gi•it•i•des
peri•an•gio•cho•li•tis
peri•aor•tal
or peri•aor•tic
peri•aor•ti•tis
peri•api•cal
peri•api•cal•ly
peri•ap•pen•di•ci•tis
peri•ar•te•ri•al
peri•ar•ter•i•tis
peri•ar•thri•tis
pl peri•ar•thri•ti•des
peri•ar•tic•u•lar
peri•au•ric•u•lar
peri•ax•i•al
peri•blast
peri•blas•tic
peri•bron•chi•al
peri•bron•chi•tis
pl peri•bron•chit•i•des
peri•car•di•ec•to•my
pl peri•car•di•ec•to•mies
peri•car•di•ot•o•my
pl peri•car•di•ot•o•mies
peri•car•dit•ic
peri•car•di•tis
pl peri•car•dit•i•des
peri•car•di•um
pl peri•car•dia
peri•cary•on
var of perikaryon
peri•ce•cal
peri•ce•ci•tis
peri•cel•lu•lar
peri•ce•ment•al
peri•ce•men•ti•tis
peri•ce•men•tum
peri•chol•an•gi•tis
pl peri•chol•an•git•i•des
peri•chon•dri•al
also peri•chon•dral
peri•chon•dri•tis
peri•chon•dri•um
pl peri•chon•dria
peri•chord
peri•chord•al
peri•co•lic
peri•co•li•tis
peri•con•chal
peri•cor•ne•al
peri•cor•o•nal
peri•cor•o•ni•tis
pl peri•cor•o•ni•tid•es
peri•cra•ni•al
peri•cra•ni•um
pl peri•cra•nia
peri•cys•tic
peri•cys•ti•tis
pl peri•cys•tit•i•des
peri•cys•ti•um
pl peri•cys•tia
peri•cyte
peri•cy•tial
peri•den•drit•ic
peri•den•tal
peri•derm
peri•der•mal
or peri•der•mic
peri•des•mic
peri•des•mi•um
peri•di•as•to•le
peri•did•y•mis
pl peri•did•y•mi•des
peri•di•ver•tic•u•li•tis
peri•du•o•de•ni•tis
peri•du•ral
peri•en•ceph•a•li•tis
pl peri•en•ceph•a•lit•i•des
peri•en•ter•ic
peri•en•ter•i•tis
pl peri•en•ter•it•i•des
or peri•en•ter•i•tis•es
peri•en•ter•on

peri·ep·en·dy·mal
peri·esoph·a·ge·al
peri·esoph·a·gi·tis
peri·fo·cal
peri·fol·lic·u·lar
peri·fol·lic·u·li·tis
peri·glot·tic
peri·glot·tis
pl peri·glot·tis·es
or peri·glot·ti·des

peri·he·pat·ic
peri·hep·a·ti·tis
pl peri·hep·a·tit·i·des

peri·kary·al
peri·kary·on
also peri·cary·on
pl peri·karya
also peri·carya

peri·la·ryn·geal
peri·lymph
peri·lym·phat·ic
peri·mas·ti·tis
pl peri·mas·tit·i·des

per·im·e·ter
peri·me·tri·tis
peri·me·tri·um
pl peri·me·tria

pe·rim·e·try
pl pe·rim·e·tries

peri·my·eli·tis
pl peri·my·e·lit·i·des

peri·my·o·si·tis
peri·my·si·al
peri·my·si·um
pl peri·my·sia

peri·na·tal

per·i·ne·al
relating to the perineum (see peritoneal, peroneal)

peri·ne·om·e·ter
peri·neo·plas·ty
pl peri·neo·plas·ties

per·i·ne·or·rha·phy
pl per·i·ne·or·rha·phies

per·i·neo·scro·tal
per·i·ne·ot·o·my
pl per·i·ne·ot·o·mies

per·i·neo·vag·i·nal
peri·neph·ric
peri·ne·phrit·ic
peri·ne·phri·tis
pl peri·ne·phrit·i·des

peri·neph·ri·um
pl peri·neph·ria

per·i·ne·um
also per·i·nae·um
pl per·i·nea
also per·i·naea
area of tissue marking the pelvic outlet (see perineurium, peritoneum)

peri·neu·ral
peri·neu·ri·al
peri·neu·ri·tis
pl peri·neu·rit·i·des
or peri·neu·ri·tis·es

peri·neu·ri·um
pl peri·neu·ria
nerve sheath of connective tissue (see perineum, peritoneum)

peri·nu·cle·ar
peri·oc·u·lar
peri·odon·tal
peri·odon·tia
peri·odon·tic
peri·odon·tics
peri·odon·tist
peri·odon·ti·tis
peri·odon·ti·um
pl peri·odon·tia

peri·odon·to·cla·sia
peri·odon·tol·o·gy
pl peri·odon·tol·o·gies

peri·odon·to·sis
pl peri·odon·to·ses

peri·om·phal·ic
peri·onych·ia
peri·onych·i·um
pl peri·onych·ia

peri·on·yx
peri·oo·pho·ri·tis
peri·oo·pho·ro·sal·pin·gi·tis
peri·ople
peri·op·lic
peri·op·tom·e·try
pl peri·op·tom·e·tries

peri·oral
peri·or·bit
peri·or·bit·al
peri·or·bi·ti·tis
peri·or·chi·tis
peri·ost
peri·os·te·al

peri·os·te·o·ma
pl peri·os·te·o·mas
or peri·os·te·o·ma·ta

peri·os·teo·phyte

peri·os·te·ot·o·my
pl peri·os·te·ot·o·mies

peri·os·te·um
pl peri·os·tea

peri·os·tit·ic

peri·os·ti·tis

peri·os·to·ma

peri·os·to·sis
pl peri·os·to·ses
or peri·os·to·sis·es

peri·otic

peri·ovu·lar

peri·pachy·men·in·gi·tis
pl peri·pachy·men·in·git·i·des

peri·pan·cre·ati·tis
pl peri·pan·cre·atit·i·des

peri·pap·il·lary

peri·pha·ci·tis

peri·pha·ryn·geal

pe·riph·er·ad

pe·riph·er·al

pe·riph·er·al·ly

pe·riph·er·a·phose

pe·riph·ery
pl pe·riph·er·ies

peri·phle·bi·tis
pl peri·phle·bit·i·des

Peri·pla·ne·ta

peri·por·tal

peri·proc·tal
or peri·proc·tic
or peri·proc·tous

peri·proc·ti·tis

peri·pros·tat·ic

peri·pros·ta·ti·tis

peri·py·le·phle·bi·tis
pl peri·py·le·phle·bit·i·des

peri·py·lo·ric

peri·rec·tal

peri·re·nal

peri·rhi·nal

peri·sal·pin·gi·tis

peri·sal·pinx
pl peri·sal·pin·ges

peri·sig·moid·itis

peri·sin·u·ous

peri·si·nus·itis

peri·sper·ma·ti·tis

peri·splen·ic

peri·sple·ni·tis

peri·spon·dyl·ic

peri·spon·dy·li·tis

peri·stal·sis
pl peri·stal·ses

peri·stal·tic

peri·stal·ti·cal·ly

peri·staph·y·line

peri·sy·no·vi·al

peri·tec·to·my
pl peri·tec·to·mies

peri·ten·din·e·um
pl peri·ten·din·ea

peri·ten·di·ni·tis

peri·ten·on

peri·ten·on·ti·tis

peri·the·li·al

peri·the·li·o·ma
pl peri·the·li·o·mas
or peri·the·li·o·ma·ta

peri·the·li·um
pl peri·the·lia

peri·thy·roid·itis

pe·rit·o·my
pl pe·rit·o·mies

peri·to·ne·al
relating to the peritoneum (*see* peri·neal, peroneal)

peri·to·ne·al·ly

peri·to·neo·cen·te·sis
pl peri·to·neo·cen·te·ses

peri·to·ne·op·a·thy
pl peri·to·ne·op·a·thies

peri·to·neo·peri·car·di·al

peri·to·neo·pexy
pl peri·to·neo·pexies

peri·to·neo·scope

peri·to·neo·scop·ic

peri·to·ne·os·co·pist

peri·to·ne·os·co·py
pl peri·to·ne·os·co·pies

peri·to·ne·ot·o·my
pl peri·to·ne·ot·o·mies

peri·to·ne·um
pl peri·to·ne·ums
or peri·to·nea
membrane lining the abdominal cavity (*see* perineum, perineurium)

peri·to·nit·ic
peri·to·ni·tis
peri·to·nize
peri·to·nized
peri·to·niz·ing
peri·ton·sil·lar
peri·ton·sil·li·tis
peri·tra·che·al
peri·typh·lic
peri·typh·li·tis
peri·um·bil·i·cal
peri·un·gual
peri·ure·ter·al
peri·ure·ter·ic
peri·ure·ter·itis
peri·ure·thral
peri·ure·thri·tis
pl peri·ure·thrit·i·des

peri·uter·ine
peri·uvu·lar
peri·vas·cu·lar
situated around a blood vessel (*see* perivesical, perivisceral)

peri·vas·cu·li·tis
peri·ve·nous
peri·ver·te·bral
peri·ves·i·cal
situated around the bladder (*see* perivascular, perivisceral)

peri·vis·cer·al
situated around the viscera (*see* perivascular, perivesical)

peri·vis·cer·i·tis
peri·vi·tel·line
per·lèche
per·lin·gual
per·lin·gual·ly
per·me·ase
per·ni·cious
per·nio
pl per·ni·o·nes

pero·bra·chi·us
pero·chi·rus
pero·cor·mus
pero·dac·ty·lus
pl pero·dac·ty·li

pero·me·lia
pe·rom·e·lus
pl pe·rom·e·li

pe·ro·ne·al
relating to the fibula (*see* perineal, peritoneal)

per·o·ne·us
pl per·o·nei

pero·pus
per·oral
per·oral·ly
per os
pe·ro·sis
pl pe·ro·ses

pero·so·mus
pl pero·so·mi
or pero·so·mus·es

pero·splanch·nia
per·os·se·ous
pe·rot·ic
per·ox·i·dase
per·oxi·som·al
per·oxi·some
per·oxy·ace·tic
per pri·mam
per·rec·tal
per·rec·tal·ly
per rec·tum
per·so·na
pl per·so·nas

per·son·al·i·ty
pl per·son·al·i·ties

per·spi·ra·tion
per·spir·a·to·ry
per·spire
per·spired
per·spir·ing
per·tus·sal
per·tus·sis
per·ver·sion
per·vert·ed
per·vi·gil·i·um
pes
pl pe·des

pes·sa·ry
pl pes·sa·ries

pes·ti·ci·dal
pes·ti·cide
pes·tif·er·ous
pes·tif·er·ous·ly
pes·ti·lence

pes·ti·lent
pes·ti·len·tial
pes·ti·len·tial·ly
pes·tis
pes·tle
pe·te·chia
pl pe·te·chi·ae

pe·te·chi·al
pe·te·chi·ate
pe·te·chi·a·tion
peth·i·dine
pet·i·o·late
also pet·i·o·lat·ed

pet·i·ole
pe·ti·o·lus
pl pe·ti·o·li

pe·tit mal
Pe·tri dish
pet·ri·fac·tion
pet·ri·fac·tive
pet·ri·fi·ca·tion
pet·ri·fy
pet·ri·fied
pet·ri·fy·ing
pe·tris·sage
pet·ro·la·tum
pet·ro·mas·toid
pet·ro-oc·cip·i·tal
pet·ro·pha·ryn·ge·us
pe·tro·sa
pl pe·tro·sae

pe·tro·sal
pet·ro·si·tis
pet·ro·sphe·noid
pet·ro·squa·mous
pet·ro·tym·pan·ic
pe·trox·o·lin
Pey·e·ri·an gland
Pey·er's patch
also Pey·er's gland

pey·o·te
or pey·otl

Pey·ro·nie's dis·ease
Pfeif·fer's ba·cil·lus
also Pfeif·fer's in·flu·en·za

phaco·er·y·sis
pha·col·y·sis
pl pha·col·y·ses

pha·com·e·ter
phaco·scle·ro·sis
pl phaco·scle·ro·ses

phage
pl phag·es
also phage

phago·cyte
phago·cyt·ic
phago·cy·tize
phago·cy·tized
phago·cy·tiz·ing
phago·cy·tose
also phago·cy·toze

phago·cy·tosed
also phago·cy·tozed

phago·cy·tos·ing
also phago·cy·toz·ing

phago·cy·to·sis
pl phago·cy·to·ses

phago·cy·tot·ic
phago·dy·na·mom·e·ter
pha·gol·y·sis
pl pha·gol·y·ses

phago·lyt·ic
phago·ma·nia
phago·some
phal·a·cro·sis
pl phal·a·cro·ses

pha·lange
pha·lan·ge·al
relating to a phalanx (*see* pharyngeal)

phal·an·gec·to·my
pl phal·an·gec·to·mies

phal·an·gette
pha·lanx
pl pha·lanx·es
or pha·lan·ges

phal·lic
phal·li·cal·ly
phal·loid
phal·loi·dine
also phal·loi·din

phal·lus
pl phal·li
or phal·lus·es

pha·nero·gam
Pha·nero·gam·ia
pha·nero·gen·ic
also pha·nero·ge·net·ic

pha·nero·ma·nia
phan·er·o·sis
pl phan·er·o·ses

pha·nero·zo·ic

pha•nero•zo•ite
pha•nero•zo•it•ic
phan•tasm
or fan•tasm

phan•tas•ma•go•ria
also phan•tas•ma•go•ry
pl phan•tas•ma•go•rias
also phan•tas•ma•go•ries

phan•tas•ma•go•ric
also phan•tas•ma•go•ri•cal

phan•tast
var of fantast

phan•ta•sy
var of fantasy

phan•tom
also fan•tom

phar•ma•cal
phar•ma•ceu•tic
phar•ma•ceu•ti•cal
phar•ma•ceu•ti•cal•ly
phar•ma•ceu•tics
phar•ma•ceu•tist
phar•ma•cist
phar•ma•co•dy•nam•ic
phar•ma•co•dy•nam•i•cal•ly
phar•ma•co•dy•nam•ics
phar•ma•co•ge•net•ic
phar•ma•co•ge•net•ics
phar•ma•cog•no•sist
phar•ma•cog•nos•tic
or phar•ma•cog•nos•ti•cal

phar•ma•cog•no•sy
pl phar•ma•cog•no•sies

phar•ma•co•ki•net•ics
phar•ma•co•log•i•cal
or phar•ma•co•log•ic

phar•ma•co•log•i•cal•ly
phar•ma•col•o•gist
phar•ma•col•o•gy
also phar•ma•co•lo•gia
pl phar•ma•col•o•gies
also phar•ma•co•lo•gias

phar•ma•co•pe•dia
phar•ma•co•pe•dic
phar•ma•co•pe•dics
phar•ma•co•poe•ia
also phar•ma•co•peia
phar•ma•co•poe•ial
phar•ma•co•poe•ist
phar•ma•co•ther•a•peu•tic
or phar•ma•co•ther•a•peu•ti•cal

phar•ma•co•ther•a•peu•tics
phar•ma•co•ther•a•py
pl phar•ma•co•ther•a•pies

phar•ma•cy
pl phar•ma•cies

pha•ryn•gal
pha•ryn•geal
relating to the pharynx (*see* phalangeal)

phar•yn•gec•to•my
pl phar•yn•gec•to•mies

phar•yn•gis•mus
pl phar•yn•gis•mi

phar•yn•gi•tis
pl phar•yn•git•i•des

pha•ryn•go•cele
pha•ryn•go•epi•glot•tic
pha•ryn•go•esoph•a•ge•al
pha•ryn•go•glos•sus
pl pha•ryn•go•glos•si

pha•ryn•go•lar•yn•gi•tis
pl pha•ryn•go•lar•yn•git•i•des
pha•ryn•go•log•i•cal
phar•yn•gol•o•gy
pl phar•yn•gol•o•gies
pha•ryn•go•na•sal
pha•ryn•go•pal•a•tine
pha•ryn•go•pal•a•ti•nus
pl pha•ryn•go•pal•a•ti•ni
pha•ryn•go•rhi•ni•tis
pl pha•ryn•go•rhi•nit•i•des
pha•ryn•go•scope
pha•ryn•go•spasm
phar•yn•got•o•my
pl phar•yn•got•o•mies
pha•ryn•go•ton•sil•li•tis
phar•ynx
pl pha•ryn•ges
also phar•ynx•es
phase-con•trast
pha•se•o•lin
Phas•mid•ia
phas•mid•i•an
phe•na•caine
or phe•no•cain
phen•ac•e•tin
phen•a•kis•to•scope
phen•an•threne
phe•nate
phe•naz•o•cine
phen•a•zone
phen•cy•cli•dine
phen•el•zine
phe•neth•i•cil•lin
phe•net•i•dine
phen•for•min
phen•met•ra•zine
phe•no•bar•bi•tal
phe•no•bar•bi•tone
phe•no•coll
phe•no•copy
pl phe•no•cop•ies
phe•nol
phe•no•lase
phe•no•late
phe•no•lat•ed
phe•no•lat•ing
phe•no•lic
phe•no•log•i•cal
also phe•no•log•ic
phe•no•log•i•cal•ly
phe•nol•o•gist
phe•nol•o•gy
pl phe•nol•o•gies
phe•nol•phtha•lein
phe•nol•sul•fone•phtha•lein
or phe•nol•sul•fon•phtha•lein
phe•no•thi•azine
phe•no•type
phe•no•typ•ic
or phe•no•typ•i•cal
phe•no•typ•i•cal•ly
phe•noxy
phen•oxy•meth•yl•pen•i•cil•lin
phen•tol•amine
phe•nyl
phen•yl•ace•tic
phe•nyl•al•a•nine
phen•yl•bu•ta•zone
phen•yl•ene•di•amine
phen•yl•eph•rine
phen•yl•hy•dra•zine
phe•nyl•ic
phe•nyl•ke•ton•uria
phe•nyl•ke•ton•uric
phen•yl•mer•cu•ric
phen•yl•pro•pa•nol•amine
phe•nyl•py•ru•vic
phen•yl•thio•car•ba•mide
phen•yl•thio•urea
phe•nyt•o•in
pheo•chrome
pheo•chro•mo•blast
also pheo•chro•mo•cy•to•blast

pheo·chro·mo·blas·to·ma
pl pheo·chro·mo·blas·to·mas
or pheo·chro·mo·blas·to·ma·ta

pheo·chro·mo·cyte

pheo·chro·mo·cy·to·ma
pl pheo·chro·mo·cy·to·mas
or pheo·chro·mo·cy·to·ma·ta

phe·ren·ta·sin

phi·al

Phi·a·loph·o·ra

philo·pro·gen·i·tive

phil·ter
or phil·tre

phil·trum
pl phil·tra

phi·mosed

phi·mo·sis
pl phi·mo·ses

phi·mot·ic

phi phe·nom·e·non

phle·bec·to·my
pl phle·bec·to·mies

phle·bit·ic

phle·bi·tis
pl phle·bit·i·des

phlebo·cly·sis
pl phlebo·cly·ses

phle·bo·gram

phle·bo·graph·ic

phle·bog·ra·phy
pl phle·bog·ra·phies

phleb·oid
also phle·boi·dal

phleb·o·lith

phlebo·li·thi·a·sis
pl phlebo·li·thi·a·ses

phle·bol·o·gy
pl phle·bol·o·gies

phlebo·scle·ro·sis
pl phlebo·scle·ro·ses

phlebo·scle·rot·ic

phlebo·throm·bo·sis
pl phlebo·throm·bo·ses

phleb·o·tom·ic
also phleb·o·tom·i·cal

phleb·o·tom·i·cal·ly

phle·bot·o·mist

phle·bot·o·mize
phle·bot·o·mized
phle·bot·o·miz·ing

phle·bo·to·mus
pl phle·bo·to·mi
also phle·bo·to·mus·es

phle·bot·o·my
pl phle·bot·o·mies

phlegm

phleg·ma·sia
pl phleg·ma·siae

phleg·ma·sia al·ba do·lens

phleg·mat·ic
or phleg·mat·i·cal

phleg·mat·i·cal·ly

phleg·mon

phleg·mon·ic

phleg·mon·ous

phleg·mon·ous·ly

phlegmy
phlegm·i·er
phlegm·i·est

phlo·gis·tic

phlog·o·ge·net·ic

phlog·o·gen·ic
also phlo·gog·e·nous

phlor·e·tin

phlo·ri·zin
or phlo·rhi·zin
or phlo·rid·zin
also phlor·rhi·zin

phlo·ro·glu·cin

phlo·ro·glu·cin·ol

phlox·ine

phlyc·te·na
or phlyc·tae·na
pl phlyc·te·nae
or phlyc·tae·nae

phlyc·te·noid

phlyc·te·nu·la
or phlyc·tae·nu·la
pl phlyc·te·nu·lae
or phyc·tae·nu·lae

phlyc·te·nu·lar

phlyc·te·nule

pho·bia

pho·bi·ac

pho·bic

pho·bism

pho·co·me·lia
also pho·ko·me·lia

pho·co·me·lic
pho·com·e·lus
pl pho·com·e·li

pho·nal
phon·as·the·nia
pho·nate
pho·nat·ed
pho·nat·ing
pho·na·tion
pho·na·to·ry
phon·au·to·graph
phon·au·to·graph·ic
phon·au·to·graph·i·cal·ly
pho·nen·do·scope
pho·ni·at·ric
pho·nism
pho·no·car·dio·gram
pho·no·car·dio·graph
pho·no·car·dio·graph·ic
pho·no·car·di·og·ra·phy
pl pho·no·car·di·og·ra·phies

pho·no·gram
pho·no·gram·mic
or pho·no·gram·ic

pho·no·gram·mi·cal·ly
or pho·no·gram·i·cal·ly

pho·no·log·i·cal
also pho·no·log·ic

pho·no·log·i·cal·ly
pho·nol·o·gist
pho·nol·o·gy
pl pho·nol·o·gies

pho·no·ma·nia
pho·nom·e·ter
pho·no·met·ric
pho·nom·e·try
pl pho·nom·e·tries

pho·nop·a·thy
pl pho·nop·a·thies

pho·no·pho·bia
pho·no·phore
pho·no·pho·to·gram
pho·no·pho·to·graph
pho·no·pho·tog·ra·phy
pl pho·no·pho·tog·ra·phies

pho·no·re·cep·tion
pho·no·re·cep·tor
pho·no·scope
pho·ria
Phor·mia
pho·rom·e·ter
phor·o·met·ric
pho·rom·e·try
pl pho·rom·e·tries

phose
phos·gene
phos·gen·ic
phos·pha·gen
phos·pha·tase
phos·phate
phos·phat·ed
phos·phat·ing
phos·pha·te·mia
phos·phat·ic
phos·pha·tide
phos·pha·tu·ria
phos·pha·tu·ric
phos·phene
phos·phide
phos·phine
phos·phite
phos·pho·ar·gi·nine
phos·pho·cre·atine
phos·pho·di·es·ter·ase
phos·pho·enol·pyr·uvate
phos·pho·enol·pyr·uvic
phos·pho·fruc·to·ki·nase
phos·pho·glu·co·mu·tase
phos·pho·glyc·er·al·de·hyde
phos·pho·glyc·er·ate
phos·pho·gly·cer·ic
phos·pho·ki·nase
phos·pho·li·pase
phos·pho·lip·id

phos·pho·mo·lyb·dic
phos·pho·mono·es·ter·ase
phos·pho·ne·cro·sis
pl phos·pho·ne·cro·ses
phos·pho·ni·um
phos·pho·pro·tein
phos·pho·py·ru·vate
phos·pho·py·ru·vic
phos·phor
also phos·phore
phos·pho·rate
phos·pho·rat·ed
phos·pho·rat·ing
phos·pho·ric
phos·pho·rism
phos·pho·rize
phos·pho·rized
phos·pho·riz·ing
phos·pho·rol·y·sis
pl phos·pho·rol·y·ses
phos·pho·ro·lyt·ic
phos·pho·rous
adjective (*see* phosphorus)
phos·pho·rus
noun (*see* phosphorous)
phos·pho·ryl
phos·phor·y·lase
phos·phor·y·late
phos·phor·y·lat·ed
phos·phor·y·lat·ing
phos·phor·y·la·tion
phos·phor·y·la·tive
phos·pho·tung·state
phos·pho·tung·stic
phos·vi·tin
pho·tal·gia
pho·tic
pho·tism
pho·to·al·ler·gy
pl pho·to·al·ler·gies
pho·to·bi·o·log·ic
or pho·to·bio·log·i·cal
pho·to·bi·ol·o·gist
pho·to·bi·ol·o·gy
pl pho·to·bi·ol·o·gies
pho·to·bi·ot·ic
pho·to·ca·tal·y·sis
pl pho·to·ca·tal·y·ses
pho·to·cat·a·lyst
pho·to·cat·a·lyt·ic
pho·to·chem·i·cal
pho·to·chem·i·cal·ly
pho·to·chem·ist
pho·to·chem·is·try
pl pho·to·chem·is·tries
pho·to·co·ag·u·la·tion
pho·to·co·ag·u·la·tive
pho·to·co·ag·u·la·tor
pho·to·de·com·po·si·tion
pho·to·dy·nam·ic
pho·to·dy·nam·i·cal·ly
pho·to·elec·tric
pho·to·elec·tric·i·ty
pl pho·to·elec·tric·i·ties
pho·to·elec·tron
pho·to·flu·o·ro·graph·ic
pho·to·flu·o·rog·ra·phy
pl pho·to·flu·o·rog·ra·phies
pho·to·flu·o·ros·co·py
pl pho·to·flu·o·ros·co·pies
pho·to·gene
pho·to·ge·nic
pho·to·in·duced
pho·to·in·duc·tion
pho·to·in·duc·tive
pho·to·ki·ne·sis
pl pho·to·ki·ne·ses
pho·to·ki·net·ic
pho·to·ky·mo·graph

pho•to•ky•mo•graph•ic
pho•to•lu•mi•nes•cence
pho•to•lu•mi•nes•cent
pho•tol•y•sis
pl pho•tol•y•ses
pho•to•lyt•ic
pho•to•lyt•i•cal•ly
pho•to•lyze
pho•to•lyzed
pho•to•lyz•ing
pho•to•mac•ro•graph
pho•to•mac•ro•graph•ic
pho•to•mac•rog•ra•phy
pl pho•to•mac•rog•ra•phies
pho•tom•e•ter
pho•to•met•ric
also pho•to•met•ri•cal
pho•to•met•ri•cal•ly
pho•tom•e•try
pl pho•tom•e•tries
pho•to•mi•cro•gram
pho•to•mi•cro•graph
pho•to•mi•crog•ra•pher
pho•to•mi•cro•graph•ic
also pho•to•mi•cro•graph•i•cal
pho•to•mi•cro•graph•i•cal•ly
pho•to•mi•crog•ra•phy
pl pho•to•mi•crog•ra•phies
pho•ton
pho•to•neg•a•tive
pho•ton•o•sus
pl pho•ton•o•si
pho•to•path•ic
pho•top•a•thy
pl pho•top•a•thies
pho•to•pe•ri•od
pho•to•pe•ri•od•ic
or pho•to•pe•ri•od•i•cal
pho•to•pe•ri•od•i•cal•ly
pho•to•pe•ri•od•ism
pho•to•phil•ic
also pho•toph•i•lous
or pho•to•phile
pho•to•pho•bia
pho•to•pho•bic
pho•to•phore
pho•to•phos•phor•y•la•tion
pho•toph•thal•mia
phot•opia
phot•opic
pho•to•pos•i•tive
pho•top•sia
phot•op•tom•e•ter
pho•to•re•ac•tion
pho•to•re•ac•ti•vat•ing
pho•to•re•ac•ti•va•tion
pho•to•re•cep•tion
pho•to•re•cep•tive
pho•to•re•cep•tor
pho•to•re•duc•tion
pho•to•scope
pho•to•sen•si•tive
pho•to•sen•si•tiv•i•ty
pl pho•to•sen•si•tiv•i•ties
pho•to•sen•si•ti•za•tion
pho•to•sen•si•tize
pho•to•sen•si•tized
pho•to•sen•si•tiz•ing
pho•to•sen•si•tiz•er
pho•to•shock
pho•to•sta•bil•i•ty
pl pho•to•sta•bil•i•ties
pho•to•sta•ble
pho•to•syn•the•sis
pl pho•to•syn•the•ses
pho•to•syn•the•size
pho•to•syn•the•sized
pho•to•syn•the•siz•ing
pho•to•syn•thet•ic

pho·to·syn·thet·i·cal·ly
pho·to·tac·tic
pho·to·tac·ti·cal·ly
pho·to·tax·is
also pho·to·taxy
pl pho·to·tax·es
also pho·to·tax·ies

pho·to·ther·a·py
pl pho·to·ther·a·pies

pho·to·ther·mal
also pho·to·ther·mic

pho·to·tim·er
pho·tot·o·nus
pho·to·troph·ic
pho·to·tro·pic
pho·to·tro·pi·cal·ly
pho·tot·ro·pism
phrag·mo·plast
phren
pl phre·nes

phren·as·the·nia
phren·em·phrax·is
pl phren·em·phrax·es

phre·net·ic
also phre·net·i·cal

phren·ic
phren·i·cec·to·my
pl phren·i·cec·to·mies

phren·i·cla·sia
or phren·i·cla·sis
pl phren·i·cla·si·as
or phren·i·cla·ses

phren·i·cot·o·my
pl phren·i·cot·o·mies

phreno·car·dia
phreno·car·di·ac
phreno·gas·tric
phreno·glot·tic
phre·no·log·i·cal
also phre·no·log·ic

phre·no·log·i·cal·ly
phre·nol·o·gist
phre·nol·o·gy
pl phre·nol·o·gies

phreno·ple·gia
phren·o·sin
phren·o·sin·ic
phreno·splen·ic
phren·sy
var of frenzy

phry·nin
phry·no·der·ma
phthal·ate
phtha·lein
phthal·ic
phthal·in
phthal·yl·sul·fa·thi·a·zole
phthi·o·col
phthi·o·ic
phthi·ri·a·sis
pl phthi·ri·a·ses

Phthir·i·us
phthis·ic
or phthis·i·cal

phthis·icky
phthis·i·ol·o·gist
phthis·i·ol·o·gy
pl phthis·i·ol·o·gies

phthis·io·ther·a·py
pl phthis·io·ther·a·pies

phthi·sis
pl phthi·ses

phthi·sis bul·bi
phy·co·bil·in
phy·co·chrome
also phy·co·chrom

phy·co·cy·a·nin
or phy·co·cy·an

phy·co·er·y·thrin
phy·co·my·cete
Phy·co·my·ce·tes
phy·co·my·ce·tous
phygo·ga·lac·tic
phyl·lo·por·phy·rin
phyl·lo·pyr·role
phyl·lo·qui·none
phy·lum
pl phy·la

phy·ma
pl phy·mas
or phy·ma·ta

phy·mat·ic
phy·ma·tor·rhy·sin
phy·ma·to·sis
pl phy·ma·to·ses

phy·sa·lis
Phy·sa·lop·tera
phys·i·an·thro·py
pl phys·i·an·thro·pies

phys·iat·rics
also phys·iat·ric

phys·iat·rist
phys·ic
phys·icked
phys·ick·ing
phys·ics
or phys·icks

phys·i·cal
phy·si·cian
phy·si·cian·ly
phys·i·cist
phys·icky
phys·i·co·chem·i·cal
phys·i·co·chem·i·cal·ly
phys·ics
phys·io·gen·ic
phys·i·og·nom·ic
also phys·i·og·nom·i·cal

phys·i·og·nom·i·cal·ly
phys·i·og·no·mist
phys·i·og·no·my
pl phys·i·og·no·mies

phys·i·o·log·i·cal
or phys·i·o·log·ic

phys·i·o·log·i·cal·ly
phys·i·ol·o·gist
phys·i·ol·o·gy
pl phys·i·ol·o·gies

phys·io·path·o·log·ic
also phys·io·path·o·log·i·cal

phys·io·pa·thol·o·gy
pl phys·io·pa·thol·o·gies

phys·io·psy·chic
phys·io·ther·a·peu·tic
phys·io·ther·a·peu·tics
phys·io·ther·a·pist
phys·io·ther·a·py
pl phys·io·ther·apies

phy·sique
Phy·so·ceph·a·lus
phy·so·stig·ma
phy·so·stig·mine
phyt·al·bu·mose
phy·tase
phy·to·be·zoar
phy·to·chem·i·cal
phy·to·chem·i·cal·ly
phy·to·chem·ist
phy·to·chem·is·try
pl phy·to·chem·is·tries

phy·to·chrome
Phy·to·fla·gel·la·ta
phy·to·flu·ene
phy·to·gen·e·sis
pl phy·to·gen·e·ses

phy·to·gen·ic

phy·to·he·mag·glu·ti·nin
also phy·to·hae·mag·glu·ti·nin

phy·to·hor·mone
phy·toid
phy·tol
Phy·to·mas·ti·gi·na
phy·to·na·di·one
phy·to·par·a·site
phy·to·patho·gen
phy·to·patho·gen·ic
phy·to·patho·gen·i·ci·ty
pl phy·to·patho·gen·i·ci·ties

phy·to·patho·log·i·cal
or phy·to·patho·log·ic

phy·to·pa·thol·o·gist
phy·to·pa·thol·o·gy
pl phy·to·pa·thol·o·gies

phy·toph·a·gous
phy·toph·a·gy
pl phy·toph·a·gies

phy·to·phar·ma·col·o·gy
pl phy·to·phar·ma·col·o·gies

phy·to·pneu·mo·co·ni·o·sis
pl phy·to·pneu·mo·co·ni·o·ses

phy·to·sis
pl phy·to·ses
phy·tos·ter·ol
phy·to·tox·ic
phy·to·tox·ic·i·ty
pl phy·to·tox·ic·i·ties
phy·to·tox·in
phy·to·tron
phy·tyl
pia
pia-arach·noid
or pi·arach·noid
pia-arach·noi·dal
pi·al
pia ma·ter
pia·ma·tral
pi·an
pi·blok·to
or pi·block·to
pi·ca
pic·e·ous
pi·chi
Pick's dis·ease
Pick·wick·ian syn·drome
pic·nom·e·ter
var of pycnometer
pi·cor·na·vi·rus
pic·rate
pic·ric
pic·ro·car·mine
pic·ro·podo·phyl·lin
pic·ro·rhi·za
pic·ro·tin
pic·ro·tox·in
pic·ro·tox·in·in
pic·ryl
pic·to·graph
pie·bald
pie·bald·ism
pie·dra
pi·ezo·chem·is·try
pl pi·ezo·chem·is·tries
pi·ezom·e·ter
pi·ezo·met·ric
pig·ment
pig·men·ta·tion
pig·men·to·phage
Pi·gnet in·dex
pig·weed
pi·lar
pi·la·ry
pi·las·ter
pi·las·tered
pi·le·ous
pi·le·us
pl pi·lei
pi·li·be·zoar
pi·li·gan
pil·lar
pil·let
pil·lion
pi·lo·car·pi·dine
pi·lo·car·pine
pi·lo·car·pus
pi·lo·cys·tic
pi·lo·erec·tion
pi·lo·mo·tor
pi·lo·ni·dal
pi·lose
pi·lo·se·ba·ceous
pi·lo·sis
pi·los·i·ty
pl pi·los·i·ties
pil·u·lar
or pil·lu·lar
pil·ule
or pil·lute
pi·lus
pl pi·li
pi·mel·ic
pim·ple
pim·pled
pim·pling
pim·ply
pi·nac·o·lone
pin·bone
pin·cers
pi·ne·al
pin·e·a·lo·ma
pl pin·e·a·lo·mas
or pin·e·a·lo·ma·ta
pi·nene
pin·guec·u·la
also pin·guic·u·la
pl pin·guec·u·lae
also pin·guic·u·lae
pink·eye
pin·na
pl pin·nae
or pin·nas
pin·nal
pi·no·cy·to·sis
pl pi·no·cy·to·ses
pi·no·cy·tot·ic
pi·no·cy·tot·i·cal·ly
pin·ta
pin·tid

pin·to
pl pin·tos

pin·worm
pi·per·a·zine
pi·per·i·dine
pip·er·ine
pi·per·o·caine
pi·per·o·nal
pip·er·ox·an
pi·pette
also pi·pet

pip·sis·se·wa
pir·i·form
var of pyriform

pir·i·for·mis
or pyr·i·for·mis

piro·plasm
or piro·plas·ma
pl piro·plasms
or piro·plas·ma·ta

Piro·plas·ma
piro·plas·mic
piro·plas·mo·sis
pl piro·plas·mo·ses

Pir·quet test
also Pir·quet re·ac·tion

pi·sci·ci·dal
pi·sci·cide
pi·si·form
pitch·blende
pithe·coid
pi·tu·i·cyte
pitu·i·ta
pl pitu·i·tae

pi·tu·itary
pl pi·tu·itar·ies

pit·y·ri·as·ic
pit·y·ri·a·sis
pl pit·y·ri·a·ses

piv·ot
pla·ce·bo
pl pla·ce·bos

pla·cen·ta
pl pla·cen·tas
also pla·cen·tae

pla·cen·tal
pla·cen·ta pre·via
pl pla·cen·tae pre·vi·ae

plac·en·ta·tion
plac·en·ti·tis
pl plac·en·tit·i·des

plac·en·tog·ra·phy
pl plac·en·tog·ra·phies

plac·en·to·ma
pl plac·en·to·mas
or plac·en·to·ma·ta

plac·ode
placque
var of plaque

pla·gio·ce·phal·ic
pla·gio·ceph·a·ly
pl pla·gio·ceph·a·lies

plague
plan·chet
pla·ni·gram
pla·ni·graph
pla·nig·ra·phy
pl pla·nig·ra·phies

pla·nim·e·ter
pla·ni·met·ric
pla·no-con·cave
pla·no-con·vex
Pla·nor·bis
plan·ta·go
plan·tar
plan·tar·is
pl plan·tar·es

plan·ta·tion
plan·ti·grade
plan·u·la
pl plan·u·lae

pla·num
pl pla·na

plaque
also placque

plas·ma
plas·ma·blast
plas·ma·cyte
plas·ma·cy·toid
plas·ma·cy·to·sis
pl plas·ma·cy·to·ses
or plas·ma·cy·to·sis·es

plas·ma·gel
plas·mal
plas·ma·lem·ma
plas·mal·o·gen
plas·ma·pher·e·sis
pl plas·ma·pher·e·ses

plas·ma·sol
plas·mat·ic
plas·ma·tor·rhex·is
pl plas·ma·tor·rhex·es

plas·mic
plas·mi·cal·ly

plas•mid
plas•min
plas•min•o•gen
plas•mo•cy•to•ma
or plas•ma•cy•to•ma
pl plas•mo•cy•to•mas
or plas•mo•cy•to•ma•ta
or plas•ma•cy•to•mas
or plas•ma•cy•to•ma•ta

plas•mo•des•ma
also plas•mo•desm
pl plas•mo•des•ma•ta
or plas•mo•des•mas
also plas•mo•desms

plas•mo•di•al
also plas•mod•ic
or plas•mo•di•ate

plas•mo•di•a•sis
also plas•mo•di•o•sis
pl plas•mo•di•a•ses
or plas•mo•di•o•ses

plas•mo•di•cide
plas•mo•di•tro•pho•blast
plas•mo•di•um
pl plas•mo•dia

plas•mog•a•my
pl plas•mog•a•mies

plas•mol•y•sis
pl plas•mol•y•ses

plas•mo•lyt•ic
plas•mo•lyt•i•cal•ly
plas•mo•lyz•abil•i•ty
pl plas•mo•lyz•abil•i•ties

plas•mo•lyz•able
plas•mo•lyze
plas•mo•lyzed
plas•mo•lyz•ing
plas•mon
also plas•mone

plas•mop•ty•sis
pl plas•mop•ty•ses

plas•mo•some
or plas•mo•so•ma
or plas•ma•some

plas•mot•o•my
pl plas•mot•o•mies

plas•tein
plas•ter of Par•is
plas•tic
plas•tic•i•ty
pl plas•tic•i•ties

plas•ti•ciz•er
plas•tics
plas•tid
plas•tid•i•al
plas•tin
plas•tog•a•my
pl plas•tog•a•mies

plas•to•qui•none
pla•teau
pl pla•teaus
or pla•teaux

plate•let
pla•tin•ic
plat•i•nous
plat•i•num
plat•ode
platy•ce•lous
or platy•coe•lous
also platy•ce•lian
or platy•coe•lian
platy•ce•phal•ic
also platy•ceph•a•lous

platy•ceph•a•ly
also platy•ceph•a•lism
pl platy•ceph•a•lies
also platy•ceph•a•lisms

plat•ycne•mia
plat•ycne mic
plat•ycne•my
pl plat•ycne•mies

platy•cra•nia
platy•hel•minth
pl platy•hel•minths

Platy•hel•minth•es
platy•hel•min•thic
platy•hi•er•ic
platy•mer•ic
platy•ope
platy•o•pia
platy•op•ic
platy•pel•lic
platy•pel•loid
platy•pel•ly
pl platy•pel•lies

platy•po•dia
plat•yr•rhine
also plat•yr•rhin•i•an
or plat•y•rhine
or plat•y•rhin•i•an

plat•yr•rhin•ic
plat•yr•rhi•ny
pl plat•yr•rhi•nies

pla•tys•ma
pl pla•tys•ma•ta
also pla•tys•mas

plat·ys·ten·ce·phal·ic
plat·ys·ten·ceph·a·ly
pl plat·ys·ten·ceph·a·lies
plec·trid·i·um
pl plec·trid·ia
pled·get
pleio·tro·pic
plei·ot·ro·pism
plei·ot·ro·py
pl plei·ot·ro·pies
pleo·chro·ic
ple·och·ro·ism
ple·och·ro·ous
pleo·cy·to·sis
pl pleo·cy·to·ses
pleo·mas·tia
pleo·mas·tic
pleo·ma·zia
pleo·mor·phic
also pleio·mor·phic
pleo·mor·phism
pleo·mor·phous
ple·o·nasm
ple·o·nex·ia
ple·oph·a·gous
ples·sor
pleth·o·ra
pleth·o·ric
ple·thys·mo·gram
ple·thys·mo·graph
ple·thys·mo·graph·ic
ple·thys·mo·graph·i·cal·ly
pleth·ys·mog·ra·phy
pl pleth·ys·mog·ra·phies
pleu·ra
pl pleu·rae
or pleu·ras
pleu·ral
pleur·apoph·y·sis
pl pleur·apoph·y·ses
pleu·ri·sy
pl pleu·ri·sies
pleu·rit·ic
pleu·ri·tis
pl pleu·rit·i·des
pleu·ro·cen·trum
pl pleu·ro·cen·trums
or pleu·ro·cen·tra
pleur·odont
pleu·ro·dyn·ia
pleu·ro·gen·ic
or pleu·rog·e·nous
pleu·rol·y·sis
pl pleu·rol·y·ses
pleu·ro·peri·car·di·tis
pl pleu·ro·peri·car·dit·i·des
pleu·ro·peri·to·ne·um
pl pleu·ro·peri·to·ne·ums
or pleu·ro·peri·to·nea
pleu·ro·pneu·mo·nia
pleu·ro·pneu·mo·nia-like or·gan·ism
pleu·ro·pul·mo·nary
pleu·ro·thot·o·nos
pleu·ro·vis·cer·al
plexi·form
plex·im·e·ter
plex·i·met·ric
plex·im·e·try
pl plex·im·e·tries
plex·or
plex·us
pli·ca
pl pli·cae
pli·ca ala·ris
pl pli·cae ala·res
pli·ca cir·cu·la·ris
pl pli·cae cir·cu·la·res
pli·cal
pli·ca po·lon·i·ca
pl pli·cae po·lon·i·cae
pli·cate
pli·cate·ly
pli·cate·ness
pli·ca·tion
ploi·dy
pl ploi·dies
plom·bage
plum·ba·gin
plum·ba·go
pl plum·ba·gos
plum·bic

plum·bism
plum·bum
Plum·mer-Vin·son syn·drome
plu·mose
plump·er
plu·ri·glan·du·lar
plu·ri·loc·u·lar
plu·rip·a·ra
pl plu·rip·a·rae

plu·rip·o·tent
plu·ri·po·ten·ti·al·i·ty
pl plu·ri·po·ten·ti·al·i·ties

plu·to·ma·nia
plu·to·nism
plu·to·ni·um
pneu·ma
pneu·mat·ic
pneu·mat·i·cal·ly
pneu·ma·tic·i·ty
pl pneu·ma·tic·i·ties

pneu·mat·ics
pneu·ma·tism
pneu·ma·ti·za·tion
pneu·ma·tized
pneu·ma·to·cele
pneu·ma·to·gram
pneu·ma·to·graph
pneu·ma·tom·e·ter
pneu·ma·tom·e·try
pl pneu·ma·tom·e·tries
pneu·ma·to·sis
pl pneu·ma·to·ses
pneu·ma·tu·ria
pneu·mec·to·my
pl pneu·mec·to·mies
pneu·mo·ba·cil·lus
pl pneu·mo·ba·cil·li
pneu·mo·cele
pneu·mo·cen·te·sis
pl pneu·mo·cen·te·ses
pneu·mo·coc·cal
also pneu·mo·coc·cic
pneu·mo·coc·ce·mia
pneu·mo·coc·cus
pl pneu·mo·coc·ci
pneu·mo·co·ni·o·sis
or pneu·mo·ko·ni·o·sis
also pneu·mo·no·co·ni·o·sis
or pneu·mo·no·ko·ni·o·sis
pl pneu·mo·co·ni·o·ses
or pneu·mo·ko·ni·o·ses
also pneu·mo·no·co·ni·o·ses
or pneu·mo·no·ko·ni·o·ses
pneu·mo·en·ceph·a·li·tis
pl pneu·mo·en·ceph·a·lit·i·des
pneu·mo·en·ceph·a·lo·gram
pneu·mo·en·ceph·a·lo·graph
pneu·mo·en·ceph·a·lo·graph·ic
pneu·mo·en·ceph·a·lo·graph·i·cal·ly
pneu·mo·en·ceph·a·log·ra·phy
pl pneu·mo·en·ceph·a·log·ra·phies

pneu·mo·en·ter·i·tis
pl pneu·mo·en·ter·it·i·des
or pneu·mo·en·ter·i·tis·es

pneu·mo·gas·tric
pneu·mo·gram
pneu·mo·graph
pneu·mo·graph·ic
pneu·mo·graph·i·cal·ly
pneu·mog·ra·phy
pl pneu·mog·ra·phies

pneu·mo·he·mo·tho·rax
also pneu·mo·hae·mo·tho·rax
pl pneu·mo·he·mo·tho·rax·es
or pneu·mo·he·mo·tho·ra·ces
also pneu·mo·hae·mo·tho·rax·es
or pneu·mo·hae·mo·tho·ra·ces

pneu·mo·hy·dro·tho·rax
pl pneu·mo·hy·dro·tho·rax·es
or pneu·mo·hy·dro·tho·ra·ces

pneu·mol·o·gy
pl pneu·mol·o·gies

pneu·mol·y·sis
pl pneu·mol·y·ses

pneu·mo·me·di·as·ti·num
pl pneu·mo·me·di·as·ti·na

pneu·mo·my·co·sis
pl pneu·mo·my·co·ses

pneu·mo·nec·to·my
pl pneu·mo·nec·to·mies

pneu·mo·nia

pneu·mon·ic

pneu·mo·ni·tis
pl pneu·mon·it·i·des

pneu·mo·no·co·ni·o·sis
var of pneumoconiosis

pneu·mo·nol·y·sis
pl pneu·mo·nol·y·ses

pneu·mo·no·ul·tra·mi·cro·scop·ic·sil·i·co·vol·ca·no·co·ni·o·sis
pl pneu·mo·no·ul·tra·mi·cro·scop·ic·sil·i·co·vol·ca·no·co·ni·o·ses

Pneu·mo·nys·sus

pneu·mo·peri·car·di·um
pl pneu·mo·peri·car·dia

pneu·mo·peri·to·ne·um
pl pneu·mo·peri·to·ne·ums
or pneu·mo·peri·to·nea

pneu·mo·peri·to·ni·tis

pneu·mo·tach·o·gram

pneu·mo·tach·o·graph

pneu·mo·tax·ic

pneu·mo·tho·rax
pl pneu·mo·tho·rax·es
or pneu·mo·tho·ra·ces

pneu·mo·tro·pic

pock·mark

po·dag·ra

po·dag·ral

po·dag·ric

po·dag·rous

po·dal·ic

po·di·at·ric

po·di·a·trist

po·di·a·try
pl po·di·a·tries

podo·derm

podo·der·ma·ti·tis
pl podo·der·ma·ti·ti·ses
or podo·der·ma·tit·i·des

po·dol·o·gy
pl po·dol·o·gies

podo·phyl·lin

podo·phyl·lo·tox·in

podo·phyl·lum
pl podo·phyl·li
or podo·phyl·lums

po·go·ni·on

poi·kilo·blast

poi·kilo·blas·tic

poi·kilo·cyte

poi·kilo·cy·to·sis
pl poi·kilo·cy·to·ses

poi·ki·lo·der·ma
pl poi·ki·lo·der·mas
or poi·ki·lo·der·ma·ta

poi·ki·lo·therm

poi·ki·lo·ther·mic
also poi·ki·lo·ther·mal
or poi·ki·lo·ther·mous

poi·ki·lo·ther·mism

poi·ki·lo·ther·my
pl poi·ki·lo·ther·mies

poin·til·lage

Poi·seuille's law

poi·son
poi·soned
poi·son·ing

poi·son·ous

po·lar·im·e·ter

po·lari·met·ric

po·lar·im·e·try
pl po·lar·im·e·tries

po·lari·scope

po•lari•scop•ic
po•lari•scop•i•cal•ly
po•lar•i•ty
pl po•lar•i•ties
po•lar•iza•tion
po•lar•ize
po•lar•ized
po•lar•iz•ing
po•lar•iz•er
po•lar•o•gram
po•laro•graph•ic
po•laro•graph•i•cal•ly
po•lar•og•ra•phy
pl po•lar•og•ra•phies
Po•len•ske val•ue
also Po•len•ske num•ber
pol•i•clin•ic
outpatient dispensary (*see* polyclinic)
po•lio
po•lio•en•ceph•a•li•tis
pl po•lio•en•ceph•a•lit•i•des
po•lio•en•ceph•a•lo•my•eli•tis
pl po•lio•en•ceph•a•lo•my•elit•i•des
po•lio•my•el•itic
po•lio•my•eli•tis
pl po•lio•my•elit•i•des
po•li•o•sis
pl po•li•o•ses
po•lio•vi•rus
po•litz•er bag
pol•len
pol•lex
pl pol•li•ces
pol•li•cal
pol•li•no•sis
or pol•len•osis
pl pol•li•no•ses
or pol•len•oses
pol•lu•tion
po•lo•cyte
po•lo•ni•um
poly
pl pol•ys
poly•ac•id
poly•acryl•amide
poly•al•co•hol
poly•am•ide
poly•amine
poly•an•dry
pl poly•an•dries
poly•ar•ter•i•tis
poly•ar•thri•tis
pl poly•ar•thri•ti•des
poly•ar•tic•u•lar
poly•ax•on
also poly•ax•one
poly•ba•sic
poly•blast
poly•blas•tic
poly•cen•tric
poly•chro•ma•sia
poly•chro•mat•ic
poly•chro•mato•phil
poly•chro•mato•phile
poly•chro•mato•phil•ia
poly•chro•mato•phil•ic
poly•chro•mia
poly•clin•ic
hospital (*see* policlinic)
poly•crot•ic
poly•cy•clic
poly•cy•e•sis
pl poly•cy•e•ses
poly•cys•tic
poly•cy•the•mia
poly•cy•the•mia ve•ra
poly•cy•the•mic
poly•dac•tyl
poly•dac•tyl•ism
poly•dac•ty•lous
poly•dac•ty•ly
pl poly•dac•ty•lies
poly•dip•sia
also poly•dyp•sia
poly•dip•sic
poly•elec•tro•lyte
poly•em•bry•o•ny
pl poly•em•bry•o•nies
poly•ene
poly•enic
poly•es•trous
poly•ga•lac•tia
poly•ga•lac•tu•ro•nase
poly•gam•ic
po•lyg•a•mist

po·lyg·a·mous
po·lyg·a·my
pl po·lyg·a·mies
poly·gas·tric
poly·gene
poly·gen·ic
poly·glan·du·lar
poly·glo·bu·lia
poly·glob·u·lism
poly·gram
poly·graph
poly·graph·ic
poly·graph·i·cal·ly
po·lyg·y·nist
po·lyg·y·nous
po·lyg·y·ny
pl po·lyg·y·nies
poly·gy·ria
poly·he·dral
poly·hi·dro·sis
also poly·idro·sis
pl poly·hi·dro·ses
also poly·idro·ses
poly·hy·brid
poly·hy·dram·ni·os
poly·mas·tia
also poly·mas·ty
pl poly·mas·tias
also poly·mas·ties
poly·mas·ti·gote
poly·me·lia
also po·lym·e·ly
pl poly·me·lias
also po·lym·e·lies
poly·men·or·rhea
also poly·men·or·rhoea

poly·mer
poly·mer·ase
poly·me·ria
poly·mer·ic
poly·mer·i·cal·ly
po·ly·mer·ism
po·ly·mer·iza·tion
po·ly·mer·ize
po·ly·mer·ized
po·ly·mer·iz·ing
poly·mi·cro·bi·al
also poly·mi·cro·bic
poly·morph
poly·mor·phic
poly·mor·phi·cal·ly
poly·mor·phism
poly·mor·pho·nu·cle·ar
poly·mor·phous
poly·mor·phous·ly
poly·my·o·si·tis
poly·myx·in
poly·neu·rit·ic
poly·neu·ri·tis
pl poly·neu·rit·i·des
or poly·neu·ri·tis·es
poly·neu·rop·a·thy
pl poly·neu·rop·a·thies
poly·nu·cle·ar
poly·nu·cle·o·sis
pl poly·nu·cle·o·ses
poly·nu·cle·o·tide
poly·odon·tia
poly·oma

poly·opia
poly·opic
poly·or·chi·dism
poly·or·chis
poly·os·tot·ic
poly·ovu·lar
poly·ovu·la·tion
pol·yp
pol·yp·ec·to·my
pl pol·yp·ec·to·mies
poly·pep·tide
poly·pha·gia
also po·lyph·a·gy
pl poly·pha·gias
also po·lyph·a·gies
po·lyph·a·gous
poly·pha·lan·gism
poly·phar·ma·cy
pl poly·phar·ma·cies
poly·pho·bia
poly·phy·let·ic
poly·phy·let·i·cal·ly
poly·phyle·tism
poly·phyle·tist
poly·phy·odont
poly·plas·tic
poly·ploid
poly·ploi·dy
pl poly·ploi·dies
po·lyp·nea
po·lyp·ne·ic
poly·pod
poly·po·dia
pol·yp·oid
or pol·yp·oi·dal
pol·yp·o·sis
pl pol·yp·o·ses

pol·yp·ous
poly·pus
pl poly·pi
or poly·pus·es
poly·ra·dic·u·li·tis
poly·ri·bo·nu·cle·o·tide
poly·ri·bo·som·al
poly·ri·bo·some
poly·sac·cha·ride
poly·scope
poly·scop·ic
poly·se·ro·si·tis
poly·some
poly·so·mic
poly·so·my
pl poly·so·mies
poly·sor·bate
poly·sper·mic
poly·sper·my
pl poly·sper·mies
poly·sty·rene
poly·syn·ap·tic
poly·syn·ap·ti·cal·ly
poly·tene
poly·the·lia
po·lyt·o·cous
poly·tro·phic
poly·trop·ic
poly·un·sat·u·rat·ed
poly·uria
poly·va·lence
or poly·va·len·cy
pl poly·va·lences
or poly·va·len·cies
poly·va·lent
poly·vi·nyl
poly·vi·nyl·pyr·rol·idone
po·made
po·man·der
po·ma·tum
pome·gran·ate
pom·pho·lyx
pon·der·a·ble
pons
pl pon·tes
pons Va·ro·lii
pl pon·tes Va·ro·lii
pon·tic
pon·tic·u·lus
pl pon·tic·u·li
pon·tile
pon·tine
pon·to·cer·e·bel·lar
pop·li·te·al
pop·lit·e·us
pl pop·lit·ei
por·ce·lain
po·ri·on
pl po·ria
or po·ri·ons
por·no·graph·ic
por·no·graph·i·cal·ly
por·nog·ra·phy
pl por·nog·ra·phies
po·ro·ceph·a·li·a·sis
pl po·ro·ceph·a·li·a·ses
Po·ro·ce·phal·i·dae
Po·ro·ceph·a·lus
po·ro·plas·tic
po·ro·sis
pl po·ro·ses
or po·ro·sis·es
po·ros·i·ty
pl po·ros·i·ties
po·rot·ic
po·rous
por·phin
also por·phine
por·pho·bi·lin·o·gen
por·phyr·ia
por·phy·rin
por·phy·rin·uria
por·phy·rop·sin
por·ta
pl por·tae
por·ta·ca·val
also por·to·ca·val
por·tio
pl porti·o·nes
po·rus
pl po·ri
or po·rus·es
po·si·tion
pos·i·tive
poso·log·ic
also poso·log·i·cal
po·sol·o·gy
pl po·sol·o·gies
post·an·es·thet·ic
post·an·ox·ic
post·ap·o·plec·tic

post·ar·te·ri·o·lar
post·ax·i·al
post·ax·i·al·ly
post·car·di·nal
post·ca·va
post·ca·val
post·cen·tral
post·ci·bal
post·cla·vic·u·lar
post·co·ital
post·com·mis·sure
post·cor·nu
post·em·bry·on·ic
also post·em·bry·o·nal
post·en·ceph·a·lit·ic
post·ep·i·lep·tic
pos·te·ri·ad
pos·te·ri·or
pos·te·ri·or·ly
pos·tero·an·te·ri·or
pos·tero·ex·ter·nal
pos·tero·in·ter·nal
pos·tero·lat·er·al
pos·tero·me·di·al
pos·tero·me·di·an
pos·tero·su·pe·ri·or
pos·tero·tem·po·ral
post·fe·brile
post·gan·gli·on·ic
post·gle·noid
also post·gle·noid·al
post·hem·or·rhag·ic
pos·thi·tis
pl pos·thit·i·des
post·hu·mous
post·hu·mous·ly
post·hyp·not·ic
post·hyp·not·i·cal·ly
post·hy·poph·y·sis
pl post·hy·poph·y·ses
post·ic·tal
post·ir·ra·di·a·tion
post·ma·tu·ri·ty
pl post·ma·tu·ri·ties
post·me·di·an
also post·me·di·al
post·meno·paus·al
post·mor·tal
post·mor·tem
post·na·ris
pl post·na·res
post·na·sal
post·na·tal
post·na·tal·ly
post·oc·u·lar
post·op·er·a·tive
post·oral
post·or·bit·al
post·pal·a·tine
post·par·tum
or post·par·tal
post·pi·tu·itary
post·pran·di·al
post·pran·di·al·ly
post·pu·ber·tal
post·py·ra·mi·dal
post·re·duc·tion
post·scap·u·la
pl post·scap·u·lae
or post·scap·u·las
post·scap·u·lar
post·syn·ap·tic
post·syn·ap·ti·cal·ly
post·trau·mat·ic
post·treat·ment
pos·tur·al
pos·ture
po·tas·sic
po·tas·si·um
po·ten·cy
pl po·ten·cies
po·tent
po·ten·tia
po·ten·tial
po·ten·ti·ate
po·ten·ti·at·ed
po·ten·ti·at·ing
po·ten·ti·a·tion
po·ten·ti·a·tor
po·ten·ti·om·e·ter
po·ten·ti·o·met·ric
po·ten·ti·o·met·ri·cal·ly
po·tion
po·to·ma·nia
Pott's dis·ease
poul·tice

Pou·part's lig·a·ment
pov·er·ty
pl pov·er·ties
po·vi·done
pow·der
pow·dery
pow·er
pox
pl pox
or poxes
pox·vi·rus
prac·ti·tio·ner
pran·di·al
pra·seo·dym·i·um
prax·e·o·log·i·cal
prax·e·ol·o·gy
also prax·i·ol·o·gy
pl prax·e·ol·o·gies
also prax·i·ol·o·gies
prax·is
pl prax·es
pre·ad·o·les·cence
pre·ad·o·les·cent
pre·ag·o·nal
pre·anal
pre·an·es·thet·ic
pre·au·ric·u·lar
pre·ax·i·al
pre·can·cer·ous
pre·cap·il·lary
pre·car·ti·lage
pre·car·ti·lag·i·nous
pre·ca·va
pl pre·ca·vae
pre·ca·val
pre·cen·tral
pre·chord·al
pre·cip·i·ta·bil·i·ty
pl pre·cip·i·ta·bil·i·ties
pre·cip·i·ta·ble
pre·cip·i·tant
pre·cip·i·tate
pre·cip·i·tat·ed
pre·cip·i·tat·ing
pre·cip·i·ta·tion
pre·cip·i·tin
pre·cip·i·tin·o·gen
pre·cip·i·tin·o·gen·ic
pre·clin·i·cal
pre·cog·ni·tion
pre·com·mis·sure
pre·con·scious
pre·con·scious·ly
pre·cop·u·la·to·ry
pre·cor·dial
pre·cor·di·um
pl pre·cor·dia
pre·cor·nu
pl pre·cor·nua
pre·cos·tal
pre·crit·i·cal
pre·cu·ne·us
pl pre·cu·nei
pre·cur·sor
pre·den·tin
pre·di·a·be·tes
pre·di·a·bet·ic
pre·di·a·stol·ic
pre·di·gest
pre·di·ges·tion
pre·dis·pose
pre·dis·posed
pre·dis·pos·ing
pre·dis·po·si·tion
pred·nis·o·lone
pred·ni·sone
pre·eclamp·sia
pre·eclamp·tic
pre·for·ma·tion
pre·fron·tal
pre·gan·gli·on·ic
also pre·gan·gli·ar
pre·gen·i·tal
preg·nan·cy
pl preg·nan·cies
preg·nane
preg·nane·di·ol
preg·nant
preg·nene
preg·nen·in·o·lone
preg·nen·o·lone
pre·hal·lux
pl pre·hal·lu·ces
pre·hen·sile
pre·hen·sil·i·ty
pl pre·hen·sil·i·ties
pre·hen·sion
pre·he·pat·ic
pre·hy·poph·y·sis
pl pre·hy·poph·y·ses
pre·in·cu·ba·tion
pre·in·duc·tion
pre·in·su·la
pl pre·in·su·lae
pre·in·va·sive
pre·leu·ke·mic

pre•ma•lig•nant
pre•mar•i•tal
pre•ma•ture
pre•ma•ture•ly
pre•ma•tu•ri•ty
pl pre•ma•tu•ri•ties
pre•max•il•la
pl pre•max•il•lae
pre•max•il•la•ry
pre•med
pre•me•di•an
pre•med•i•cal
pre•med•i•cate
pre•med•i•cat•ed
pre•med•i•cat•ing
pre•med•i•ca•tion
pre•meno•paus•al
pre•meno•pause
pre•men•stru•al
pre•men•stru•al•ly
pre•men•stru•um
pl pre•men•stru•ums
or pre•men•strua
pre•mo•lar
pre•mon•i•to•ry
also pre•mon•i•tary
pre•mune
pre•mu•ni•tion
also pre•mu•ni•ty
pl pre•mu•ni•tions
also pre•mu•ni•ties
pre•mu•nize
pre•mu•nized
pre•mu•niz•ing
pre•my•elo•cyte

pre•na•ris
pl pre•na•res
pre•na•tal
pre•na•tal•ly
pre•oc•cip•i•tal
pre•op•er•a•tive
pre•op•er•a•tive•ly
pre•op•tic
pre•oral
pre•oral•ly
pre•ovu•la•to•ry
prep
prepped
prep•ping
pre•pal•a•tal
pre•par•a•tor
pre•par•tum
also pre•par•tal
pre•pa•tel•lar
pre•pa•tent
pre•per•cep•tion
pre•per•cep•tive
pre•phe•nic
pre•pla•cen•tal
pre•pon•tine
pre•po•ten•cy
pl pre•po•ten•cies
pre•po•tent
pre•po•tent•ly
pre•psy•chot•ic
pre•pu•ber•tal
or pre•pu•ber•al
pre•pu•ber•tal•ly
or pre•pu•ber•al•ly
pre•pu•ber•ty
pl pre•pu•ber•ties
pre•pu•bes•cence

pre•pu•bes•cent
pre•pu•bic
also pre•pu•bian
pre•puce
pre•pu•tial
also pre•pu•cial
pre•pu•ti•um
pl pre•pu•tia
pre•py•lo•ric
pre•rec•tal
pre•re•pro•duc•tive
pre•ret•i•nal
pre•sa•cral
pres•by•cu•sis
or pres•by•a•cu•sia
also pres•by•a•cou•sia
pl pres•by•cu•ses
or pres•by•a•cu•sias
also pres•by•a•cou•sias
pres•by•ope
pres•by•o•phre•nia
pres•by•o•phren•ic
pres•by•opia
pres•by•opic
pres•byt•ic
pre•scribe
pre•scribed
pre•scrib•ing
pre•scrip•tion
pre•se•nile
pre•se•nil•i•ty
pl pre•se•nil•i•ties
pre•serv•a•tive
pre•so•mite
pre•sphe•noid

pre·sphyg·mic
pres·sor
pres·so·re·cep·tor
pres·so·sen·si·tive
pre·sup·pu·ra·tive
pres·sure
pre·ster·nal
pre·ster·num
pl pre·ster·nums
or pre·ster·na

pre·su·bic·u·lum
pl pre·su·bic·u·la

pre·sump·tive
pre·syl·vi·an
pre·syn·ap·tic
pre·syn·ap·ti·cal·ly
pre·sys·to·le
pre·sys·tol·ic
pre·tem·po·ral
pre·ter·mi·nal
pre·tib·i·al
pre·treat·ment
pre·tu·ber·cu·lous
pre·ven·ta·tive
pre·ven·tive
pre·ven·to·ri·um
pl pre·ven·to·ria
also pre·ven·to·ri·ums

pre·ves·i·cal
pre·vil·lous
pre·zone
pri·a·pism
pri·a·pis·mic
pri·a·pus
pl pri·a·pi
or pri·a·pus·es

pri·ma·quine
pri·mi·grav·i·da
pl pri·mi·grav·i·das
or pri·mi·grav·i·dae

pri·mip·a·ra
pl pri·mip·a·ras
or pri·mip·a·rae

pri·mi·par·i·ty
pl pri·mi·par·i·ties

pri·mip·a·rous
pri·mite
pri·mi·ti·ae
pri·mor·di·al
pri·mor·di·al·ly
pri·mor·di·um
pl pri·mor·dia

prin·ceps
prin·ci·ple
pro·ac·cel·er·in
pro·ac·tive
pro·al
pro·am·ni·on
pl pro·am·ni·ons
or pro·am·nia

pro·am·ni·ot·ic
pro·at·las
pro·bac·te·rio·phage
pro·band
pro·bang
pro·ben·e·cid
pro·bos·cis
pl pro·bos·cis·es
or pro·bos·ci·des

pro·caine
pro·cary·ote
var of prokaryote

pro·cary·otic
var of prokaryotic

pro·cat·arc·tic
pro·ce·phal·ic
pro·cer·coid
pro·ces·sus
pl pro·ces·sus

pro·chord·al
proci·den·tia
pro·con·ver·tin
proct·al·gia
proc·tec·to·my
pl proc·tec·to·mies

proc·ti·tis
proc·to·cly·sis
pl proc·to·cly·ses

proc·to·co·li·tis
proc·to·dae·um
or proc·to·de·um
pl proc·to·daea
or proc·to·dae·ums
or proc·to·dea
or proc·to·de·ums

proc·to·dyn·ia
proc·to·log·ic
or proc·to·log·i·cal

proc·tol·o·gist
proc·tol·o·gy
pl proc·tol·o·gies

proc·to·scope
proc·to·scop·ic
proc·to·scop·i·cal·ly
proc·tos·co·py
pl proc·tos·co·pies

proc·to·sig·moid·ec·to·my
pl proc·to·sig·moid·ec·to·mies

proc·to·sig·moid·o·scope
proc·to·sig·moi·do·scop·ic
proc·to·sig·moid·os·co·py
pl proc·to·sig·moid·os·co·pies

proc·tos·to·my
pl proc·tos·to·mies

pro·cum·bent
pro·dig·i·o·sin
pro·dro·mal
or pro·drom·ic

pro·drome
pl pro·dro·ma·ta
or pro·dromes

pro·emi·al
pro·en·zyme
pro·eryth·ro·blast
pro·eryth·ro·cyte
pro·es·trus
or pro·es·trum
pl pro·es·trus·es
or pro·es·trums

pro·fi·bri·nol·y·sin
pro·fla·vine
pro·fun·da
pl pro·fun·dae

pro·fun·dus
pro·ge·ria
pro·ges·ta·tion·al
pro·ges·ter·one
pro·ges·ter·on·ic
pro·ges·tin
pro·ges·to·gen
pro·glot·tid
pro·glot·tid·e·an
pro·glot·tis
pl pro·glot·ti·des

prog·na·thic
prog·na·thism
also prog·na·thy
pl prog·na·thisms
also prog·na·thies

prog·na·thous
prog·no·sis
pl prog·no·ses

prog·nos·tic
prog·nos·ti·cate
prog·nos·ti·cat·ed
prog·nos·ti·cat·ing
pro·grav·id
pro·ji·cient
pro·ji·cient·ly
pro·kary·ote
or pro·cary·ote

pro·kary·otic
or pro·cary·otic

pro·la·bi·um
pl pro·la·bia

pro·lac·tin
pro·la·min
or pro·la·mine

pro·lan
pro·lapse
pro·lapsed
pro·laps·ing
pro·lap·sus
pro·lep·sis
pl pro·lep·ses

pro·lep·tic
also pro·lep·ti·cal

pro·leu·co·cyte
or pro·leu·ko·cyte

pro·lif·er·ate
pro·lif·er·at·ed
pro·lif·er·at·ing
pro·lif·er·a·tion
pro·lif·er·a·tive
pro·lig·er·ous
pro·line
pro·lo·ther·a·py
pl pro·lo·ther·a·pies

pro·lym·pho·cyte
pro·ma·zine
pro·meg·a·lo·blast
pro·meta·phase
pro·meth·a·zine
pro·me·thi·um
pro·mono·cyte
prom·on·to·ry
pl prom·on·to·ries

pro·mo·tor
pro·my·elo·cyte
pro·nase
pro·nate
pro·nat·ed
pro·nat·ing
pro·na·tion
pro·na·tor
pro·na·tor qua·dra·tus
pro·na·tor te·res
pro·neph·ros
also pro·neph·ron
pl pro·neph·roi
also pro·neph·ra

pro·neth·a·lol

pro·no·grade
pro·nor·mo·blast
pro·nu·cle·us
pl pro·nu·clei
also pro·nu·cle·us·es
pro·otic
prop·a·gate
prop·a·gat·ed
prop·a·gat·ing
prop·a·ga·tion
prop·a·ga·tive
pro·pal·i·nal
pro·pam·i·dine
pro·pane
pro·pa·no·ic
pro·pa·nol
pro·pene
pro·pe·nyl
pro·per·din
pro·peri·to·ne·al
pro·phage
pro·phase
pro·phy·lac·tic
pro·phy·lac·ti·cal·ly
pro·phy·lax·is
pl pro·phy·lax·es
pro·pi·o·nate
pro·pi·oni·bac·te·ri·um
pl pro·pi·oni·bac·te·ria
pro·pi·on·ic
pro·pos·i·tus
pl pro·pos·i·ti
pro·pran·o·lol
pro·pri·etary
pl pro·pri·etar·ies
pro·prio·cep·tion
pro·prio·cep·tive
pro·prio·cep·tor
pro·prio·spi·nal
pro·pto·sis
pl pro·pto·ses
pro·pyl
pro·pyl·ene
pro·pyl·par·a·ben
pro·pyl·thio·ura·cil
pro·sco·lex
pl pro·sco·li·ces
pro·sect
pro·sec·tion
pro·sec·tor
pros·en·ce·phal·ic
pros·en·ceph·a·lon
pl pros·en·ceph·a·la
proso·coel
also proso·cele
or proso·coele
pros·o·dem·ic
pro·sop·ic
pro·sop·i·cal·ly
proso·pla·sia
pros·o·pos·chi·sis
pl pros·o·pos·chi·ses
or pros·o·pos·chi·sis·es
pros·ta·glan·din
pros·tate
pros·ta·tec·to·my
pl pros·ta·tec·to·mies
pros·tat·ic
pros·tat·i·co·ves·i·cal
or pros·ta·to·ves·i·cal
pros·ta·tism
pros·ta·ti·tis
pros·ta·to·cys·ti·tis
pl pros·ta·to·cys·tit·i·des
pros·ta·tog·ra·phy
pl pros·ta·tog·ra·phies
pros·tato·lith
pros·ta·to·ve·sic·u·li·tis
pros·ter·na·tion
pros·the·sis
pl pros·the·ses
pros·thet·ic
pros·thet·i·cal·ly
pros·thet·ics
pros·the·tist
pros·thi·on
prosth·odon·tia
prosth·odon·tics
prosth·odon·tist
Pros·tho·gon·i·mus
pros·tra·tion
prot·ac·tin·i·um
or pro·to·ac·tin·i·um
pro·ta·gon
prot·amine
prot·anom·a·ly
pl prot·anom·a·lies
pro·ta·nope
pro·ta·no·pia

pro·te·an
pro·te·ase
pro·teid
also pro·teide

pro·tein
pro·tein·aceous
pro·tein·ase
pro·tein·ate
pro·tein·oid
pro·tein·uria
pro·teo·clas·tic
pro·teo·lip·id
pro·te·ol·y·sis
pl pro·te·ol·y·ses

pro·teo·lyt·ic
pro·te·ose
pro·te·us
pl pro·tei

proth·e·sis
pl proth·e·ses

pro·throm·bin
pro·tide
pro·tist
Pro·tis·ta
pro·tis·tan
pro·tis·tol·o·gist
pro·tis·tol·o·gy
pl pro·tis·tol·o·gies

pro·ti·um
pro·to·blast
pro·to·blas·tic
pro·to·cat·e·chu·ic
pro·to·cone
pro·to·co·nid
pro·to·derm
pro·to·der·mal
pro·to·gen
pro·to·heme
pro·tom·er·ite
pro·to·path·ic
pro·to·pec·tin
pro·to·plasm
pro·to·plas·mal
or pro·to·plas·mat·ic

pro·to·plas·mic
pro·to·plast
pro·to·por·phy·rin
pro·to·pro·te·ose
pro·to·spasm
Pro·to·stron·gy·lus
pro·to·troph
pro·to·tro·phic
pro·tot·ro·py
pl pro·tot·ro·pies

pro·to·ve·ra·trine
pro·to·ver·te·bra
pl pro·to·ver·te·brae
or pro·to·ver·te·bras

pro·to·ver·te·bral
prot·ox·ide
Pro·to·zoa
pro·to·zo·al
pro·to·zo·an
pro·to·zo·i·a·sis
pl pro·to·zo·i·a·ses

pro·to·zo·ol·o·gist
pro·to·zo·ol·o·gy
pl pro·to·zo·ol·o·gies

pro·trac·tion
pro·trac·tor
pro·tu·ber·ance
pro·tu·ber·ant
pro·ven·tric·u·lus
pl pro·ven·tric·u·li

pro·vi·ral
pro·vi·rus
pro·vi·ta·min
prov·o·ca·tion
pro·voc·a·tive
pro·voke
pro·voked
pro·vok·ing
prox·i·mad
prox·i·mal
prox·i·mal·ly
prox·i·mate
prox·i·mate·ly
prox·i·mo·atax·ia
prox·i·mo·buc·cal
prox·i·mo·la·bi·al
prox·i·mo·lin·gual
pro·zone
pru·i·nate
pru·rig·i·nous
pru·ri·go
pru·rit·ic
pru·ri·tus
prus·si·ate
prus·sic
psal·te·ri·al
psal·te·ri·um
pl psal·te·ria

psam·mo·ma
pl psam·mo·mas
or psam·mo·ma·ta

psam·moma·tous

pseud·ar·thro·sis
also pseu·do·ar·thro·sis
pl pseud·ar·thro·ses
also pseu·do·ar·thro·ses

pseud·es·the·sia

pseu·do·acon·i·tine
or pseud·acon·i·tine
also pseu·do·acon·i·tin

pseu·do·ag·glu·ti·na·tion

pseu·do·ane·mia

pseu·do·an·gi·na

pseu·do·bul·bar

pseu·do·cho·lin·es·ter·ase

pseu·do·chrom·es·the·sia

pseu·do·cir·rho·sis
pl pseu·do·cir·rho·ses

pseu·do·cop·u·la·tion

pseu·do·croup

pseu·do·cy·e·sis
pl pseu·do·cy·e·ses

pseu·do·cyst

pseu·do·diph·the·ria

pseu·do·ephed·rine

pseu·do·far·cy
pl pseu·do·far·cies

pseu·do·glan·ders

pseu·do·glob·u·lin

pseu·do·hal·lu·ci·na·tion

pseu·do·he·mo·phil·ia

pseu·do·her·maph·ro·dite

pseu·do·her·maph·ro·dit·ism

pseu·do·hy·o·scy·a·mine

pseu·do·hy·per·tro·phic

pseu·do·hy·per·tro·phy
pl pseu·do·hy·per·tro·phies

pseu·do·hy·po·para·thy·roid·ism

pseu·do·iso·chro·mat·ic

pseu·do·ker·a·tin

pseu·do·leu·ke·mia

pseu·do·ma·nia

pseu·do·mel·a·no·sis
pl pseu·do·mel·a·no·ses

pseu·do·mem·brane

pseu·do·mem·bra·nous

pseu·do·men·stru·a·tion

pseu·do·mo·nad

pseu·do·mo·nas
pl pseu·do·mon·a·des

pseu·do·neu·ro·ma
pl pseu·do·neu·ro·mas
or pseu·do·neu·ro·ma·ta

pseu·do·pa·ral·y·sis
pl pseu·do·pa·ral·y·ses

pseu·do·par·a·site

Pseu·do·phyl·lid·ea

pseu·do·pod

pseu·do·po·di·um
pl pseu·do·po·dia

pseu·do·preg·nan·cy
pl pseu·do·preg·nan·cies

pseu·do·preg·nant

pseu·dop·sia

pseu·do·pto·sis
pl pseu·do·pto·ses

pseu·do·ra·bies
pl pseu·do·ra·bies

pseu·do·re·ac·tion

pseu·do·scle·ro·sis
pl pseu·do·scle·ro·ses

pseu·dos·to·ma
pl pseu·dos·to·ma·ta
also pseu·dos·to·mas

pseu·do·tro·pine

pseu·do·trun·cus ar·ter·i·o·sus
pseu·do·tu·ber·cle
pseu·do·tu·ber·cu·lo·sis
pl pseu·do·tu·ber·cu·lo·ses

pseu·do·ven·tri·cle
pseu·do·vom·it·ing
pseu·do·xan·tho·ma e·las·ti·cum
psi·lo·cin
psi·lo·cy·bin
psit·ta·co·sis
pl psit·ta·co·ses

pso·as
pl pso·ai
or pso·ae

pso·mo·pha·gia
pso·ra
Psor·er·gates
pso·ri·a·si·form
pso·ri·a·sis
pl pso·ri·a·ses

pso·ri·at·ic
Pso·rop·tes
psy·cha·go·gy
pl psy·cha·go·gies

psy·chal·gia
psych·as·the·nia
psych·as·then·ic
psy·che
psy·chi·at·ric
also psy·chi·at·ri·cal

psy·chi·at·ri·cal·ly
psy·chi·a·trist
psy·chi·a·try
pl psy·chi·a·tries

psy·chic
psy·chi·cal
psy·cho·acous·tic
psy·cho·acous·tics
psy·cho·ac·tive
psy·cho·anal·y·sis
also psych·anal·y·sis
pl psy·cho·anal·y·ses
also psych·anal·y·ses

psy·cho·an·a·lyst
also psych·an·a·lyst

psy·cho·an·a·lyt·ic
or psy·cho·an·a·lyt·i·cal
also psych·an·a·lyt·ic
or psych·an·a·lyt·i·cal

psy·cho·an·a·lyze
psy·cho·an·a·lyzed
psy·cho·an·a·lyz·ing
psy·cho·bi·o·log·ic
or psy·cho·bi·o·log·i·cal

psy·cho·bi·ol·o·gist
psy·cho·bi·ol·o·gy
pl psy·cho·bi·ol·o·gies

psy·cho·ca·thar·sis
pl psy·cho·ca·thar·ses

psy·cho·chem·i·cal
psy·cho·cor·ti·cal
psy·cho·di·ag·no·sis
pl psy·cho·di·ag·no·ses

psy·cho·di·ag·nos·tic
psy·cho·di·ag·nos·tics
Psy·chodi·dae
psy·cho·dra·ma
psy·cho·dy·nam·ic
psy·cho·dy·nam·i·cal·ly
psy·cho·dy·nam·ics
psy·cho·gal·van·ic
psy·cho·gal·va·nom·e·ter
psy·cho·gen·e·sis
pl psy·cho·gen·e·ses

psy·cho·ge·net·ic
psy·cho·gen·ic
psy·cho·gen·i·cal·ly
psy·chog·e·ny
pl psy·chog·e·nies

psy·chog·no·sis
also psy·chog·no·sy
pl psy·chog·no·ses
also psy·chog·no·sies

psy·chog·nos·tic
psy·cho·gram
psy·cho·graph·ic
psy·cho·graph·i·cal·ly
psy·chog·ra·phy
pl psy·chog·ra·phies

psy·cho·ki·ne·sia
psy·cho·ki·ne·sis
pl psy·cho·ki·ne·ses

psy·cho·lep·sy
pl psy·cho·lep·sies

psy·cho·lep·tic
psy·cho·log·i·cal
also psy·cho·log·ic

psy·cho·log·i·cal·ly
psy·chol·o·gist
psy·chol·o·gize
psy·chol·o·gized
psy·chol·o·giz·ing
psy·chol·o·gy
pl psy·chol·o·gies

psy·cho·met·ric
psy·cho·met·ri·cal·ly
psy·chom·e·tri·cian
psy·cho·met·rics
psy·chom·e·try
pl psy·chom·e·tries

psy·cho·mo·tor
psy·cho·neu·ro·sis
pl psy·cho·neu·ro·ses

psy·cho·neu·rot·ic
psy·cho·nom·ics
psy·chon·o·my
pl psy·chon·o·mies

psy·cho·path
psy·cho·path·ia
psy·cho·path·ic
psy·cho·path·i·cal·ly
psy·cho·patho·log·ic
or psy·cho·patho·log·i·cal

psy·cho·pa·thol·o·gist
psy·cho·pa·thol·o·gy
pl psy·cho·pa·thol·o·gies

psy·chop·a·thy
pl psy·chop·a·thies

psy·cho·phar·ma·ceu·ti·cal
psy·cho·phar·ma·co·log·i·cal
or psy·cho·phar·ma·co·log·ic

psy·cho·phar·ma·col·o·gist
psy·cho·phar·ma·col·o·gy
pl psy·cho·phar·ma·col·o·gies

psy·cho·phon·as·the·nia
psy·cho·phys·i·cal
psy·cho·phys·i·cal·ly
psy·cho·phys·i·cist
psy·cho·phys·ics
psy·cho·phys·i·o·log·i·cal
or psy·cho·phys·i·o·log·ic

psy·cho·phys·i·ol·o·gy
pl psy·cho·phys·i·ol·o·gies

psy·cho·quack
psy·cho·quack·ery
pl psy·cho·quack·er·ies

psy·cho·sen·so·ri·al
psy·cho·sen·so·ry
psy·cho·sex·u·al
psy·cho·sex·u·al·i·ty
pl psy·cho·sex·u·al·i·ties

psy·cho·sex·u·al·ly
psy·cho·sis
pl psy·cho·ses

psy·cho·so·cial
psy·cho·so·cial·ly
psy·cho·so·mat·ic
psy·cho·so·mat·i·cal·ly
psy·cho·so·mat·ics
psy·cho·sur·geon

psy·cho·sur·gery
pl psy·cho·sur·ger·ies
psy·cho·sur·gi·cal
psy·cho·syn·the·sis
pl psy·cho·syn·the·ses
psy·cho·ther·a·peu·tic
psy·cho·ther·a·peu·ti·cal·ly
psy·cho·ther·a·peu·tics
psy·cho·ther·a·pist
psy·cho·ther·a·py
pl psy·cho·ther·a·pies
psy·chot·ic
psy·chot·i·cal·ly
psy·chot·o·gen
psy·choto·gen·ic
psy·choto·mi·met·ic
psy·choto·mi·met·cal·ly
psy·cho·tox·ic
psy·cho·trop·ic
psy·chro·es·the·sia
psy·chrom·e·ter
psy·chrom·e·try
pl psy·chrom·e·tries
psy·chro·ther·a·py
pl psy·chro·ther·a·pies
psyl·li·um
ptar·mic
ptar·mus
pteri·on
pte·ryg·i·um
pl pte·ryg·i·ums
or pte·ryg·ia
pter·y·goid
also pter·y·goi·dal
pter·y·go·man·dib·u·lar
pter·y·go·pal·a·tine
pti·lo·sis
pl pti·lo·ses
pto·maine
ptosed
or ptot·ic
pto·sis
pl pto·ses
pty·al·a·gogue
pty·a·lin
pty·a·lism
pty·a·log·ra·phy
pl pty·a·log·ra·phies
pu·ber·tal
or pu·ber·al
pu·ber·tas
pu·ber·ty
pl pu·ber·ties
pu·ber·u·lic
pu·bes
pl pu·bes
pu·bes
pl of pubis
pu·bes·cence
pu·bes·cent
pu·bic
pu·bi·ot·o·my
pl pu·bi·ot·o·mies
pu·bis
pl pu·bes
pu·bo·coc·cy·geal
pu·bo·fem·o·ral
pu·bo·pros·tat·ic
pu·den·dal
pu·den·dum
pl pu·den·da
pu·dic
pu·er·pera
pl pu·er·per·ae
pu·er·per·al
pu·er·pe·ri·um
pl pu·er·pe·ria
Pu·lex
Pu·lic·i·dae
pu·li·ci·dal
pu·li·cide
pul·lo·rum dis·ease
pul·mo·gas·tric
pul·mom·e·ter
pul·mom·e·try
pl pul·mom·e·tries
pul·mo·nary
pul·mo·nate
pul·mo·nec·to·my
pl pul·mo·nec·to·mies
pul·mon·ic
pul·mo·tor
pulp·al
also pulp·ar
pulp·al·ly

pulp·ec·to·my
pl pulp·ec·to·mies

pulp·ot·o·my
pl pulp·ot·o·mies

pulp·stone
pul·que
pul·sate
pul·sat·ed
pul·sat·ing
pul·sa·tile
Pul·sa·til·la
pul·sa·tion
pul·sa·tor
pul·sa·to·ry
pulse
pulsed
puls·ing
pul·sion
pul·sion di·ver·tic·u·lum
pul·sus
pl pul·sus

pul·ta·ceous
pul·ver·i·za·tion
pul·ver·ize
pul·ver·ized
pul·ver·iz·ing
pul·ver·u·lent
pul·vi·nar
pul·vi·nate
or pul·vi·nat·ed

pum·ice
pu·na
punc·tate
punc·ti·form
punc·tum
pl punc·ta

punc·ture
punc·tured
punc·tur·ing
pu·pil
pu·pil·la
pl pu·pil·lae

pu·pil·lary
pu·pil·lom·e·ter
pu·pil·lom·e·try
pl pu·pil·lom·e·tries

pu·pil·lo·mo·tor
pu·pil·lo·sta·tom·e·ter
pur·ga·tion
pur·ga·tive
pu·ri·form
pu·rine
Pur·kin·je af·ter·im·age
Pur·kin·je·an
Pur·kin·je cell
Pur·kin·je fi·ber
Pur·kin·je phe·nom·e·non
or Pur·kin·je shift
also Pur·kin·je ef·fect

Pur·kin·je's fig·ure
or Pur·kin·je fig·ure

Pur·kin·je's net·work
or Pur·kin·je's sys·tem
or Pur·kin·je's tis·sue

pu·ro·my·cin
pur·pu·ra
pur·pu·ra hem·or·rhag·i·ca
pur·pu·ric
pur·pu·rin
pu·ru·lence
also pu·ru·len·cy
pl pu·ru·lenc·es
also pu·ru·len·cies

pu·ru·lent
pu·ru·loid
pus·sy
pus·si·er
pus·si·est
pus·tu·lant
pus·tu·lar
pus·tu·late
pus·tu·lat·ed
pus·tu·lat·ing
pus·tu·la·tion
pus·tule
pus·tu·li·form
pus·tu·lo·sis
pl pus·tu·lo·ses
or pus·tu·lo·sis·es

pu·ta·men
pl pu·tam·i·na

pu·tres·cine
py·ae·mia
var of pyemia

py·ar·thro·sis
pl py·ar·thro·ses

pyc·nic
var of pyk·nic

pyc·nom·e·ter
also pic·nom·e·ter
or pyk·nom·e·ter

pyc·no·mor·phic
also pyc·no·mor·phous

pyc·no·sis
or pyk·no·sis

pyc·not·ic
or pyk·not·ic

py·el·ec·ta·sis
pl py·el·ec·ta·ses

py·el·ic

py·elit·ic

py·eli·tis

py·elo·cys·ti·tis
pl py·elo·cys·tit·i·des

py·elo·gram
also py·elo·graph

py·elo·graph·ic

py·elog·ra·phy
pl py·elog·ra·phies

py·elo·li·thot·o·my
pl py·elo·li·thot·o·mies

py·elo·ne·phrit·ic

py·elo·ne·phri·tis
pl py·elo·ne·phrit·i·des

py·elo·ne·phro·sis
pl py·elo·ne·phro·ses

py·elos·to·my
pl py·elos·to·mies

py·elo·ure·ter·o·gram

py·elo·ve·nous

py·emia
or py·ae·mia

py·emic

py·esis

py·gal

py·gal·gia

pyg·ma·lion·ism

py·gop·a·gus
pl py·gop·a·gi

pyk·nic
also pyc·nic

pyk·no·ep·i·lep·sy
pl pyk·no·ep·i·lep·sies

pyk·no·lep·sy
pl pyk·no·lep·sies

pyk·nom·e·ter
var of pycnometer

pyk·no·sis
var of pycnosis

pyk·not·ic
var of pycnotic

py·la
pl py·las
or py·lae

py·lar

py·le·phle·bec·ta·sis
pl py·le·phle·bec·ta·ses

py·le·phle·bi·tis
pl py·le·phle·bit·i·des

py·le·throm·bo·sis
pl py·le·throm·bo·ses

py·lic

py·lon

py·lor·ic

py·lo·ri·tis

py·lo·ro·gas·trec·to·my
pl py·lo·ro·gas·trec·to·mies

py·lo·ro·my·ot·o·my
pl py·lo·ro·my·ot·o·mies

py·lo·ro·plas·ty
pl py·lo·ro·plas·ties

py·lo·ro·spasm

py·lo·rot·o·my
pl py·lo·rot·o·mies

py·lo·rus
pl py·lo·ri
also py·lo·rus·es

pyo·cele

pyo·coc·cus
pl pyo·coc·ci

pyo·col·pos

pyo·cy·a·nase

pyo·cy·a·nin
or pyo·cy·a·nine

pyo·der·ma
also pyo·der·mia

pyo·gen

pyo·gen·ic

pyo·he·mo·tho·rax
pl pyo·he·mo·tho·rax·es
or pyo·he·mo·tho·ra·ces

py·oid

pyo·me·tra

pyo·ne·phri·tis
pl pyo·ne·phrit·i·des

pyo·ne·phro·sis
pl pyo·ne·phro·ses

pyo·ne·phrot·ic

pyo·pneu·mo·tho·rax
pl pyo·pneu·mo·tho·rax·es
or pyo·pneu·mo·tho·ra·ces

pyo·poi·e·sis
pl pyo·poi·e·ses

py·or·rhea
also py·or·rhoea

py·or·rhea al·ve·o·lar·is
pyo·sal·pinx
pl pyo·sal·pin·ges

pyo·sep·ti·ce·mia
pyo·stat·ic
pyo·tho·rax
pl pyo·tho·rax·es
or pyo·tho·ra·ces

pyo·xan·those
pyr·a·mid
py·ram·i·dal
py·ram·i·da·le
py·ram·i·da·lis
pl py·ram·i·da·les
or py·ram·i·da·lis·es

pyr·a·mi·dot·o·my
pl pyr·a·mi·dot·o·mies

pyr·a·mis
pl py·ra·mi·des

py·ra·nose
pyr·a·zin·amide
py·re·thrum
py·ret·ic
pyr·e·to·gen·ic
also pyr·e·tog·e·nous

pyr·e·to·ther·a·py
pl pyr·e·to·ther·a·pies

py·rex·ia
py·rex·i·al
py·rex·ic
py·rex·in
pyr·i·dox·al
pyr·i·dox·amine
pyr·i·dox·ic
pyr·i·dox·ine
also pyr·i·dox·in

pyr·i·form
or pir·i·form

pyr·i·for·mis
var of piriformis

py·ril·amine
py·ri·meth·amine
py·rim·i·dine
py·ro·cat·e·chin
py·ro·cat·e·chol
py·ro·gal·lol
py·ro·gen
py·ro·gen·ic
py·ro·lig·ne·ous
py·rol·y·sis
pl py·rol·y·ses

py·ro·ma·nia
py·ro·ma·ni·ac
py·ro·ma·ni·a·cal
py·rone
py·ro·nine
py·ro·pho·bia
py·ro·phos·pha·tase
py·ro·phos·phate
py·ro·phos·pho·ric
py·ro·sis
py·ro·tox·in
py·ru·vate
py·ru·vic
pytho·gen·ic
py·uria

Q

qat
var of kat

quack·ery
pl quack·eries

quack·sal·ver
quad·rate
qua·dra·tus
pl qua·dra·ti

quad·ri·ceps
also quad·ri·ceps ex·ten·sor
or quad·ri·ceps fem·o·ris

quad·ri·cip·i·tal
quad·ri·gem·i·nal
quad·ri·gem·i·nate
quad·ri·lat·er·al
qua·drip·a·rous
quad·ri·ple·gia
quad·ri·ple·gic
quad·ri·sect
qua·droon
quad·ru·ped
qua·dru·pe·dal
qua·dru·plet
quan·ta·some

quan·tim·e·ter
quar·an·tine
quar·tan
quat
  var of kat

qua·ter·na·ry
quer·ce·tin
  also quer·ci·tin

quer·u·lent
  also quer·u·lant

quick·en
  quick·ened
  quick·en·ing
quick·lime
quick·sil·ver
qui·es·cent
qui·na
quin·a·crine
  also chin·a·crin
  or chin·a·crine

quin·al·dine
quin·i·cine
quin·i·dine
qui·nine
quin·oid
quin·o·line
  also chin·o·line

qui·nol·o·gist
qui·nol·o·gy
  pl qui·nol·o·gies

qui·none
quin·o·vin
qui·no·vose
quin·qui·na
quin·sy
  pl quin·sies

quin·tan
quin·tu·plet
quit·tor
quo·tid·i·an

R

rab·bet·ing
ra·bic
ra·bid
ra·bies
  pl ra·bies

ra·bi·form
ra·ce·mase
ra·ce·mate
ra·ceme
ra·ce·mic
ra·ce·mose
ra·chi·al
  or ra·chid·i·al

ra·chi·cen·te·sis
  pl ra·chi·cen·te·ses

ra·chid·i·an
ra·chi·om·e·ter
ra·chis
  pl ra·chis·es
  or ra·chi·des

ra·chis·chi·sis
  pl ra·chis·chi·ses

ra·chit·ic
ra·chi·tis
  also rha·chi·tis
  pl ra·chit·i·des
  also rha·chit·i·des

rach·i·to·gen·ic
ra·clage
ra·dec·to·my
  pl ra·dec·to·mies

ra·di·abil·i·ty
  pl ra·di·abil·i·ties

ra·di·al
ra·di·a·le
  pl ra·di·a·lia

ra·di·a·lis
ra·di·al·ly
ra·di·an
ra·di·ant
Ra·di·a·ta
ra·di·ate
  ra·di·at·ed
  ra·di·at·ing
ra·di·a·tion
rad·i·cal
ra·di·ces
  pl of radix

rad·i·cle
ra·dic·u·lar
ra·dic·u·lec·to·my
  pl ra·dic·u·lec·to·mies

ra·dic·u·li·tis
ra·dif·er·ous
ra·dii
  pl of radius

ra·dio·ac·tin·i·um
ra·dio·ac·tive
ra·dio·ac·tive·ly
ra·dio·ac·tiv·i·ty
  pl ra·dio·ac·tiv·i·ties

ra·dio·au·to·gram
ra·dio·au·to·graph
ra·dio·au·to·graph·ic

ra·dio·au·tog·ra·phy
pl ra·dio·au·tog·ra·phies

ra·dio·bi·o·log·i·cal
or ra·dio·bi·o·log·ic

ra·dio·bi·o·log·i·cal·ly
ra·dio·bi·ol·o·gist
ra·dio·bi·ol·o·gy
pl ra·dio·bi·ol·o·gies

ra·dio·car·bon
ra·dio·chem·i·cal
ra·dio·chem·i·cal·ly
ra·dio·chem·ist
ra·dio·chem·is·try
pl ra·dio·chem·is·tries

ra·dio·chro·mato·graph·ic
ra·dio·chro·ma·tog·ra·phy
pl ra·dio·chro·ma·tog·ra·phies

ra·dio·co·balt
ra·dio·col·loid
ra·dio·der·ma·ti·tis
pl ra·dio·der·ma·ti·ti·ses
or ra·dio·der·ma·tit·i·des

ra·di·odon·tia
ra·di·odon·tic
ra·di·odon·tist
ra·dio·ecol·o·gist
ra·dio·ecol·o·gy
pl ra·dio·ecol·o·gies

ra·dio·el·e·ment
ra·dio·gen·ic
ra·dio·gram
ra·dio·graph
ra·di·og·ra·pher
ra·dio·graph·ic
ra·dio·graph·i·cal·ly
ra·di·og·ra·phy
pl ra·di·og·ra·phies

ra·dio·hu·mer·al
ra·dio·im·mu·no·as·say
ra·dio·io·dine
ra·dio·iron
ra·dio·iso·tope
ra·dio·iso·to·pic
ra·dio·iso·to·pi·cal·ly
ra·dio·lead
ra·dio·log·i·cal
or ra·dio·log·ic

ra·dio·log·i·cal·ly
ra·di·ol·o·gist
ra·di·ol·o·gy
pl ra·di·ol·o·gies

ra·dio·lu·cen·cy
pl ra·dio·lu·cen·cies

ra·dio·lu·cent
ra·dio·lu·mi·nes·cence
ra·di·om·e·ter
ra·dio·met·ric
ra·dio·met·ri·cal·ly
ra·di·om·e·try
pl ra·di·om·e·tries

ra·dio·mi·crom·e·ter
ra·dio·mi·met·ic
ra·dio·ne·cro·sis
pl ra·dio·ne·cro·ses

ra·dio·ne·crot·ic
ra·di·opac·i·ty
pl ra·di·opac·i·ties

ra·di·opaque
ra·dio·phar·ma·ceu·ti·cal
ra·dio·phos·pho·rus
ra·dio·pro·tec·tion
ra·dio·pro·tec·tive
ra·dio·pro·tec·tor
ra·dio·re·sis·tance
ra·dio·re·sis·tant
ra·dio·scope
ra·dio·scop·ic
or ra·dio·scop·i·cal

ra·di·os·co·py
pl ra·di·os·co·pies

ra·dio·sen·si·tive
ra·dio·sen·si·tiv·i·ty
pl ra·dio·sen·si·tiv·i·ties

ra·dio·so·di·um
ra·dio·ster·il·iza·tion
ra·dio·ster·il·ized
ra·dio·stron·tium

ra·dio·sur·gery
pl ra·dio·sur·ger·ies
ra·dio·tele·met·ric
ra·dio·te·lem·e·try
pl ra·dio·te·lem·e·tries
ra·dio·ther·a·peu·tic
ra·dio·ther·a·peu·tics
ra·dio·ther·a·pist
ra·dio·ther·a·py
pl ra·dio·ther·a·pies
ra·dio·ther·my
pl ra·dio·ther·mies
ra·dio·tho·ri·um
ra·dio·tro·pic
ra·di·um
ra·di·us
pl ra·dii
also ra·di·us·es
ra·dix
pl ra·di·ces
or ra·dix·es
raf·fi·nose
Rail·lie·ti·na
Rain·ey's cor·pus·cle
ra·mal
Ra·man ef·fect
ram·i·fi·ca·tion
ram·i·fy
ram·i·fied
ram·i·fy·ing
ra·mose

Rams·den eye·piece
ram·u·lus
pl ram·u·li
ra·mus
pl ra·mi
ra·mus com·mu·ni·cans
pl ra·mi com·mu·ni·can·tes
ran·cid·i·fi·ca·tion
ran·cid·i·fy
ran·cid·i·fied
ran·cid·i·fy·ing
ran·cid·i·ty
pl ran·cid·i·ties
ra·nine
Ran·kine scale
ran·u·la
Ran·vier's node
Ra·oult's law
ra·phe
or rha·phe
rap·id eye move·ment
rap·ture of the deep
rap·tus
rar·efac·tion
rar·efy
also rar·i·fy
rar·efied
also rar·ified
rar·efy·ing
also rar·ify·ing
ra·sce·ta
noun pl

ras·pa·to·ry
pl ras·pa·to·ries
rat-bite fe·ver
Rath·ke's pouch
also Rath·ke's pock·et
ra·tio
pl ra·tios
ra·tion
ra·tioned
ra·tion·ing
ra·tio·nal
ra·tio·nal·i·ty
pl ra·tio·nal·i·ties
ra·tio·nal·iza·tion
ra·tio·nal·ize
ra·tio·nal·ized
ra·tio·nal·iz·ing
rats·bane
rat·tle·snake
Rat·tus
rau·wol·fia
Ray·leigh equa·tion
Ray·naud's dis·ease
re·ab·sorb
re·ab·sorp·tion
re·act
re·ac·tance
re·ac·tant
re·ac·tion
re·ac·ti·vate
re·ac·ti·vat·ed
re·ac·ti·vat·ing
re·ac·ti·va·tion
re·ac·tive

re·ac·tiv·i·ty
pl re·ac·tiv·i·ties

re·ac·tor
re·agent
re·ag·gre·ga·tion
re·agin
re·agin·ic
re·al·gar
re·al·i·ty
pl re·al·i·ties

ream·er
re·am·pu·ta·tion
re·at·tach·ment
Re·au·mur scale
Re·au·mur ther·mom·e·ter
re·bel·lion
re·branch
re·cal·ci·fi·ca·tion
re·cal·ci·trant
re·can·a·li·za·tion
re·ca·pit·u·la·tion
re·cep·tac·u·lum
pl re·cep·tac·u·la

re·cep·tor
re·ces·sus
re·cid·i·va·tion
re·cid·i·vism
re·cid·i·vist
re·cid·i·vis·tic
rec·i·pe
re·cip·ro·cal
re·cip·ro·ca·tion
Reck·ling·hau·sen's dis·ease
re·com·bi·nant
re·com·bi·na·tion
re·com·pres·sion
re·con·di·tion
re·con·sti·tute
re·con·sti·tut·ed
re·con·sti·tut·ing
re·con·sti·tu·tion
re·con·struct
re·con·struc·tion
re·con·struc·tive
re·cov·er
re·cov·ered
re·cov·er·ing
re·cov·ery
pl re·cov·eries

rec·re·ment
rec·re·men·ti·tious
re·cru·des·cence
re·cru·des·cent
re·cruit·ment
rec·tal
rec·tal·ly
rec·ti·fi·ca·tion
rec·ti·fi·er
rec·ti·fy
rec·ti·fied
rec·ti·fy·ing
rec·to·cele
rec·toc·ly·sis
pl rec·toc·ly·ses

rec·to·coc·cyg·e·us
pl rec·to·coc·cyg·ei

rec·to·scope
rec·to·sig·moid
rec·to·sig·moid·o·scope
rec·to·sig·moid·o·scop·ic
rec·to·sig·moid·os·co·py
pl rec·to·sig·moid·os·co·pies

rec·to·uter·ine
rec·to·ves·i·cal
rec·tum
pl rec·tums
or rec·ta

rec·tus
pl rec·ti

re·cum·ben·cy
pl re·cum·ben·cies

re·cum·bent
re·cu·per·ate
re·cu·per·at·ed
re·cu·per·at·ing
re·cu·per·a·tion
re·cu·per·a·tive
re·cur
re·curred
re·cur·ring
re·cur·rence
re·cur·rent
re·cur·va·tion
Red Cross
red-green blind·ness
re·dia
pl re·di·ae
also re·di·as

re·di·al
re·dif·fer·en·ti·a·tion

red·in·te·gra·tion
red·in·te·gra·tive
red·out
re·dox
re·duce
  re·duced
  re·duc·ing
re·duc·er
re·duc·ibil·i·ty
  pl re·duc·ibil·i·ties
re·duc·ible
re·duc·tant
re·duc·tase
re·duc·tic
re·duc·tion
re·duc·tone
re·du·pli·cate
  re·du·pli·cat·ed
  re·du·pli·cat·ing
re·du·pli·ca·tion
Red·u·vi·idae
Re·du·vi·us
re·ed·u·ca·tion
re·en·try
  pl re·en·tries
re·fec·tion
re·fer
  re·ferred
  re·fer·ring
re·fer·ral
re·fill
re·flect
re·flec·tion
re·flec·tor
re·flex
re·flexo·gen·ic
  or re·flex·og·e·nous
re·flexo·log·ic
re·flexo·log·i·cal·ly
re·flex·ol·o·gist
re·flex·ol·o·gy
  pl re·flex·ol·o·gies
re·flux
re·fract
re·frac·tile
re·frac·tion
re·frac·tion·ist
re·frac·tive
re·frac·tive·ness
re·frac·tiv·i·ty
  pl re·frac·tiv·i·ties
re·frac·tom·e·ter
re·frac·to·met·ric
re·frac·tom·e·try
  pl re·frac·tom·e·tries
re·frac·to·ri·ness
re·frac·to·ry
re·frac·ture
re·fran·gi·bil·i·ty
  pl re·fran·gi·bil·i·ties
re·fran·gi·ble
re·frig·er·ant
re·frig·er·ate
  re·frig·er·at·ed
  re·frig·er·at·ing
re·frig·er·a·tion
re·frin·gen·cy
  also re·frin·gence
  pl re·frin·gen·cies
  also re·frin·gen·ces
re·frin·gent
re·fu·sion
re·gen·er·ate
  re·gen·er·at·ed
  re·gen·er·at·ing
re·gen·er·a·tion
reg·i·men
re·gion
re·gion·al
reg·is·ter
  reg·is·tered
  reg·is·ter·ing
reg·is·trant
reg·is·trar
reg·is·tra·tion
reg·is·try
  pl reg·is·tries
reg·nan·cy
  pl reg·nan·cies
re·gress
re·gres·sion
re·gres·sive
re·grow
  re·grew
  re·grown
  re·grow·ing
reg·u·lar
reg·u·lar·i·ty
  pl reg·u·lar·i·ties
reg·u·late
  reg·u·lat·ed
  reg·u·lat·ing
reg·u·la·tion
reg·u·la·tive
reg·u·la·tor
re·gur·gi·tant

re·gur·gi·tate
re·gur·gi·tat·ed
re·gur·gi·tat·ing
re·gur·gi·ta·tion
re·gur·gi·ta·tive
re·ha·bil·i·tant
re·ha·bil·i·tate
re·ha·bil·i·tat·ed
re·ha·bil·i·tat·ing
re·ha·bil·i·ta·tion
re·ha·bil·i·ta·tive
re·ha·bil·i·ta·tor
re·ha·bil·i·tee
re·ha·la·tion
Reh·fuss tube
re·hy·drate
re·hy·drat·ed
re·hy·drat·ing
re·hy·dra·tion
Rei·chert-Meissl num·ber
or Rei·chert-Meissl val·ue

Rei·chert val·ue
or Rei·chert num·ber

re·in·fec·tion
re·in·force
re·in·forced
re·in·forc·ing
re·in·force·ment
re·in·forc·er
re·in·ner·va·tion
re·in·oc·u·la·tion
re·in·te·grate
re·in·te·grat·ed
re·in·te·grat·ing
re·in·te·gra·tion
re·in·te·gra·tive
Reiss·ner's fi·ber
Rei·ter's dis·ease
also Rei·ter's syn·drome

re·ject
re·jec·tion
re·ju·ve·nate
re·ju·ve·nat·ed
re·ju·ve·nat·ing
re·ju·ve·na·tion
re·ju·ve·nes·cence
re·ju·ve·nes·cent
re·lapse
re·lapsed
re·laps·ing
re·late
re·lat·ed
re·lat·ing
re·la·tion
re·la·tion·ship
re·lax
re·lax·ant
re·lax·a·tion
re·lax·in
re·leas·er
re·lief
re·lieve
re·lieved
re·liev·ing
re·line
re·lined
re·lin·ing
Re·mak's fi·ber
re·me·di·a·ble
re·me·di·al
re·me·di·al·ly
rem·e·dy
pl rem·e·dies

re·mis·sion
re·mit
re·mit·ted
re·mit·ting
re·mit·tent
re·mit·tent·ly
re·move
re·moved
re·mov·ing
REM sleep
re·nal
re·na·tur·ation
re·na·ture
re·na·tured
re·na·tur·ing
re·ni·fleur
re·ni·form
re·nin
re·ni·por·tal
ren·net
ren·nin
re·no·gram
re·no·graph·ic
re·nog·ra·phy
pl re·nog·ra·phies

re·no·tro·phic
re·no·tro·pic

re•no•vas•cu•lar
reo•vi•rus
re•par•a•tive
re•pel•lent
also re•pel•lant
re•pel•ler
re•per•co•la•tion
re•per•cus•sion
rep•e•ti•tion com•pul•sion
re•place•ment
re•plan•ta•tion
re•ple•tion
rep•li•ca•ble
rep•li•case
rep•li•cate
rep•li•cat•ed
rep•li•cat•ing
rep•li•ca•tion
rep•li•ca•tive
re•po•si•tion
re•po•si•tioned
re•po•si•tion•ing
re•pos•i•to•ry
pl re•pos•i•to•ries
re•press
re•press•ibil•i•ty
pl re•press•ibil•i•ties
re•press•ible
re•pres•sion
re•pres•sor
re•pro•duce
re•pro•duced
re•pro•duc•ing
re•pro•duc•tion
re•pro•duc•tive
re•pro•duc•tive•ly
Rep•til•ia
re•pul•lu•la•tion
re•pul•sion
re•search
re•sect
re•sect•abil•i•ty
pl re•sect•abil•i•ties
re•sect•able
re•sec•tion
re•sec•to•scope
re•ser•pine
re•ser•pin•iza•tion
re•ser•pi•nized
re•serve
res•er•voir
res•i•den•cy
pl res•i•den•cies
res•i•dent
re•sid•u•al
res•i•due
re•sid•u•um
pl re•sid•ua
re•sil•ience
re•sil•ient
res•in
re•si•na
re•sin•oid
res•in•ous
re•sis•tance
re•sis•tant
also re•sis•tent
res•o•lu•tion
re•solve
re•solved
re•solv•ing
re•sol•vent
res•o•nance
res•o•nant
res•o•na•tor
re•sorb
res•or•cin
res•or•cin•ol
re•sorp•tion
re•sorp•tive
re•spi•ra•ble
res•pi•ra•ting
res•pi•ra•tion
res•pi•ra•tor
re•spi•ra•to•ry
re•spire
re•spired
re•spir•ing
res•pi•rom•e•ter
res•pi•ro•met•ric
res•pi•rom•e•try
pl res•pi•rom•e•tries
re•spon•dent
re•sponse
res•ti•form
res•ti•tu•tion
res•to•ra•tion
re•stor•ative
re•store
re•stored
re•stor•ing
re•strain
re•straint
re•sult•ant
re•su•pi•nate
also re•su•pi•nat•ed
re•su•pi•na•tion
res•ur•rec•tion•ism

res·ur·rec·tion·ist
re·sus·ci·tate
re·sus·ci·tat·ed
re·sus·ci·tat·ing
re·sus·ci·ta·tion
re·sus·ci·ta·tive
re·sus·ci·ta·tor
re·tain·er
re·tar·date
re·tar·da·tion
re·tard·ed
re·te
pl re·tia
re·te mi·rab·i·le
pl re·tia mir·a·bil·ia
re·ten·tion
re·ti·al
re·tic·u·lar
re·tic·u·late
or re·tic·u·lat·ed
re·tic·u·la·tion
re·tic·u·lin
re·tic·u·lo·cyte
re·tic·u·lo·cyt·ic
re·tic·u·lo·cy·to·sis
pl re·tic·u·lo·cy·to·ses
re·tic·u·lo·en·do·the·li·al
re·tic·u·lo·en·do·the·li·o·sis
pl re·tic·u·lo·en·do·the·li·o·ses
re·tic·u·lo·en·do·the·li·um
pl re·tic·u·lo·en·do·the·lia
re·tic·u·lo·sis
pl re·tic·u·lo·ses
re·tic·u·lum
pl re·tic·u·la
ret·i·form
ret·i·na
pl ret·i·nas
or ret·i·nae
ret·i·nac·u·lum
pl ret·i·nac·u·la
ret·i·nal
ret·i·nene
ret·i·ni·tis
pl reti·nit·i·des
ret·i·no·blas·to·ma
pl ret·i·no·blas·to·mas
or ret·i·no·blas·to·ma·ta
ret·i·no·cho·roid·i·tis
ret·i·noid
ret·i·nol
ret·i·no·pap·il·li·tis
ret·i·nop·a·thy
pl ret·i·nop·a·thies
ret·i·no·scope
ret·i·no·scop·ic
ret·i·nos·co·py
pl ret·i·nos·co·pies
re·tort
re·tract
re·trac·tile
re·trac·tion
re·trac·tor
re·trad
re·tra·hent
re·trench·ment
ret·ro·ac·tion
ret·ro·bul·bar
ret·ro·ca·val
ret·ro·ce·cal
or ret·ro·cae·cal
ret·ro·cede
ret·ro·ced·ed
ret·ro·ced·ing
ret·ro·ces·sion
ret·ro·dis·place·ment
ret·ro·flex
or ret·ro·flexed
ret·ro·flex·ion
or ret·ro·flec·tion
ret·ro·grade
ret·ro·grade·ly
ret·ro·gres·sion
ret·ro·ject
ret·ro·jec·tion
ret·ro·len·tal
ret·ro·len·tic·u·lar
ret·ro·lin·gual
ret·ro·mo·lar
ret·ro-oc·u·lar
ret·ro·peri·to·ne·al
ret·ro·peri·to·ne·al·ly
ret·ro·posed
ret·ro·pu·bic
ret·ro·pul·sion
ret·ro·spec·tion
ret·ro·spec·tive

ret·ro·stal·sis
pl ret·ro·stal·ses

ret·ro·vac·cin·a·tion
ret·ro·ver·sion
ret·ro·vert·ed
re·trude
re·trud·ed
re·trud·ing
re·tru·sion
re·tru·sive
Ret·zi·us's vein
re·vel·lent
rev·er·ie
or rev·ery
pl rev·er·ies

re·ver·sal
re·verse tran·scrip·tase
re·vers·ible
re·ver·sion
re·vert
re·ver·tant
re·vive
re·vived
re·viv·ing
re·viv·i·fi·ca·tion
re·viv·i·fy
re·viv·i·fied
re·viv·i·fy·ing
rev·o·lute
re·vul·sion
re·vul·sive
Rhab·di·tis
rhab·doid
rhab·dom
or rhab·dome

rhab·do·mere
rhab·do·my·o·ma
pl rhab·do·my·o·mas
or rhab·do·my·o·ma·ta

rhab·do·myo·sar·co·ma
pl rhab·do·myo·sar·co·mas
or rhab·do·myo·sar·co·ma·ta

rha·gad·i·form
rhag·e·des
rham·ni·nose
rham·nose
rham·no·side
Rham·nus
rha·phe
var of raphe

rhat·a·ny
pl rhat·a·nies

rha·thy·mia
rhe·a·dine
or rhoe·a·dine

rhe·in
rhe·ni·um
rheo·base
rheo·ba·sic
rhe·ol·o·gist
rhe·ol·o·gy
pl rhe·ol·o·gies

rhe·om·e·ter
rhe·om·e·try
pl rhe·om·e·tries

rhe·o·stat
rheo·tax·is
pl rheo·tax·es

rheo·trope
rhe·ot·ro·pism
rhe·sus mon·key
or rhe·sus
also rhe·sus ma·caque

rheum
Rhe·um
rheu·mat·ic
rheu·mat·i·cal·ly
rheu·ma·tism
rheu·ma·toid
rheu·ma·tol·o·gist
rheu·ma·tol·o·gy
pl rheu·ma·tol·o·gies

rhex·is
pl rhex·es

Rh fac·tor
rhi·nal
rhi·nal·gia
rhin·en·ce·phal·ic
also rhin·en·ceph·a·lous

rhin·en·ceph·a·lon
pl rhin·en·ceph·a·la

rhi·nen·chy·sis
rhin·i·on
rhi·ni·tis
pl rhi·nit·i·des

rhi·no·gen·ic
or rhi·nog·e·nous

rhi·no·la·lia
rhi·no·lar·yn·gol·o·gy
pl rhi·no·lar·yn·gol·o·gies

rhi·no·lar·yn·go·scope

rhi·no·lith
rhi·no·lith·ic
rhi·no·log·ic
or rhi·no·log·i·cal
rhi·nol·o·gist
rhi·nol·o·gy
pl rhi·nol·o·gies
rhi·no·phar·yn·gi·tis
pl rhi·no·phar·yn·git·i·des
rhi·no·phar·ynx
pl rhi·no·pha·ryn·ges
also rhi·no·phar·ynx·es
rhi·no·pho·nia
rhi·no·phy·ma
pl rhi·no·phy·mas
or rhi·no·phy·ma·ta
rhi·no·plas·ty
pl rhi·no·plas·ties
rhi·nor·rha·gia
rhi·nor·rhea
or rhi·nor·rhoea
rhi·no·scle·ro·ma
pl rhi·no·scle·ro·ma·ta
rhi·no·scope
rhi·no·scop·ic
rhi·nos·co·py
pl rhi·nos·co·pies
rhi·no·spo·rid·i·o·sis
pl rhi·no·spo·rid·i·o·ses
rhi·no·spo·rid·i·um
pl rhi·no·spo·rid·ia
rhi·no·vi·rus
Rhipi·ceph·a·lus
rhi·zo·bi·um
pl rhi·zo·bia
rhi·zoid
rhi·zome
rhi·zo·pod
Rhi·zop·o·da
rhi·zop·ter·in
rhi·zot·o·my
pl rhi·zot·o·mies
Rh-neg·a·tive
rho·da·mine
rho·dan·ate
rho·da·nese
rho·dan·ic
rho·di·um
rho·dop·sin
rhoe·a·dine
var of rheadine
rhomb·en·ceph·a·lon
pl rhomb·en·ceph·a·la
rhom·boid
rhom·boi·dal
rhom·boi·de·us
pl rhom·boi·dei
rhon·chi·al
rhon·chus
pl rhon·chi
rho·ta·cism
also rho·ta·cis·mus
or ro·ta·cism
Rh-pos·i·tive
rhus
pl rhus·es
or rhus
rhus gla·bra
rhythm
rhyth·mic
or rhyth·mi·cal
rhyth·mi·cal·ly
rhyth·mic·i·ty
pl rhyth·mic·i·ties
rhyt·i·do·plas·ty
pl rhyt·i·do·plas·ties
rib·bon
ri·bi·tol
ri·bo·fla·vin
also ri·bo·fla·vine
ri·bo·nu·cle·ase
ri·bo·nu·cle·ic
ri·bo·nu·cleo·pro·tein
ri·bo·nu·cle·o·side
ri·bo·nu·cle·o·tide
ri·bose
ri·bo·side
ri·bo·som·al
ri·bo·som·al RNA
ri·bo·some
ri·bo·syl
ri·bu·lose
Ric·co's law
ri·cin
ric·i·nine
ri·cin·ole·ate
ri·cin·ole·ic
ric·i·nus
rick·ets
rick·ett·sia
pl rick·ett·si·as
or rick·ett·si·ae
rick·ett·si·al
rick·ett·si·al·pox

rick·ett·si·o·sis
pl rick·ett·si·o·ses

rick·ett·sio·stat·ic
rick·ety
ric·tal
ric·tus
pl ric·tus
or ric·tus·es

rid·er's bone
ridge·ling
or ridg·ling

ri·fam·pi·cin
ri·fa·my·cin
Riggs' dis·ease
right-eyed
right-hand
adj

right-hand·ed
ri·gid·i·ty
ri·gid·i·ties
rig·or mor·tis
ri·ma
pl ri·mae

ri·ma glot·ti·dis
ri·mose
or ri·mous

rim·u·la
pl rim·u·lae

rin·der·pest
ring·bone
ring·boned
Ring·er's so·lu·tion
or Ring·er so·lu·tion

ring·worm
ri·par·i·an
ri·so·ri·us
pl ri·so·rii

ri·sus sar·do·ni·cus
riz·i·form
RNase
or RNA·ase

roar·er
roar·ing
ro·bo·rant
Ro·chelle salt
Rocky Moun·tain spot·ted fe·ver
Ro·den·tia
ro·den·ti·cide
roent·gen
also rönt·gen

roent·gen·iza·tion
also rönt·gen·iza·tion

roent·gen·ize
also rönt·gen·ize

roent·gen·ized
also rönt·gen·ized

roent·gen·iz·ing
also rönt·gen·iz·ing

roent·gen·ky·mo·gram
roent·gen·ky·mo·graph·ic
roent·gen·ky·mog·ra·phy
pl roent·gen·ky·mog·ra·phies

roent·gen·o·gram
roent·gen·o·graph
roent·gen·o·graph·ic
roent·gen·o·graph·i·cal·ly
roent·gen·og·ra·phy
pl roent·gen·og·ra·phies

roent·gen·o·log·ic
or roent·gen·o·log·i·cal

roent·gen·o·log·i·cal·ly
roent·gen·ol·o·gist
roent·gen·ol·o·gy
pl roent·gen·ol·o·gies

roent·gen·om·e·ter
roent·gen·om·e·try
pl roent·gen·om·e·tries

roent·gen·o·scope
roent·gen·o·scop·ic
roent·gen·o·scop·i·cal·ly
roent·gen·os·co·py
pl roent·gen·os·co·pies

roent·gen·o·ther·a·py
pl roent·gen·o·ther·a·pies

roent·gen·ther·a·py
pl roent·gen·ther·a·pies

Ro·lan·dic

Ro·lan·dic ar·ea
Ro·ma·now·sky stain
Rom·berg sign
or Rom·berg's sign
ron·geur
ron·nel
rönt·gen
var of roentgen
rönt·gen·iza·tion
var of roentgenization
rönt·gen·ize
var of roentgenize
Ror·schach test
also Ror·schach ink·blot test
ro·sa·cea
ros·an·i·line
ro·sa·ry
pl ro·sa·ries
rose ben·gal
also rose ben·gale
ro·se·o·la
ro·se·o·la in·fan·tum
ro·sette
ros·in
ro·so·lic
ros·tel·lar
ros·tel·late
ros·tel·lum
ros·trad
ros·tral
ros·trate
ros·trum
pl ros·trums
or ros·tra

ro·ta·cism
var of rhotacism
ro·ta·me·ter
ro·ta·ry
ro·tate
ro·tat·ed
ro·tat·ing
ro·ta·tion
ro·ta·tor
pl ro·ta·tors
or ro·ta·to·res
ro·ta·to·ry
ro·te·none
rott·lera
rot·u·lar
Rou·get cell
rough·age
rou·leau
pl rou·leaux
or rou·leaus
round-shoul·dered
round·worm
roup
Rous sar·co·ma
Ru·barth's dis·ease
rub·ber dam
ru·be·do
ru·be·fa·cient
ru·be·fac·tion
ru·bel·la
ru·be·o·la
ru·be·o·lar
ru·bes·cence
ru·bes·cent
ru·bid·i·um

ru·big·i·nous
Ru·bin test
ru·bor
ru·bro·spi·nal
Ru·bus
ru·di·ment
ru·di·men·ta·ry
ru·fous
ru·ga
pl ru·gae
ru·gal
ru·gose
ru·gose·ly
ru·gos·i·ty
pl ru·gos·i·ties
ru·gous
ru·men
pl ru·mi·na
or ru·mens
ru·men·itis
ru·men·ot·o·my
pl ru·men·ot·o·mies
Ru·mex
ru·mi·nant
ru·mi·nate
ru·mi·nat·ed
ru·mi·nat·ing
ru·mi·na·tion
ru·mi·na·tive
run·around
or run·round
ru·pia
ru·pi·al
rup·ture
rup·tured
rup·tur·ing
Rus·sell's vi·per

ru·the·ni·um
ruth·er·ford
ru·tin
ru·tin·ose

S

sab·a·dil·la
also ceb·a·dil·la

sab·u·lous
also sab·u·lose
or sab·u·line

sa·bur·ra
sa·bur·ral
sac·cade
sac·cad·ic
sac·cate
sac·cha·rase
sac·cha·rate
sac·cha·rat·ed
sac·char·ic
sac·cha·ride
sac·cha·rif·er·ous
sac·char·i·fi·ca·tion
sac·char·i·fy
sac·char·i·fied
sac·char·i·fy·ing
sac·cha·rim·e·ter
sac·char·i·met·ric
or sac·char·i·met·ri·cal

sac·cha·rim·e·try
pl sac·cha·rim·e·tries

sac·cha·rin
sac·cha·rine
sac·cha·rin·i·ty
pl sac·cha·rin·i·ties

sac·cha·ro·lyt·ic
sac·cha·rom·e·ter
sac·cha·ro·met·ric
sac·cha·rom·e·try
pl sac·cha·rom·e·tries

Sac·cha·ro·my·ces
Sac·cha·ro·my·ce·ta·ce·ae
sac·cha·ro·my·ce·ta·ceous
Sac·cha·ro·my·ce·ta·les
sac·cha·ro·my·cete
sac·cha·ro·my·ce·tic
sac·cha·rose
sac·cha·rum
sac·ci·form
sac·cu·lar
sac·cu·late
or sac·cu·lat·ed

sac·cu·la·tion
sac·cule
sac·cu·lus
pl sac·cu·li

sac·cus
pl sac·ci

sa·crad
sa·cral
sa·cral·iza·tion
sa·crec·to·my
pl sa·crec·to·mies

sa·cro·coc·cy·geal
sa·cro·coc·cyg·e·us
pl sa·cro·coc·cyg·ei

sa·cro·dyn·ia
sa·cro·il·i·ac
sa·cro·lum·ba·lis
sa·cro·sci·at·ic
sa·cro·spi·na·lis
sa·cro·spi·nous
sa·cro·tu·ber·ous
sa·crum
pl sa·cra

sa·dism
sa·dist
sa·dis·tic
sa·dis·ti·cal·ly
sa·do·mas·och·ism
sa·do·mas·och·ist
sa·do·mas·och·is·tic
sa·git·ta
sag·it·tal
sag·it·tal·ly
Saint An·tho·ny's fire
Saint Lou·is en·ceph·a·li·tis
Saint Vi·tus' dance
or Saint Vi·tus's dance

sal·i·cin
sal·i·cyl·al·de·hyde

sal·i·cyl·am·ide
sal·i·cyl·an·i·lide
sa·lic·y·late
sa·lic·y·lat·ed
sal·i·cyl·azo·sul·fa·pyr·i·dine
sal·i·cyl·ic
sal·i·cyl·ism
sal·i·cyl·iza·tion
sal·i·cyl·ize
  sal·i·cyl·ized
  sal·i·cyl·iz·ing
sal·i·cyl·uric ac·id
sa·lient
sal·i·fi·able
sal·i·fi·ca·tion
sal·i·fy
  sal·i·fied
  sal·i·fy·ing
sal·i·gen·in
sa·lim·e·ter
sa·line
sa·li·nom·e·ter
sa·li·va
sal·i·vant
sal·i·vary
sal·i·vate
  sal·i·vat·ed
  sal·i·vat·ing
sal·i·va·tion
Salk vac·cine
sal·mine
sal·mo·nel·la
  pl sal·mo·nel·lae
  or sal·mo·nel·las
  or sal·mo·nel·la
sal·mo·nel·lo·sis
  pl sal·mo·nel·lo·ses
sal·ol
sal·pin·gec·to·my
  pl sal·pin·gec·to·mies
sal·pin·gian
sal·pin·gi·tis
  pl sal·pin·gi·tis·es
sal·pin·go·cath·e·ter·ism
sal·pin·go·cele
sal·pin·go·cy·e·sis
  pl sal·pin·go·cy·e·ses
sal·pin·gog·ra·phy
  pl sal·pin·gog·ra·phies
sal·pin·go-oo·pho·rec·to·my
  pl sal·pin·go-oo·pho·rec·to·mies
sal·pin·go-oo·pho·ri·tis
sal·pin·go·pal·a·tine
sal·pin·go·peri·to·ni·tis
sal·pin·go·pexy
  pl sal·pin·go·pexies
sal·pin·go·pha·ryn·geal
sal·pin·go·plas·ty
  pl sal·pin·go·plas·ties
sal·pin·gos·to·my
  pl sal·pin·gos·to·mies
sal·pin·gys·tero·cy·e·sis
  pl sal·pin·gys·tero·cy·e·ses
sal·pinx
  pl sal·pin·ges
sal·ta·tion
sal·ta·to·ry
salt·pe·ter
  also salt·pe·tre
sa·lu·bri·ous
sa·lu·bri·ous·ly
sa·lu·bri·ty
  pl sa·lu·bri·ties
sal·uret·ic
sal·u·ret·i·cal·ly
sal·u·tari·ly
sal·u·tary
sal·via
sal vo·la·ti·le
Sam·bu·cus
san·a·tar·i·um
  pl san·a·tar·i·ums
  or san·a·tar·ia
san·a·tive
san·a·to·ri·um
  pl san·a·to·ri·ums
  or san·a·to·ria
san·a·to·ry
sand-blind
sand crack
sand·fly fe·ver
san·guic·o·lous
san·gui·fi·ca·tion
san·gui·nar·ia
san·guin·a·rine
san·guine
san·guine·ly

san·guin·e·ous
san·guin·o·lent
san·gui·no·pu·ru·lent
san·gui·nous
san·guis
san·guiv·o·rous
san·i·cle
sa·ni·es
pl sa·ni·es
sa·ni·ous
san·i·tar·i·an
san·i·tari·ly
san·i·tar·i·um
pl san·i·tar·i·ums
also san·i·tar·ia
san·i·tary
san·i·tate
san·i·tat·ed
san·i·tat·ing
san·i·ta·tion
san·i·ta·tion·ist
san·i·ti·za·tion
san·i·tize
san·i·tized
san·i·tiz·ing
san·i·tiz·er
san·i·to·ri·um
pl san·i·to·ri·ums
or san·i·to·ria
san·i·ty
pl san·i·ties
san·ton·i·ca
san·to·nin
San·to·ri·ni's car·ti·lage
sa·phe·na
sa·phe·nous
sa·po
pl sa·pos
sa·po·ge·nin
sap·o·na·ceous
sa·pon·i·fi·able
sa·pon·i·fi·ca·tion
sa·pon·i·fi·er
sa·pon·i·fy
sa·pon·i·fied
sa·pon·i·fy·ing
sa·po·nin
sa·po·ta
sap·o·tox·in
sap·pan·wood
or sa·pan·wood
also sap·pan
sap·phic
sap·phism
sa·pre·mia
sa·pre·mic
sap·ro·gen
sap·ro·gen·ic
sap·ro·ge·nic·i·ty
pl sap·ro·ge·nic·i·ties
sa·prog·e·nous
sa·proph·a·gous
sa·proph·i·lous
also sap·ro·phile
sap·ro·phyte
sap·ro·phyt·ic
sap·ro·phyt·i·cal·ly
sar·a·pus
sar·ci·na
pl sar·ci·nas
or sar·ci·nae
sar·co·cele
sar·co·cys·tis
pl sar·co·cys·tis
or sar·co·cys·tis·es
Sar·co·di·na
sar·co·din·i·an
sar·co·glia
sar·coid
sar·coid·osis
pl sar·coid·o·ses
sar·co·lac·tic
sar·co·lem·ma
sar·co·lem·mal
sar·col·y·sis
pl sar·col·y·ses
sar·co·ma
pl sar·co·mas
or sar·co·ma·ta
sar·co·ma·gen·ic
sar·co·ma·toid
sar·co·ma·to·sis
p sar·co·ma·to·ses
sar·co·ma·tous
sar·co·mere
sar·co·mer·ic
sar·co·plasm
sar·co·plas·ma
pl sar·co·plas·ma·ta
sar·co·plas·mat·ic
sar·co·plas·mic
sar·co·poi·et·ic
Sar·cop·tes
sar·co·sine
sar·co·som·al
sar·co·some

sar·co·spo·rid·i·o·sis
pl sar·co·spo·rid·i·o·ses
sar·co·style
sar·cous
sa·rin
sar·sa·pa·ril·la
sar·to·ri·us
pl sar·to·rii
sas·sa·fras
sa·tan·o·pho·bia
sat·el·lite
sat·el·lit·osis
pl sat·el·lit·oses
sa·ti·ate
sa·ti·at·ed
sa·ti·at·ing
sa·ti·a·tion
sa·ti·ety
pl sa·ti·eties
sat·u·rate
sat·u·rat·ed
sat·u·rat·ing
sat·u·ra·tion
sat·ur·nine
sat·urn·ism
sa·ty·ri·a·sis
pl sa·ty·ri·a·ses
sau·cer·iza·tion
sau·cer·ize
sau·cer·ized
sau·cer·iz·ing
sau·na
sau·ri·a·sis
saxi·tox·in
scab
scabbed
scab·bing
scab·by
scab·bi·er
scab·bi·est
scab·i·ci·dal
scab·i·cide
or sca·bi·et·i·cide
sca·bies
pl sca·bies
sca·bi·et·ic
also sca·bet·ic
sca·bi·ous
sca·bri·ti·es
sca·la
pl sca·lae
sca·la me·dia
pl sca·lae me·di·ae
sca·la tym·pa·ni
pl sca·lae tym·pa·no·rum
sca·la ves·tib·u·li
pl sca·lae ves·tib·u·lo·rum
sca·lene
sca·le·nec·to·my
pl sca·le·nec·to·mies
sca·le·not·o·my
pl sca·le·not·o·mies
sca·le·nus
pl sca·le·ni
scal·er
sca·lo·gram
scal·pel
scal·pri·form
scal·prum
pl scal·pra
scam·mo·ny
pl scam·mo·nies
scan·di·um
scan·ning elec·tron mi·cro·scope
Scan·zo·ni's ma·neu·ver
sca·pha
scaph·o·ce·phal·ic
or scaph·o·ceph·a·lous
scaph·o·ceph·a·lism
scaph·o·ceph·a·ly
pl scaph·o·ceph·a·lies
scaph·oid
scap·u·la
pl scap·u·lae
or scap·u·las
scap·u·lar
scap·u·lary
pl scap·u·laries
sca·pus
pl sca·pi
scarf·skin
scar·i·fi·ca·tion
scar·i·fi·ca·tor
scar·i·fi·er
scar·i·fy
scar·i·fied
scar·i·fy·ing
scar·la·ti·na
scar·la·ti·nal
scar·la·ti·ni·form
scar·la·ti·no·gen·ic

scar·la·ti·noid
Scar·pa's fas·cia
Scar·pa's fo·ra·men
Scar·pa's tri·an·gle
also Scar·pa's tri·gone
sca·tole
var of ska·tole
scat·o·log·i·cal
also scat·o·log·ic
sca·tol·o·gy
also ska·tol·o·gy
pl sca·tol·o·gies
also ska·tol·o·gies
sca·to·ma
pl sca·to·mas
or sca·to·ma·ta
sca·toph·a·gous
sca·toph·a·gy
pl sca·toph·a·gies
scat·u·la
pl scat·u·lae
Scheib·ler's re·agent
sche·mato·graph
Schick test
Schiff base
Schiff re·ac·tion
Schiff re·agent
Schil·der's dis·ease
Schil·ling in·dex
schin·dy·le·sis
pl schin·dy·le·ses
schir·rhus
var of scirrhus
schis·to·cyte
schis·to·cy·to·sis
pl schis·to·cy·to·ses
or schis·to·cy·to·sis·es
schis·to·glos·sia
schis·tom·e·lus
pl schis·tom·e·li
schis·tor·rha·chis
schis·to·so·ma
schis·to·some
schis·to·so·mi·a·sis
pl schis·to·so·mi·a·ses
schis·to·so·mi·a·sis ja·pon·i·ca
schis·to·so·mi·a·sis man·soni
schiz·ax·on
schizo
pl schiz·os
schizo-af·fec·tive
schizo·gen·e·sis
pl schizo·gen·e·ses
schizo·ge·net·ic
or schizo·gen·ic
schizo·ge·net·i·cal·ly
schi·zog·e·nous
schi·zog·e·nous·ly
schi·zog·o·nous
also schizo·gon·ic
schi·zog·o·ny
pl schi·zog·o·nies
schiz·oid
schiz·oid·man·ic
also schizo·man·ic
schizo·my·cete
Schizo·my·ce·tes
schizo·my·cet·ic
schizo·my·ce·tous
schiz·ont
schi·zon·ti·ci·dal
schi·zon·ti·cide
schizo·pha·sia
schizo·phre·nia
schizo·phren·ic
schizo·phren·i·cal·ly
schizo·thy·mic
also schizo·thy·mous
Schiz·o·tryp·a·num
Schlemm's ca·nal
Schnei·de·ri·an mem·brane
Schnei·der in·dex
Schuff·ner's dots
Schül·ler-Chris·tian dis·ease
Schultz-Dale re·ac·tion
Schwann cell
Schwann·ian
Schwann's sheath
or Schwann tube
sci·age
sci·at·ic
sci·at·i·ca
scil·la
scin·ti·gram
scin·ti·graph·ic
scin·tig·ra·phy
pl scin·tig·ra·phies

scin·til·late
scin·til·lat·ed
scin·til·lat·ing

scin·til·la·tion

scin·til·la·tor

scin·til·lom·e·ter

scin·ti·scan

scin·ti·scan·ner

scin·ti·scan·ning

sci·on
also ci·on

scir·rhoid

scir·rhous

scir·rhus
also schir·rhus
pl scir·rhi
also scir·rhus·es
or schir·rhi
or schir·rhus·es

scis·sile

scis·sion

scis·si·par·i·ty
pl scis·si·par·i·ties

scis·su·ra
pl scis·su·rae

sclera
pl scler·as
or scler·ae

scler·al

scler·ec·ta·sia

scle·rec·to·iri·dec·to·my
pl scle·rec·to·iri·dec·to·mies

scle·rec·to·my
pl scle·rec·to·mies

scler·ede·ma
pl scler·ede·mas
or scler·ede·ma·ta

scle·re·ma ad·ul·to·rum

scle·re·ma neo·na·to·rum

scle·ri·tis
pl scle·ri·tis·es

sclero·blas·tem
or sclero·blas·te·ma
pl sclero·blas·tems
or sclero·blas·te·mas
or sclero·blas·te·ma·ta

sclero·blas·te·mic

sclero·con·junc·ti·val

sclero·cor·nea

sclero·cor·ne·al

sclero·dac·tyl·ia
or sclero·dac·ty·ly
pl sclero·dac·tyl·ias
or sclero·dac·ty·lies

sclero·der·ma
pl sclero·der·mas
or sclero·der·ma·ta

sclero·der·ma·ti·tis
pl sclero·der·ma·ti·tis·es
or sclero·der·ma·tit·i·des

sclero·der·ma·tous

scle·rog·e·nous
also sclero·gen·ic

scler·oid

sclero·ker·a·ti·tis
pl sclero·ker·a·tit·i·des

scle·ro·ma
pl scle·ro·mas
or scle·ro·ma·ta

scle·ro·ma·la·cia

sclero·me·ninx
pl sclero·me·nin·ges

sclero·mere

scle·rom·e·ter

scle·ro·nych·ia

scle·ro·plas·ty
pl scle·ro·plas·ties

sclero·pro·tein

scle·rose
scle·rosed
scle·ros·ing

scle·ro·sis
pl scle·ro·ses

sclero·ste·no·sis
pl sclero·ste·no·ses

scle·ros·to·my
pl scle·ros·to·mies

sclero·ther·a·py
pl sclero·ther·a·pies

scle·rot·ic

scle·rot·i·ca

sclero·ti·tis
pl sclero·ti·tis·es

scle·ro·tium
pl scle·ro·tia

sclero·tome

sclero·tomic

scle·rot·o·my
pl scle·rot·o·mies

scler·ous

sco·le·coid

sco·lex
pl sco·li·ces
also scol·e·ces
or sco·lex·es

sco·li·o·sis
pl sco·li·o·ses

sco·li·ot·ic
sco·pa·rin
sco·par·i·us
sco·pine
sco·po·la
also sco·po·lia

sco·pol·amine
sco·po·phil·ia
or scop·to·phil·ia

sco·po·phil·i·ac
or scop·to·phil·i·ac

sco·po·phil·ic
or scop·to·phil·ic

scor·bu·tic
scor·bu·ti·cal·ly
scor·bu·ti·gen·ic
scor·bu·tus
scor·pi·on
Scor·pi·on·i·da
sco·to·din·ia
sco·to·graph
sco·to·ma
pl sco·to·mas
or sco·to·ma·ta

sco·to·ma·graph
sco·to·ma·tous
sco·tom·e·ter
sco·to·pia
sco·to·pic
scra·pie
screw·worm
scro·bic·u·late
scrof·u·la
scrof·u·lo·der·ma
scrof·u·lo·der·mic
scrof·u·lo·sis
pl scrof·u·lo·ses

scrof·u·lous
scro·tal
scro·tec·to·my
pl scro·tec·to·mies

scro·to·cele
scro·tum
pl scro·ta
or scro·tums

scrub ty·phus
scru·ple
scru·pu·los·i·ty
pl scru·pu·los·i·ties

scur·vy
pl scur·vies

scu·ti·form
Scu·tig·era
scu·tu·lum
pl scu·tu·la

scu·tum
pl scu·ta

scyb·a·lous
scyb·a·lum
pl scyb·a·la

sea·sick·ness
seat·worm
se·ba·ceous
se·bip·a·rous
seb·or·rhea
or seb·or·rhoea

seb·or·rhe·ic
or seb·or·rhoe·ic

se·bum
se·cern·ent
se·clu·sion
seco·bar·bi·tal
sec·odont

sec·ond-de·gree burn
se·cre·ta
se·cre·ta·gogue
also sec·re·to·gogue

se·crete
se·cret·ed
se·cret·ing
se·cre·tin
se·cre·tion
sec·re·to·mo·tor
se·cre·tor
se·cre·to·ry
sec·tar·i·an
sec·to·ri·al
se·cun·di·grav·i·da
pl se·cun·di·grav·i·das
or se·cun·di·grav·i·dae

se·cun·dines
or se·con·dines

sec·un·dip·a·ra
pl sec·un·dip·a·ras
or sec·un·dip·a·rae

sec·un·dip·a·rous
se·cure
se·cur·er
se·cur·est
se·cu·ri·ty
pl se·cu·ri·ties

se·date
se·dat·ed
se·dat·ing
se·da·tion
sed·a·tive
sed·en·tary

sed·i·ment
sed·i·men·ta·tion
se·do·hep·tu·lose
seg·men·tal
seg·men·ta·tion
seg·men·tec·to·my
pl seg·men·tec·to·mies
seg·ment·er
seg·re·gant
seg·re·gate
seg·re·gat·ed
seg·re·gat·ing
seg·re·ga·tion
Seid·litz pow·ders
Sei·gnette salt
or Sei·gnette's salt
sei·zure
se·junc·tion
sel·a·chyl
se·lec·tion
se·le·nic
se·le·ni·um
se·len·odont
sel·e·no·sis
self-abuse
self-ac·cu·sa·tion
self-anal·y·sis
pl self-anal·y·ses
self-an·a·lyt·i·cal
also self-an·a·lyt·ic
self-aware
self-aware·ness
self-con·cept
self-con·cep·tion
self-dif·fer·en·ti·a·tion
self-di·ges·tion
self-hyp·no·sis
pl self-hyp·no·ses
self-iden·ti·fi·ca·tion
self-im·age
self-in·duc·tance
self-in·flict·ed
self-lim·it·ed
or self-lim·it·ing
self-per·cep·tion
self-rep·li·cat·ing
self-re·pres·sion
self-re·pro·duc·ing
self-stim·u·la·tion
self-treat·ment
sel·la
pl sel·las
or sel·lae
sel·lar
sel·la tur·ci·ca
pl sel·lae tur·ci·cae
se·mei·ot·ic
also se·mei·ot·i·cal
se·mei·ot·ics
se·men
pl se·mi·na
or se·mens
semi·car·ti·lag·i·nous
semi·cir·cu·lar
semi·co·ma
semi·co·ma·tose
semi·con·scious
semi·con·scious·ly
semi·con·scious·ness
semi·dom·i·nant
semi·le·thal
semi·lu·nar
semi·mem·bra·no·sus
pl semi·mem·bra·no·si
semi·mem·bra·nous
sem·i·nal
sem·i·nal·ly
sem·i·nate
sem·i·nat·ed
sem·i·nat·ing
sem·i·na·tion
sem·i·nif·er·ous
also sem·i·nif·er·al
sem·i·no·ma
pl sem·i·no·mas
or sem·i·no·ma·ta
semi·nu·ria
se·mi·og·ra·phy
also se·mei·og·ra·phy
pl se·mi·og·ra·phies
or se·mei·og·ra·phies
se·mi·o·log·i·cal
also se·mei·o·log·i·cal
se·mi·ol·o·gy
also se·mei·ol·o·gy
pl se·mi·ol·o·gies
also se·mei·ol·o·gies
semi·per·me·able
semi·pri·vate
semi·pro·na·tion

semi·qui·none
semi·spi·na·lis
pl semi·spi·na·les
semi·syn·thet·ic
sem·i·ten·di·no·sus
pl sem·i·ten·di·no·si
semi·ten·di·nous
se·ne·cio
pl se·ne·cios
se·ne·ci·osis
pl se·ne·ci·oses
sen·e·ga
or sen·e·ca
sen·e·gin
se·nes·cence
se·nes·cent
se·nile
se·nile·ly
se·nil·i·ty
pl se·nil·i·ties
se·ni·um
sen·na
se·no·pia
sen·sa·tion
sen·sa·tion·al
sense-da·tum
pl sense-da·ta
sen·si·bil·ia
sen·si·bil·i·ty
pl sen·si·bil·i·ties
sen·si·ble
sen·si·tive
sen·si·tive·ly
sen·si·tive·ness
sen·si·tiv·i·ty
pl sen·si·tiv·i·ties
sen·si·ti·za·tion
sen·si·tize
sen·si·tized
sen·si·tiz·ing
sen·sor
sen·so·ri·al
sen·so·ri·al·ly
sen·so·ri·mo·tor
also sen·si·mo·tor
or sen·so·mo·tor
sen·so·ri·neu·ral
sen·so·ri·um
pl sen·so·ri·ums
or sen·so·ria
sen·so·ry
pl sen·so·ries
sen·su·al
sen·su·al·ism
sen·su·al·i·ty
pl sen·su·al·i·ties
sen·su·al·ly
sen·sum
pl sen·sa
sen·tient
sep·a·ra·tor
sep·sis
pl sep·ses
sep·ta
pl of septum
sep·tal
sep·tate
also sep·tat·ed
sep·ta·tion
sep·tic
sep·ti·ce·mia
or sep·ti·cae·mia
sep·ti·ce·mic
or sep·ti·cae·mic
sep·ti·co·py·emia
sep·ti·co·py·emic
sep·tile
sep·to·mar·gin·al
sep·tom·e·ter
sep·to·na·sal
sep·to·tome
sep·tu·lum
pl sep·tu·la
sep·tum
pl sep·ta
or sep·tums
sep·tum pel·lu·ci·dum
pl sep·ta pel·lu·ci·da
sep·tum trans·ver·sum
pl sep·ta trans·ver·sa
sep·tup·let
se·quela
pl se·quel·ae
se·ques·ter
se·ques·tered
se·ques·ter·ing
se·ques·tra·tion
se·ques·trec·to·my
pl se·ques·trec·to·mies
se·ques·trum
pl se·ques·trums
also se·ques·tra
se·ra
pl of serum
Sere·noa
se·ri·al·o·graph
or se·rio·graph
ser·i·cin

se•ries
pl se•ries

ser•ine

se•ro•di•ag•no•sis
pl se•ro•di•ag•no•ses

se•ro•di•ag•nos•tic

se•ro•fi•bri•nous

se•ro•log•i•cal
or se•ro•log•ic

se•ro•log•i•cal•ly

se•rol•o•gist

se•rol•o•gy
pl se•rol•o•gies

se•ro•mu•cous

se•ro•mus•cu•lar

se•ro•neg•a•tive

se•ro•neg•a•tiv•i•ty
pl se•ro•neg•a•tiv•i•ties

se•ro•pos•i•tive

se•ro•pos•i•tiv•i•ty
pl se•ro•pos•i•tiv•i•ties

se•ro•pu•ru•lent

se•ro•re•ac•tion

se•ro•re•sis•tance

se•ro•re•sis•tant

se•ro•sa
pl se•ro•sas
also se•ro•sae

se•ro•sal

se•ro•san•gui•nous
or se•ro•san•guin•e•ous

se•ro•si•tis
pl se•ro•si•tis•es

se•ros•i•ty
pl se•ros•i•ties

se•ro•sy•no•vi•tis

se•ro•ther•a•py
pl se•ro•ther•a•pies

se•ro•to•nin

se•ro•type

se•rous

ser•pen•tar•ia

ser•pig•i•nous

ser•pig•i•nous•ly

ser•rate

ser•rat•ed

Ser•ra•tia

ser•ra•tion

ser•ra•tus
pl ser•ra•ti

serre•fine

ser•ru•late
also ser•ru•lat•ed

ser•ru•la•tion

Ser•to•li cell
also Ser•to•li's cell

se•rum
pl se•rums
or se•ra

se•rum•al

ser•vo•mech•a•nism

ses•a•me

ses•a•moid

ses•a•moid•itis
pl ses•a•moid•itis•es

ses•sile

se•ta
pl se•tae

se•ta•ceous

se•ta•ceous•ly

se•tal

Se•tar•ia

set•fast
var of sitfast

se•tig•er•ous

se•ton

set•up

se•vum

sex•dig•i•tal
or sex•dig•i•tate
or sex•dig•i•tat•ed

sex-in•ter•grade

sex-lim•it•ed

sex-link•age

sex-linked

sex•o•log•i•cal

sex•ol•o•gist

sex•ol•o•gy
pl sex•ol•o•gies

sex•tip•a•ra
pl sex•tip•a•ras
or sex•tip•a•rae

sex•tu•plet

sex•u•al

sex•u•al•i•ty
pl sex•u•al•i•ties

sex•u•al•iza•tion

sex•u•al•ize
sex•u•al•ized
sex•u•al•iz•ing

sex•u•al•ly

shad•ow-cast•ing

shark-liv•er oil

Shar•pey's fi•ber

sheath of Schwann

shel•lac
also shel•lack

shell-shock
Shi·ga ba·cil·lus
also Shi·ga dys·en·tery ba·cil·lus
shi·gel·la
pl shi·gel·lae *also* shi·gel·las
shig·el·lo·sis
pl shig·el·lo·ses
shi·kim·ic
shin·bone
shin·gles
shin·splints
shiv·er
shiv·ered
shiv·er·ing
Shope pap·il·lo·ma
also Shope's pap·il·lo·ma
short sight
short·sight·ed
short·sight·ed·ly
short·sight·ed·ness
short-wind·ed
shoul·der
shoul·der blade
Shrap·nell's mem·brane
si·al·a·gog·ic
si·al·a·gogue
si·al·ic
si·alo·ad·e·ni·tis
si·alo·do·chi·tis
si·a·log·e·nous
si·al·o·gogue
si·al·o·gram
si·a·log·ra·phy
pl si·a·log·ra·phies
si·a·loid
si·al·o·lith
si·al·o·li·thi·a·sis
pl si·al·o·li·thi·a·ses
si·al·or·rhea
also si·al·or·rhoea
Si·a·mese twin
sib·i·lant
sib·ling
sib·ship
sic·cant
sic·ca·tive
sic·cus
sick·en
sick·ened
sick·en·ing
sick·le
sick·led
sick·ling
sick·le-cell ane·mia
sick·le-hammed
sick·le-hocked
sickl·emia
also sickl·aemia
sick·le·mic
sick·ness
sick·room
sid·er·ism
sid·er·o·cyte
sid·ero·fi·bro·sis
pl sid·ero·fi·bro·ses
sid·ero·pe·nia
sid·er·o·phile
also sid·er·o·phil
sid·er·oph·i·lin
sid·er·o·sis
pl sid·er·o·sis·es
sid·er·ot·ic
sig·ma·tism
sig·moid
also sig·moi·dal
sig·moi·dal·ly
sig·moid·ec·to·my
pl sig·moid·ec·to·mies
sig·moid·itis
sig·moid·o·scope
sig·moid·o·scop·ic
sig·moid·os·co·py
pl sig·moid·os·co·pies
sig·moid·os·to·my
pl sig·moid·os·to·mies
sig·na·ture
si·lex
sil·i·ca
sil·i·cate
si·li·ceous
or si·li·cious
si·lic·ic
sil·i·co·flu·o·ride
sil·i·con
sil·i·cone
si·li·co·si·der·o·sis
sil·i·co·sis
pl sil·i·co·ses
sil·i·cot·ic

sil·i·co·tu·ber·cu·lo·sis
pl sil·i·co·tu·ber·cu·lo·ses

sil·i·quose
or sil·i·quous

Sil·ves·ter meth·od
or Sil·ves·ter's meth·od

sim·i·an
Sim·monds' dis·ease
sim·u·la·tion
sim·u·la·tor
Si·mu·li·um
si·nal
si·na·pis
sin·a·pism
sin·cip·i·tal
sin·ci·put
pl sin·ci·puts
or sin·cip·i·ta

sin·ew
sin·gle-blind
sin·gul·tus
sin·i·grin
sin·is·ter
si·nis·trad
si·nis·tral
si·nis·tral·i·ty
pl si·nis·tral·i·ties

si·nis·tral·ly
sin·is·tro·cer·e·bral
sin·is·troc·u·lar
sin·is·troc·u·lar·i·ty
pl sin·is·troc·u·lar·i·ties

sin·is·tro·gy·ra·tion
sin·is·tro·man·u·al
sin·is·trop·e·dal
sin·is·trorse
sin·is·trorse·ly
also sin·is·tror·sal·ly

sin·is·tro·tor·sion
si·nis·trous
si·no·atri·al
also si·nu·atri·al

si·no·au·ric·u·lar
or si·nu·au·ric·u·lar

sin·u·ous
sin·u·ous·ly
si·nus
si·nus·itis
si·nu·soid
si·nu·soi·dal
si·nu·soi·dal·ly
si·nus·ot·o·my
pl si·nus·ot·o·mies

si·phon·age
Si·phon·ap·tera
si·phon·ap·ter·ous
Sip·py di·et
or Sip·py reg·i·men

si·re·nom·e·lus
pl si·re·nom·e·li

si·ri·a·sis
pl si·ri·a·ses

sit·fast
or set·fast

si·tol·o·gy
pl si·tol·o·gies

si·to·ma·nia
si·tos·ter·ol
si·tu
sit·u·a·tion
sit·u·a·tion·al
si·tus
pl si·tus

si·tus in·ver·sus
sitz bath
six-o-six *or* 606
ska·tole
also ska·tol
or sca·tole

ska·tol·o·gy
var of scatology

skel·e·tal
skel·e·tal·ly
skel·e·ti·za·tion
skel·e·tog·e·nous
skel·e·to·mus·cu·lar
skel·e·ton
ske·nei·tis
or ske·ni·tis

Skene's gland
skia·gram
skia·graph
ski·ag·ra·pher
ski·ag·ra·phy
pl ski·ag·ra·phies

ski·am·e·try
pl ski·am·e·tries

skia·scope

ski•as•co•py
pl ski•as•co•pies
Skin•ner box
Skin•ner•ian
skull•cap
sleep•ing pill
sleep•walk
sleep•walk•er
slime mold
slit lamp
sliv•er
slob•ber
slob•bered
slob•ber•ing
slough
or sluff
slow vi•rus
slur•ry
pl slur•ries
small•pox
smeg•ma
smi•lax
Smith-Pe•ter•son nail
snake•bite
snake•root
sneeze
sneezed
sneez•ing
Snel•len test
snif•fle
snif•fled
snif•fling
snow-blind
or snow-blind•ed
snow blind•ness
snuf•fles
soap•stone
so•cial
so•cial•iza•tion
so•cial•ize
so•cial•ized
so•cial•iz•ing
so•cial•ly
so•cio•cen•tric
so•cio•cen•tric•i•ty
pl so•cio•cen•tric•i•ties
so•cio•cen•trism
so•cio•gen•e•sis
pl so•cio•gen•e•ses
so•cio•ge•net•ic
so•cio•gen•ic
so•cio•gram
so•cio•log•i•cal
also so•cio•log•ic
so•ci•ol•o•gist
so•ci•ol•o•gy
pl so•ci•ol•o•gies
so•cio•med•i•cal
so•cio•met•ric
so•ci•om•e•trist
so•ci•om•e•try
pl so•ci•om•e•tries
so•cio•path
so•cio•path•ic
so•ci•op•a•thy
pl so•ci•op•a•thies
so•cio•sex•u•al
so•cio•sex•u•al•i•ty
pl so•cio•sex•u•al•i•ties
sock•et
so•di•um
so•do•ku
sod•om•ite
sod•omy
pl sod•omies
soil•borne
soja
also soja bean
or soia
So•la•na•ce•ae
so•la•na•ceous
so•lan•i•dine
so•la•nine
or so•la•nin
so•la•num
so•lar
so•lar•i•um
pl so•lar•ia
also so•lar•i•ums
so•lar•iza•tion
so•lar•ize
so•lar•ized
so•lar•iz•ing
so•lar plex•us
sol•ation
so•le•no•glyph
So•le•nog•ly•pha
so•le•nog•ly•phous
or so•le•no•glyph•ic
sole•plate
sole•print
so•le•us
pl so•lei
also so•le•us•es
sol•i•da•go
pl sol•i•da•gos
sol•id•un•gu•late

sol•i•dus
pl sol•i•di

soli•ped

sol•u•bil•i•ty
pl sol•u•bil•i•ties

sol•u•bi•li•za•tion

sol•u•bi•lize
sol•u•bi•lized
sol•u•bi•liz•ing

sol•u•ble

sol•u•bly

sol•ute

so•lu•tion

sol•vate
sol•vated
sol•vat•ing

sol•va•tion

sol•vent

sol•vol•y•sis
pl sol•vol•y•ses

sol•vo•lyt•ic

so•ma
pl so•ma•ta
also so•mas

so•mas•the•nia

so•ma•tes•the•sia

so•ma•tic

so•mat•i•cal•ly

so•mat•i•co•vis•cer•al

so•ma•tist

so•ma•ti•za•tion

so•mato•chrome

so•mato•gen•ic
or so•mato•ge•net•ic

so•ma•to•log•i•cal

so•ma•tol•o•gy
pl so•ma•tol•o•gies

so•ma•tome

so•mato•met•ric

so•ma•tom•e•try
pl so•ma•tom•e•tries

so•ma•tom•ic

so•mato•path•ic

so•mato•plasm

so•mato•plas•tic

so•mato•pleure

so•mato•pleu•ric

so•mato•psy•chic

so•mato•sen•so•ry

so•mato•splanch•nic

so•mato•ther•a•pist

so•mato•ther•a•py
pl so•mato•ther•a•pies

so•mato•to•nia

so•mato•top•ic
also so•mato•top•i•cal

so•mato•tro•phic

so•mato•trop•ic

so•mato•tro•pin

so•mato•type

so•mato•typ•ic

so•mato•typ•i•cal•ly

so•mato•ty•pol•o•gy
pl so•mato•ty•pol•o•gies

som•es•the•sia
also som•es•the•sis
pl som•es•the•sias
also som•es•the•sis•es

so•mite

som•nam•bu•lant

som•nam•bu•lar

som•nam•bu•late
som•nam•bu•lat•ed
som•nam•bu•lat•ing

som•nam•bu•la•tion

som•nam•bu•la•tor

som•nam•bu•lism

som•nam•bu•list

som•nam•bu•lis•tic

som•nam•bu•lis•ti•cal•ly

som•ni•fa•cient

som•nif•er•ous

som•nif•er•ous•ly

som•nif•ic

som•nif•u•gous

som•nil•o•quist

som•nil•o•quy
pl som•nil•o•quies

som•nip•a•thist

som•nip•a•thy
pl som•nip•a•thies

som•no•cin•e•mat•o•graph

som·no·lence
also som·no·len·cy
pl som·no·lenc·es
also som·no·len·cies

som·no·lent
som·no·lent·ly
son·ic
son·i·cate
son·i·cat·ed
son·i·cat·ing
son·i·ca·tion
son·i·ca·tor
so·nom·e·ter
so·no·rous
so·phis·ti·cate
so·phis·ti·cat·ed
so·phis·ti·cat·ing
so·phis·ti·ca·tion
so·pho·ra
soph·o·rine
so·por
so·po·rif·er·ous
so·po·rif·er·ous·ness
so·po·rif·ic
so·po·rose
sor·be·fa·cient
sor·bic
sor·bi·tan
sor·bi·tol
sor·bose
sor·des
pl sor·des

sore·head
sore·muz·zle
so·ro·ri·a·tion
sorp·tion
souf·fle
soya
soy·bean
spa·cial
var of spatial

spall·ation
Span·ish fly
Span·ish in·flu·en·za
spar·ga·no·sis
pl spar·ga·no·ses

spar·ga·num
pl spar·ga·na
also spar·ga·nums

spar·go·sis
pl spar·go·ses
or spar·go·sis·es

spar·te·ine
spasm
spas·mat·ic
or spas·mat·i·cal

spas·mod·ic
or spas·mod·i·cal

spas·mod·i·cal·ly
spas·mo·gen·ic
spas·mol·y·sis
pl spas·mol·y·ses

spas·mo·lyt·ic
spas·mo·lyt·i·cal·ly
spas·mo·phil·ia
spas·mo·phil·ic
or spas·mo·phile

spas·mus
spas·tic
spas·ti·cal·ly
spas·tic·i·ty
pl spas·tic·i·ties

spa·tial
or spa·cial

spa·tial·ly
spa·tial sum·ma·tion
spa·ti·um
pl spa·tia

spat·u·la
spat·u·late
spat·u·lat·ed
spat·u·lat·ing
spat·u·la·tion
spa·tule
spav·in
also spav·ine

spav·ined
spay
spayed
spay·ing
spe·cial·ism
spe·cial·ist
spe·cial·iza·tion
spe·cial·ize
spe·cial·ized
spe·cial·iz·ing
spe·cial·ty
pl spe·cial·ties

spe·cies
pl spe·cies

spe·cies-spe·cif·ic
spe·cies-spec·i·fic·i·ty
pl spe·cies-spec·i·fic·i·ties

spe·cif·ic
spe·cif·i·cal·ly
spec·i·fic·i·ty
pl spec·i·fic·i·ties

spec·i·men
spec·ta·cles
spec·tral
spec·tral·ly
spec·tro·chem·i·cal
spec·tro·chem·is·try
pl spec·tro·chem·is·tries

spec·tro·gram
spec·tro·graph
spec·trog·ra·pher
spec·tro·graph·ic
spec·tro·graph·i·cal·ly
spec·trog·ra·phy
pl spec·trog·ra·phies

spec·trom·e·ter
spec·trom·e·try
pl spec·trom·e·tries

spec·tro·pho·tom·e·ter
spec·tro·pho·to·met·ric
or spec·tro·pho·to·met·ri·cal

spec·tro·pho·to·met·ri·cal·ly
spec·tro·pho·tom·e·try
pl spec·tro·pho·tom·e·tries

spec·tro·po·lar·im·e·ter
spec·tro·scope
spec·tro·scop·ic
also spec·tro·scop·i·cal

spec·tro·scop·i·cal·ly
spec·tros·co·pist
spec·tros·co·py
pl spec·tros·co·pies

spec·trum
pl spec·tra
or spec·trums

spec·u·lar
spec·u·lum
pl spec·u·la
also spec·u·lums

speedy cut
or speedy cut·ting

sperm
sper·ma·ce·ti
sper·ma·ry
pl sper·ma·ries

sper·ma·te·li·o· sis
sper·mat·ic
sper·mat·i·cal·ly
sper·ma·tid
sper·ma·tin
sper·mato·blast
sper·mato·blas·tic
sper·mato·cele
sper·mato·cid·al
or sper·mi·cid·al

sper·mato·cide
or sper·mi·cide

sper·mato·cyst
sper·mato·cys·tic
sper·mato·cy·tal
sper·mato·cyte
sper·mato·gen·e·sis
pl sper·mato·gen·e·ses

sper·mato·ge·net·ic
or sper·mato·gen·ic

sper·ma·tog·e·nous
sper·ma·tog·e·ny
pl sper·ma·tog·e·nies

sper·mato·go·ni·al
also sper·mato·gon·ic

sper·mato·go·ni·um
pl sper·mato·go·nia

sper·ma·toid
sper·ma·tol·y·sis
pl sper·ma·tol·y·ses

sper·mato·lyt·ic
sper·ma·top·a·thy
pl sper·ma·top·a·thies

sper·mato·phore
sper·mator·rhea
or sper·mator·rhoea

sper·ma·tox·in
sper·ma·to·zo·al
sper·ma·to·zo·an
sper·ma·to·zo·id
sper·ma·to·zo·on
pl sper·ma·to·zoa

sper·ma·tu·ria

sper·mi·a·tion
sper·mi·cid·al
var of spermatocidal
sper·mi·cide
var of spermatocide
sper·mi·dine
sperm·ine
sper·mio·gen·e·sis
pl sper·mio·gen·e·ses
sperm·ism
sperm·ist
sper·mi·um
pl sper·mia
sper·mo·lith
sper·mol·y·sis
pl sper·mol·y·ses
sper·mo·tox·in
spes phthis·i·ca
sphac·e·late
sphac·e·lat·ed
sphac·e·lat·ing
sphac·e·la·tion
sphac·e·lo·der·ma
pl sphac·e·lo·der·mas *or* sphac·e·lo·der·ma·ta
sphac·e·lus
sphaer·oid
var of spheroid
Sphae·roph·o·rus
sphen·eth·moid
sphe·ni·on
sphe·no·bas·i·lar
also sphe·no·bas·i·lic
sphe·no·ce·phal·ic
or sphe·no·ceph·a·lous
sphe·no·ceph·a·ly
pl sphe·no·ceph·a·lies
sphe·no·eth·moid
sphe·no·fron·tal
sphe·noid
also sphe·noi·dal
sphe·noid·itis
sphe·no·man·dib·u·lar
sphe·no·max·il·lary
sphe·no-oc·cip·i·tal
sphe·no·pal·a·tine
sphe·no·pa·ri·etal
sphe·no·pe·tro·sal
sphe·no·sis
sphe·no·squa·mo·sal
sphen·otic
sphe·no·tur·bi·nal
spher·i·cal
sphe·ro·cyte
sphe·ro·cyt·ic
sphe·ro·cy·to·sis
spher·oid
or sphaer·oid
sphe·roi·dal
sphe·rom·e·ter
Sphe·roph·o·rus
sphe·ro·plast
spher·ule
sphinc·ter
sphinc·ter·al
sphinc·ter·al·gia
sphinc·ter·ec·to·my
pl sphinc·ter·ec·to·mies
sphinc·ter·ic
sphinc·ter of Od·di
sphinc·ter·ol·y·sis
pl sphinc·ter·ol·y·ses
sphinc·ter·ot·o·my
pl sphinc·ter·ot·o·mies
sphinc·ter pu·pil·lae
sphinc·ter va·gi·nae
sphin·go·lip·id
also sphin·go·lip·ide
sphin·go·my·elin
sphin·go·sine
sphyg·mic
sphyg·mo·chro·no·graph
sphyg·mo·gram
sphyg·mo·graph
sphyg·mo·graph·ic
sphyg·mog·ra·phy
pl sphyg·mog·ra·phies
sphyg·moid
sphyg·mo·ma·nom·e·ter
sphyg·mo·mano·met·ric
sphygo·mo·mano·met·ri·cal·ly
sphyg·mo·ma·nom·e·try
pl sphyg·mo·ma·nom·e·tries
sphyg·mom·e·ter

sphyg•mo-os•cil•lom•e•ter
spi•ca
pl spi•cae
or spi•cas
spic•u•lar
spic•u•late
or spic•u•lat•ed
spic•u•la•tion
spic•ule
spic•u•lum
pl spic•u•la
Spi•ge•lia
spi•ge•lian
spi•lo•ma
spi•lus
spi•na
pl spi•nae
spi•na bi•fi•da
spina•cene
spi•nal
spi•na•lis
pl spi•na•les
spi•nal•ly
spi•nate
spin•dle
spine•less
spi•no•cer•e•bel•lar
spi•no-ol•i•vary
spi•nose
spi•nose•ly
spi•no•tec•tal
spi•no•tha•lam•ic
spi•nous
spin•thar•i•scope
spin•ther•ism
spiny-head•ed worm
spi•ra•cle
spi•reme
also spi•rem
Spi•ril•la•ce•ae
spi•ril•la•ceous
spi•ril•li•ci•dal
spi•ril•lo•sis
pl spi•ril•lo•ses
or spi•ril•lo•sis•es
spi•ril•lum
pl spi•ril•la
spir•i•tu•ous
spir•i•tus
spir•i•tus fru•men•ti
Spi•ro•cer•ca
spi•ro•chae•ta
or spi•ro•che•ta
pl spi•ro•chae•tae
or spi•ro•che•tae
Spi•ro•chae•ta•ce•ae
Spi•ro•chae•ta•les
spi•ro•chet•al
or spi•ro•chaet•al
spi•ro•chete
or spi•ro•chaete
spi•ro•chet•emia
spi•ro•che•ti•ci•dal
spi•ro•che•ti•cide
or spi•ro•chae•ti•cide
spi•ro•chet•osis
or spi•ro•chaet•osis
pl spi•ro•chet•oses
or spi•ro•chaet•oses
spi•ro•gram
spi•ro•graph
spi•ro•graph•ic
spi•rom•e•ter
spi•ro•met•ric
spi•rom•e•try
pl spi•rom•e•tries
spi•rono•lac•tone
spis•si•tude
spit•al
spit•tle
splanch•nec•to•pia
splanch•nes•the•sia
splanch•nic
splanch•ni•cec•to•my
pl splanch•ni•cec•to•mies
splanch•ni•cot•o•my
pl splanch•ni•cot•o•mies
splanch•no•coele
or splanch•no•coel
splanch•nol•o•gy
pl splanch•nol•o•gies
splanch•no•meg•a•ly
pl splanch•no•meg•a•lies
splanch•no•pleure
splanch•no•pleu•ric
splanch•nop•to•sis
pl splanch•nop•to•ses
splanch•nos•co•py
pl splanch•nos•co•pies

splay·foot
pl splay·feet
spleen
sple·nal·gia
sple·nal·gic
sple·nec·to·mize
sple·nec·to·mized
sple·nec·to·miz·ing
sple·nec·to·my
pl sple·nec·to·mies
sple·ne·o·lus
pl sple·ne·o·li
sple·net·ic
sple·net·i·cal·ly
sple·ni·al
sple·nic
also sple·ni·cal
sple·ni·fi·ca·tion
sple·ni·form
sple·ni·tis
pl sple·ni·tis·es
sple·ni·um
pl sple·nia
sple·ni·us
pl sple·nii
sple·ni·za·tion
sple·no·cyte
sple·no·dyn·ia
sple·no·gen·ic
sple·no·hep·ato·meg·a·ly
pl sple·no·hep·ato·meg·a·lies
sple·noid
sple·no·ma·la·cia
sple·no·meg·a·ly
pl sple·no·meg·a·lies
sple·nop·a·thy
pl sple·nop·a·thies
sple·no·pexy
pl sple·no·pex·ies
sple·nop·to·sis
pl sple·nop·to·ses
sple·not·o·my
pl sple·not·o·mies
splen·u·lus
or sple·nun·cu·lus
pl splen·u·li
or sple·nun·cu·li
splint·age
splin·ter
splint·ered
splin·ter·ing
split-brain
spoke·shave
spon·dy·lit·ic
spon·dy·li·tis
spon·dy·lo·dyn·ia
spon·dy·lo·lis·the·sis
spon·dy·lol·y·sis
pl spon·dy·lol·y·ses
spon·dy·lop·a·thy
pl spon·dy·lop·a·thies
spon·dy·lo·sis
pl spon·dy·lo·ses
or spon·dy·lo·sis·es
spon·dy·lo·syn·de·sis
spon·dy·lot·o·my
pl spon·dy·lot·o·mies
spon·dyl·ous
spon·gin
spon·gio·blast
spon·gio·blas·to·ma
pl spon·gio·blas·to·mas
or spon·gio·blas·to·ma·ta
spon·gio·cyte
spon·gio·plasm
spon·gio·plas·mic
spon·gi·o·sa
spon·gi·o·sis
spon·ta·ne·ous
spon·ta·ne·ous·ly
spoo·ner·ism
spo·ran·gio·phore
spo·ran·gio·spore
spo·ran·gi·um
pl spo·ran·gia
spo·ri·cid·al
spo·ri·cide
spo·rid·i·um
pl spo·rid·ia
spo·ro·blast
spo·ro·cyst
spo·ro·cys·tic
spo·ro·gen·e·sis
pl spo·ro·gen·e·ses
spo·ro·gen·ic
spo·rog·e·nous
spo·rog·e·ny
pl spo·rog·e·nies
spo·ro·gon·ic
also spo·rog·o·nous
spo·rog·o·ny
pl spo·rog·o·nies
spo·ront

spo·ro·phore
spo·ro·phyte
spo·ro·plasm
spo·ro·tri·cho·sis
pl spo·ro·tri·cho·ses

spo·rot·ri·chum
pl spo·rot·ri·cha

Spo·ro·zoa
spo·ro·zo·an
spo·ro·zo·ite
spo·ro·zo·on
pl spo·ro·zoa

spor·u·lar
spor·u·late
spor·u·lat·ed
spor·u·lat·ing
spor·u·la·tion
spor·u·la·tive
spor·ule
spread·er
sprue
spu·tum
pl spu·ta

squa·lene
squa·ma
pl squa·mae

squa·mate
also squa·mat·ed

squame
squa·mo·co·lum·nar
squa·moid
squa·mo-oc·cip·i·tal
squa·mo·sa
pl squa·mo·sas
or squa·mo·sae

squa·mo·sal
squa·mose
squa·mous
squar·rose
also squar·rous

squill
squint-eyed
stab·i·lim·e·ter
stac·ca·to
pl stac·ca·tos
or stac·ca·ti

stach·y·drine
stach·y·ose
stac·tom·e·ter
Sta·der splint
sta·di·um
pl sta·dia
or sta·di·ums

staff of Aes·cu·la·pi·us
stag·gers
stag·na·tion
stain·abil·i·ty
pl stain·abil·i·ties

stal·ag·mom·e·ter
stale
staled
stal·ing
stam·mer
stam·mered
stam·mer·ing
stand·still
Stan·ford-Bi·net test
stan·nate
stan·nic
stan·nous

stan·num
sta·pe·dec·to·mized
sta·pe·dec·to·my
pl sta·pe·dec·to·mies

sta·pe·di·al
sta·pe·dio·ves·tib·u·lar
sta·pe·di·us
pl sta·pe·dii

sta·pes
pl sta·pes
or sta·pe·des

staph·y·lec·to·my
pl staph·y·lec·to·mies

staph·yl·ede·ma
pl staph·yl·ede·mas
or staph·yl·ede·ma·ta

sta·phyl·i·on
staph·y·li·tis
staph·y·lo·coc·cal
staph·y·lo·coc·ce·mia
staph·y·lo·coc·ce·mic
staph·y·lo·coc·cic
staph·y·lo·coc·cus
pl staph·y·lo·coc·ci

staph·y·lo·der·ma·ti·tis
pl staph·y·lo·der·ma·ti·ti·ses
or staph·y·lo·der·ma·tit·i·des

staph·y·lo·ma
staph·y·lo·plas·ty
pl staph·y·lo·plas·ties

staph·y·lot·o·my
pl staph·y·lot·o·mies

starch•i•ness
starchy
starch•i•er
starch•i•est
Star•ling's law
sta•sis
pl sta•ses
stoppage of flow of a bodily fluid (see staxis)
stat•im
stato•cyst
stato•ki•net•ic
stato•lith
stato•lith•ic
stat•ure
sta•tus
sta•tus asth•mat•i•cus
sta•tus ep•i•lep•ti•cus
sta•tus lym•phat•i•cus
sta•tus thy•mi•co•lym•phat•i•cus
stau•ri•on
stax•is
a dripping (see stasis)
ste•ap•sin
stea•rate
stea•ric ac•id
stea•rin
stea•rop•tene
also stea•rop•ten
ste•atite
ste•atit•ic
ste•ati•tis
ste•atog•e•nous
ste•atol•y•sis
pl ste•atol•y•ses
ste•ato•ma
pl ste•ato•mas
or ste•ato•ma•ta
ste•atoma•tous
ste•ato•py•gia
also ste•ato•py•ga
ste•ato•py•gic
or ste•ato•py•gous
ste•at•or•rhea
or ste•at•or•rhoea
ste•ato•sis
pl ste•ato•ses
stego•my•ia
Stein•mann pin
stel•late
stel•late•ly
stel•lec•to•my
pl stel•lec•to•mies
Sten•der dish
steni•on
pl stenia
steno•car•dia
steno•car•di•ac
steno•ce•phal•ic
steno•ceph•a•ly
also steno•ce•phal•ia
pl steno•ceph•a•lies
also steno•ce•phal•ias
steno•cho•ria
steno•co•ri•a•sis
steno•mer•ic
steno•pa•ic
also steno•pe•ic
or steno•pae•ic
Ste•no's duct
ste•nose
ste•nosed
ste•nos•ing
ste•no•sis
pl sten•o•ses
steno•therm
steno•ther•mal
also steno•ther•mic
steno•ther•my
pl steno•ther•mies
steno•tho•rax
pl steno•tho•rax•es
or steno•tho•ra•ces
ste•not•ic
Sten•sen's duct
also Sten•son's duct
ste•pha•ni•on
Steph•a•no•fi•lar•ia
steph•a•no•fil•a•ri•a•sis
pl steph•a•no•fil•a•ri•a•ses
Steph•a•nu•rus
step•page
ste•ra•di•an
also ste•rad
ster•co•bi•lin
ster•co•bi•lin•o•gen
ster•co•ra•ceous
ster•co•ral
ster•co•ro•ma
pl ster•co•ro•mas
or ster•co•ro•ma•ta
ster•cu•lia
ster•cus
pl ster•co•ra

ste•reo•blas•tu•la
pl ste•reo•blas•tu•las
or ste•reo•blas•tu•lae

ste•reo•cam•pim•e•ter
ste•reo•chem•i•cal
ste•reo•chem•is•try
pl ste•reo•chem•is•tries

ste•reo•cil•i•um
pl ste•reo•cil•ia

stere•og•no•sis
stere•og•nos•tic
ste•reo•gram
ste•reo•graph
ste•reo•iso•mer
ste•reo•iso•mer•ic
ste•reo•isom•er•ism
ste•re•om•e•ter
ste•reo•met•ric
ste•re•om•e•try
pl ste•re•om•e•tries

ste•reo•pho•to•mi•cro•graph
ste•re•op•sis
ste•reo•ra•dio•graph
ste•reo•ra•dio•graph•ic
ste•reo•ra•di•og•ra•phy
pl ste•reo•ra•di•og•ra•phies

ste•reo•scope
ste•reo•scop•ic
also ste•reo•scop•i•cal
ste•reo•scop•i•cal•ly
ste•re•os•co•py
pl ste•re•os•co•pies

ste•reo•spe•cif•ic
ste•reo•spe•cif•i•cal•ly
ste•reo•spec•i•fic•i•ty
pl ste•reo•spec•i•fic•i•ties

ste•reo•tac•tic
ste•reo•tac•ti•cal•ly
ste•reo•tax•ic
ste•reo•tax•i•cal•ly
ste•reo•tax•is
pl ste•reo•tax•es

ste•re•ot•ro•pism
ste•reo•type
ste•reo•ty•py
pl ste•reo•ty•pies

ste•rid
also ste•ride

ste•rig•ma
pl ste•rig•ma•ta
also ste•rig•mas

ster•ile
ster•ile•ly
ste•ril•i•ty
pl ste•ril•i•ties

ster•il•iza•tion
ster•il•ize
ster•il•ized
ster•il•iz•ing
ster•il•iz•er
ster•nad
ster•nal
ster•na•lis
pl ster•na•les

Stern•berg cell
also Stern•berg-Reed cell

ster•ne•bra
pl ster•ne•brae

ster•no•cla•vic•u•lar
ster•no•clei•do•mas•toid
ster•no•cos•tal
ster•no•fa•ci•a•lis
pl ster•no•fa•ci•a•les

ster•no•hy•oid
ster•no•mas•toid
ster•no•thy•roid
ster•not•o•my
pl ster•not•o•mies

ster•num
pl ster•nums
or ster•na

ster•nu•ta•tion
ster•nu•ta•tor
ster•nu•ta•to•ry
or ster•nu•ta•tive

ste•roid
ste•roi•dal
ste•roido•gen•e•sis
pl ste•roido•gen•e•ses

ste•roido•gen•ic
ste•rol
ster•tor
ster•to•rous
ster•to•rous•ly
stetho•graph

stetho·graph·ic
ste·thom·e·ter
stetho·met·ric
stetho·scope
stetho·scop·ic
or stetho·scop·i·cal

stetho·scop·i·cal·ly
ste·thos·co·py
pl ste·thos·co·pies

sthen·ic
stib·amine
stib·i·um
sti·bo·ni·um
stib·o·phen
stig·ma
pl stig·ma·ta
or stig·mas

stig·mal
stig·mas·ter·ol
stig·mat·ic
stig·ma·tism
stig·ma·ti·za·tion
stig·ma·tize
stig·ma·tized
stig·ma·tiz·ing
stilb·am·i·dine
stil·bene
stil·bes·trol
also stil·boes·trol

sti·let
also sti·lette

sti·let·ted
still·birth
still·born
Still's dis·ease

sti·lus
var of stylus

stim·u·lant
stim·u·late
stim·u·lat·ed
stim·u·lat·ing
stim·u·la·tion
stim·u·la·tive
stim·u·la·tor
also stim·u·lat·er

stim·u·la·to·ry
stim·u·lus
pl stim·u·li

stip·pling
stir·rup
stock·i·nette
or stock·i·net

stoi·chio·met·ric
also stoi·chio·met·ri·cal

stoi·chio·met·ri·cal·ly
stoi·chi·om·e·try
pl stoi·chi·om·e·tries

sto·ma
pl sto·ma·ta
also sto·mas

stom·ach
stom·ach·ache
stom·ach·al
sto·mach·ic
also sto·mach·i·cal

sto·mach·i·cal·ly
sto·mal
sto·ma·tal
sto·mat·ic

sto·ma·ti·tis
pl sto·ma·tit·i·des
or sto·ma·ti·tis·es

sto·mato·gas·tric
sto·ma·to·log·i·cal
also sto·ma·to·log·ic

sto·ma·tol·o·gist
sto·ma·tol·o·gy
pl sto·ma·tol·o·gies

sto·mat·o·my
pl sto·mat·o·mies

sto·ma·to·sis
pl sto·ma·to·ses
or sto·ma·to·sis·es

sto·mo·dae·al
or sto·mo·de·al

sto·mo·dae·um
or sto·mo·de·um
pl sto·mo·daea
also sto·mo·dae·ums
or sto·mo·dea
also sto·mo·de·ums

Sto·mox·ys
stone-blind
stone-blind·ness
stone-deaf
stone-deaf·ness
stop·cock
stop·page
sto·rax
stra·bis·mal
stra·bis·mal·ly
stra·bis·mic
stra·bis·mom·e·ter
stra·bis·mom·e·try
pl stra·bis·mom·e·tries

stra·bis·mus
strain·er
strait·jack·et
or straight·jack·et
stra·mo·ni·um
strand·ed
strand·ed·ness
stran·gle
stran·gled
stran·gling
stran·gles
stran·gu·late
stran·gu·lat·ed
stran·gu·lat·ing
stran·gu·la·tion
stran·gu·ry
pl stran·gu·ries
stra·tum
pl stra·ta
also stra·tums
stra·tum cor·ne·um
pl stra·ta cor·nea
stra·tum ger·mi·na·ti·vum
pl stra·ta ger·mi·na·ti·va
stra·tum gran·u·lo·sum
pl stra·ta gran·u·lo·sa
stra·tum lu·ci·dum
pl stra·ta lu·ci·da
straw·ber·ry mark
strepho·sym·bo·lia
strepho·sym·bol·ic
strepo·gen·in
strep·ti·dine
strep·to·ba·cil·la·ry
strep·to·ba·cil·lus
pl strep·to·ba·cil·li
strep·to·bi·o·sa·mine
strep·to·coc·cal
or strep·to·coc·cic
strep·to·coc·ce·mia
strep·to·coc·co·sis
strep·to·coc·cus
pl strep·to·coc·ci
strep·to·dor·nase
strep·to·ki·nase
strep·to·ly·sin
strep·to·my·ces
pl strep·to·my·ces
or strep·to·my·ce·tes
strep·to·my·cin
strep·to·ni·grin
strep·tose
strep·to·thri·cin
strep·to·thrix
pl strep·to·thri·ces
strep·to·tri·cho·sis
also strep·to·thri·cho·sis
stress·or
stretch·er
stria
pl stri·ae
stria lon·gi·tu·di·na·lis
pl stri·ae lon·gi·tu·di·na·les
stri·a·tal
stri·ate
stri·at·ed
stri·a·tion
stri·a·tum
pl stri·a·ta
strick·en
stric·ture
stri·dent
stri·dent·ly
stri·dor
strid·u·lous
string·halt
string·halt·ed
strip·per
stro·bi·la
pl stro·bi·lae
stro·bi·lar
stro·bi·la·tion
also stro·bi·li·za·tion
stro·bile
also stro·bil
strob·i·loid
stro·bi·lus
pl stro·bi·li
stro·bo·scope
stro·bo·scop·ic
stro·bo·scop·i·cal·ly
stro·ma
pl stro·ma·ta
stro·mal
stro·ma·tal

stro·mat·ic
stro·ma·tin
stro·muhr
stron·gyle
also stron·gyl
Stron·gy·loi·dea
Stron·gy·loi·des
stron·gy·loi·di·a·sis
also stron·gy·loi·do·sis
stron·gy·lo·sis
Stron·gy·lus
stron·tium
stro·phan·thin
stro·phan·thus
stroph·u·lus
pl stroph·u·li
stru·ma
pl stru·mae
or stru·mas
stru·mi·form
stru·mi·tis
stru·mous
strych·nine
strych·nin·ism
strych·nin·iza·tion
Strych·nos
stu·pe·fa·cient
stu·pe·fac·tion
stu·pe·fac·tive
stu·pe·fy
stu·pe·fied
stu·pe·fy·ing
stu·por
stu·por·ous
stur·dy
pl stur·dies
stur·ine
also stur·in
stut·ter
stut·tered
stut·ter·ing
sty·let
sty·li·form
sty·lo·glos·sus
pl sty·lo·glos·si
sty·lo·hy·al
sty·lo·hy·oid
sty·lo·hy·oi·de·us
pl sty·lo·hy·oi·dei
sty·loid
sty·lo·man·dib·u·lar
sty·lo·mas·toid
sty·lo·pha·ryn·ge·us
pl sty·lo·pha·ryn·gei
sty·lus
also sti·lus
pl sty·li
also sty·lus·es
or sti·li
styp·sis
styp·tic
sty·ra·cin
sty·rax
sty·rene
sty·rol
sub·ab·dom·i·nal
sub·acro·mi·al
sub·acute
sub·acute·ly
sub·al·i·men·ta·tion
sub·api·cal
sub·api·cal·ly
sub·apo·neu·rot·ic
sub·arach·noid
sub·are·o·lar
sub·ar·cu·ate
also sub·ar·cu·at·ed
sub·as·trin·gent
sub·au·ric·u·lar
sub·ax·il·lary
also sub·ax·il·lar
sub·bas·al
sub·brach·i·al
also sub·bra·chi·an
sub·brachy·ce·phal·ic
sub·cal·ca·rine
sub·cal·lo·sal
sub·cap·su·lar
sub·car·bon·ate
sub·car·ti·lag·i·nous
sub·cel·lu·lar
sub·chlo·ride
sub·chon·dral
sub·cho·ri·on·ic
sub·cla·vi·an
sub·cla·vi·us
pl sub·cla·vii
sub·clin·i·cal
sub·clin·i·cal·ly
sub·col·lat·er·al
sub·co·ma
sub·con·junc·ti·val

sub•con•junc•ti•val•ly
sub•con•scious
sub•con•scious•ly
sub•con•scious•ness
sub•cor•a•coid
sub•cor•tex
pl sub•cor•ti•ces
or sub•cor•tex•es
sub•cor•ti•cal
sub•cor•ti•cal•ly
sub•cos•tal
sub•crep•i•tant
sub•crep•i•ta•tion
sub•cul•ture
sub•cu•ra•tive
sub•cu•ta•ne•ous
sub•cu•ta•ne•ous•ly
sub•cu•tic•u•lar
sub•cu•tis
pl sub•cu•tes
or sub•cu•tis•es
sub•del•toid
sub•der•mal
sub•di•a•phrag•mat•ic
sub•dol•i•cho•ce•phal•ic
also sub•dol•i•cho•ceph•a•lous
sub•dor•sal
sub•dor•sal•ly
sub•duct
sub•duc•tion
sub•du•ral
sub•du•ral•ly

sub•en•ceph•a•lon
pl sub•en•ceph•a•la
sub•en•do•car•di•al
sub•en•do•the•li•al
sub•epi•car•di•al
sub•epi•der•mal
sub•ep•i•the•li•al
su•ber•in
su•ber•iza•tion
su•ber•ized
su•ber•yl•ar•gi•nine
sub•gal•late
sub•gin•gi•val
sub•gle•noid
sub•glos•si•tis
sub•glot•tic
sub•he•pat•ic
sub•ic•ter•ic
su•bic•u•lar
su•bic•u•lum
pl su•bic•u•la
sub•in•ci•sion
sub•in•fec•tion
sub•in•gui•nal
sub•in•teg•u•men•tal
sub•in•ti•mal
sub•in•vo•lu•tion
sub•ja•cent
sub•ja•cent•ly
sub•jec•tive
sub•ject•ive•ly
sub•la•tion
sub•le•thal

sub•le•thal•ly
sub•leu•ke•mic
sub•li•mate
sub•li•mat•ed
sub•li•mat•ing
sub•li•ma•tion
sub•lime
sub•limed
sub•lim•ing
sub•lim•i•nal
sub•lim•i•nal•ly
sub•li•mis
sub•lin•gual
sub•lob•u•lar
sub•lob•u•lar•ly
sub•lux•a•tion
sub•man•dib•u•lar
sub•mar•gin•al
sub•max•il•la
pl sub•max•il•lae
or sub•max•il•las
sub•max•il•lary
sub•me•di•al
sub•me•di•al•ly
sub•me•di•an
sub•men•tal
sub•mi•cro•scop•ic
sub•mil•i•ary
sub•min•i•mal
sub•mi•to•chon•dri•al
sub•mu•co•sa
sub•mu•co•sal
sub•mu•cous
sub•nar•cot•ic
sub•na•sal
sub•neu•ral

sub·nor·mal
sub·nor·mal·ly
sub·nu·cle·us
pl sub·nu·clei
or sub·nu·cle·us·es
sub·nu·tri·tion
sub·oc·cip·i·tal
sub·oc·cip·i·tal·ly
sub·op·ti·mal
sub·op·ti·mum
sub·or·bit·al
sub·pec·to·ral
sub·pe·dun·cu·lar
sub·peri·os·te·al
sub·phren·ic
sub·pi·al
sub·pla·cen·ta
pl sub·pla·cen·tas
or sub·pla·cen·tae
sub·pla·cen·tal
sub·plan·ti·grade
sub·pleu·ral
sub·pleu·ral·ly
sub·po·ten·cy
pl sub·po·ten·cies
sub·po·tent
sub·pu·bic
sub·ros·tral
sub·scap·u·lar
sub·scap·u·lar·is
sub·scler·al
sub·scle·rot·ic
sub·scrip·tion
sub·se·ro·sa
sub·se·rous
sub·spi·nous
sub·stage
sub·stance of Schwann
sub·stan·tia
pl sub·stan·ti·ae
sub·stan·tia ni·gra
pl sub·stan·ti·ae ni·grae
sub·stan·tia pro·pria
pl sub·stan·ti·ae pro·pri·ae
sub·ster·nal
sub·strate
sub·stra·tum
pl sub·stra·ta
sub·struc·ture
sub·sul·fate
sub·sul·tus
sub·ten·to·ri·al
sub·ter·mi·nal
sub·te·tan·ic
sub·tha·lam·ic
sub·thal·a·mus
pl sub·thal·a·mi
sub·thresh·old
sub·ti·lin
sub·til·i·sin
sub·tro·chan·ter·ic
sub·un·gual
also sub·un·gui·al
sub·vag·i·nal
sub·vi·ral
sub·vo·la
sub·vo·lu·tion
suc·ce·da·ne·ous
suc·ce·da·ne·um
pl suc·ce·da·ne·ums
or suc·ce·da·nea
suc·cen·tu·ri·ate
suc·ci·nate
suc·cin·chlor·im·ide
suc·cin·ic
suc·cin·ox·i·dase
suc·ci·nyl·cho·line
suc·ci·nyl·sul·fa·thi·a·zole
suc·cor·ance
suc·cor·ant
suc·cor·rhea
or suc·cor·rhoea
suc·cus
pl suc·ci
suc·cus en·ter·i·cus
suc·cus·sion
suck·le
suck·led
suck·ling
su·crase
su·crate
su·crose
su·cros·uria
suc·to·ri·al
su·da·men
pl su·dam·i·na
su·dam·i·nal
Su·dan
su·dan·o·phil
or su·dan·o·phil·ic
su·dan·o·phil·ia

su·da·tion
su·da·to·ri·um
pl su·da·to·ria
su·do·mo·tor
su·do·rif·er·ous
su·do·rif·ic
su·do·rip·a·rous
suf·fo·cate
suf·fo·cat·ed
suf·fo·cat·ing
suf·fo·ca·tion
suf·fuse
suf·fused
suf·fus·ing
suf·fu·sion
sug·gil·la·tion
sui·cid·al
sui·cid·al·ly
sui·cide
sui·cid·ol·o·gist
sui·cid·ol·o·gy
pl sui·cid·ol·o·gies
sui·gen·der·ism
su·int
sul·cal
also sul·car
sul·cate
also sul·cat·ed
sul·cu·lus
pl sul·cu·li
sul·cus
pl sul·ci
sul·cus lu·na·tus
pl sul·ci lu·na·ti
sul·cus of Ro·lan·do
sul·cus ter·mi·na·lis
pl sul·ci ter·mi·na·les
sul·fa
also sul·pha
sul·fa·cet·a·mide
also sul·fa·cet·i·mide
sul·fa·di·a·zine
sul·fa·gua·ni·dine
sul·fa·mer·a·zine
sul·fa·meth·a·zine
sul·fa·mez·a·thine
sul·fa·nil·amide
sul·fan·i·late
sul·fa·nil·ic
sul·fa·pyr·azine
sul·fa·pyr·i·dine
sul·fa·qui·nox·a·line
sulf·ars·phen·a·mine
sul·fa·tase
sul·fate
or sul·phate
sul·fat·ed
or sul·phat·ed
sul·fat·ing
or sul·phat·ing
sul·fa·thi·a·zole
sulf·he·mo·glo·bin
sulf·he·mo·glo·bi·ne·mia
sulf·hy·drate
also sul·phy·drate
sulf·hy·dryl
also sul·phy·dryl
sul·fide
or sul·phide
sul·fi·sox·a·zole
sul·fite
or sul·phite
sul·fit·ic
sul·fo ac·id
sul·fo·cy·a·nate
sul·fon·amide
sul·fo·nate
also sul·pho·nate
sul·fo·nat·ed
also sul·pho·nat·ed
sul·fo·nat·ing
also sul·pho·nat·ing
sul·fone
sul·fon·eth·yl·meth·ane
sul·fon·ic
sul·fon·meth·ane
sul·fo·nyl
sul·fo·nyl·urea
sul·fo·sal·i·cyl·ic
sulf·ox·ide
sulf·ox·one
sul·fur
or sul·phur
sul·fured
or sul·phured
sul·fur·ing
or sul·phur·ing

sul·fu·rate
or sul·phu·rate
sul·fu·rat·ed
or sul·phu·rat·ed
sul·fu·rat·ing
or sul·phu·rat·ing
sul·fu·ret
sul·fu·ret·ed
or sul·fu·ret·ted
sul·fur·ret·ing
or sul·fur·ret·ting
sul·fu·ric
sul·fu·rize
or sul·phu·rize
sul·fu·rized
or sul·phu·rized
sul·fu·riz·ing
or sul·phu·riz·ing
sul·fu·rous
or sul·phu·rous
sul·fu·ryl
sul·fy·drate
sul·lage
sul·pha
var of sulfa
sul·phate
var of sulfate
sul·phide
var of sulfide
sul·phite
var of sulfite
sul·pho·nate
var of sulfonate
sul·phur
var of sulfur
sul·phu·rate
var of sulfurate
sul·phu·rize
var of sulfurize
sul·phu·rous
var of sulfurous
sul·phy·drate
var of sulfhydrate
sul·phy·dryl
var of sulfhydryl
sum·mate
sum·mat·ed
sum·mat·ing
sum·ma·tion
sun·burn
sun·burned
or sun·burnt
sun·burn·ing
sun·stroke
su·per·ab·duc·tion
su·per·acute
su·per·al·i·men·ta·tion
su·per·cen·tral
su·per·cil·i·ary
su·per·cil·i·um
pl su·per·cil·ia
su·per·ego
su·per·ex·ci·ta·tion
su·per·ex·ten·sion
su·per·fe·cun·da·tion
su·per·fe·ta·tion
su·per·fi·cial
su·per·gene
su·per·im·preg·nate
su·per·im·preg·nat·ed
su·per·im·preg·nat·ing
su·per·im·preg·na·tion
su·per·in·duce
su·per·in·duced
su·per·in·duc·ing
su·per·in·duc·tion
su·per·in·fect
su·per·in·fec·tion
su·pe·ri·or
su·pe·ri·or·ly
su·per·lac·ta·tion
su·per·mo·lec·u·lar
su·per·mol·e·cule
su·per·na·tant
su·per·nate
su·per·nor·mal
su·per·nu·mer·ary
pl su·per·nu·mer·ar·ies
su·per·ovu·late
su·per·ovu·lat·ed
su·per·ovu·lat·ing
su·per·ovu·la·tion
su·per·par·a·sit·ism
su·per·phos·phate
su·per·pig·men·ta·tion

su·per·po·ten·cy
pl su·per·po·ten·cies

su·per·po·tent
su·per·sat·u·rate
su·per·sat·u·rat·ed
su·per·sat·u·rat·ing
su·per·sat·u·ra·tion
su·per·scrip·tion
su·per·sen·si·tive
su·per·sen·si·ti·za·tion
su·per·sep·tal
su·per·son·ic
su·per·son·i·cal·ly
su·per·struc·ture
su·per·tem·po·ral
su·per·ven·tion
su·per·vi·sor
su·per·volt·age
su·pi·nate
su·pi·nat·ed
su·pi·nat·ing
su·pi·na·tion
su·pi·na·tor
su·pine
sup·ple·ment
sup·ple·men·tal
sup·ple·men·ta·ry
sup·port·er
sup·pos·i·to·ry
pl sup·pos·i·to·ries

sup·press
sup·pres·sant
sup·pres·sion
sup·pres·sor
sup·pu·rate
sup·pu·rat·ed
sup·pu·rat·ing
sup·pu·ra·tion
sup·pu·ra·tive
su·pra-au·ric·u·lar
su·pra·cel·lu·lar
su·pra·cer·vi·cal
su·pra·cho·roid
or su·pra·cho·roi·dal

su·pra·cho·roi·dea
su·pra·cil·i·ary
su·pra·cla·vic·u·lar
su·pra·com·mis·sure
su·pra·con·dy·lar
su·pra·di·a·phrag·mat·ic
su·pra·di·a·phrag·mat·i·cal·ly
su·pra·gle·noid
su·pra·glot·tal
or su·pra·glot·tic

su·pra·he·pat·ic
su·pra·hy·oid
su·pra·lim·i·nal
su·pra·lim·i·nal·ly
su·pra·man·dib·u·lar
su·pra·mar·gin·al
su·pra·mas·toid
su·pra·max·il·la
pl su·pra·max·il·lae
or su·pra·max·il·las

su·pra·max·il·lary
su·pra·me·a·tal
su·pra·men·tal
su·pra·na·sal
su·pra·nu·cle·ar
su·pra·oc·cip·i·tal
su·pra·oc·clu·sion
su·pra·op·tic
su·pra·or·bit·al
su·pra·pa·tel·lar
su·pra·pu·bic
su·pra·re·nal
su·pra·re·nal·ec·to·my
pl su·pra·re·nal·ec·to·mies

su·pra·scap·u·la
pl su·pra·scap·u·lae
or su·pra·scap·u·las

su·pra·scap·u·lar
su·pra·sel·lar
su·pra·spi·nal
su·pra·spi·na·tus
su·pra·spi·nous
su·pra·sta·pe·di·al
su·pra·ster·nal
su·pra·tem·po·ral
su·pra·ten·to·ri·al
su·pra·ton·sil·lar
su·pra·troch·le·ar
su·pra·ven·tric·u·lar
su·pra·ver·gence
su·pra·ver·sion

su·pra·vi·tal
su·ra
su·ral
sur·al·i·men·ta·tion
sur·a·min
sur·cin·gle
sur·di·ty
pl sur·di·ties
sur·ex·ci·ta·tion
sur·face-ac·tive
sur·fac·tant
sur·geon
sur·geon apoth·e·cary
pl sur·geon apoth·e·car·ies
sur·geon gen·er·al
pl sur·geons gen·er·al
sur·gery
pl sur·ger·ies
sur·gi·cal
sur·gi·cal·ly
sur·ra
also sur·rah
sur·ro·gate
sur·sum·duc·tion
sur·sum·ver·gence
sur·sum·ver·sion
sur·veil·lance
sus·cep·ti·bil·i·ty
pl sus·cep·ti·bil·i·ties
sus·cep·ti·ble
sus·cep·ti·bly
sus·ci·tate
sus·ci·tat·ed
sus·ci·tat·ing
sus·ci·ta·tion
sus·pen·sion
sus·pen·soid
sus·pen·so·ri·um
pl sus·pen·so·ria
sus·pen·so·ry
pl sus·pen·so·ries
sus·ten·tac·u·lar
sus·ten·tac·u·lum
pl sus·ten·tac·u·la
su·sur·rus
su·ture
su·tured
su·tur·ing
sved·berg
or sved·berg unit
swal·low
sway·back
sway·backed
swee·ny
also swee·ney
or swin·ney
pl swee·nies
also swee·neys
or swin·neys
sweet·bread
swell·head
swim·mer's itch
sy·co·sis
pl sy·co·ses
inflammatory disease of the hair follicles (see psychosis)
Sy·den·ham's cho·rea
syl·lep·si·ol·o·gy
pl syl·lep·si·ol·o·gies
syl·lep·sis
pl syl·lep·ses
Syl·vi·an aq·ue·duct
Syl·vi·an fis·sure
sym·bal·lo·phone
sym·bi·on
sym·bi·ont
sym·bi·o·sis
pl sym·bi·o·ses
sym·bi·ote
also sym·bi·ot
sym·bi·ot·ic
also sym·bi·ot·i·cal
sym·bi·ot·i·cal·ly
sym·bleph·a·ron
sym·bol·ism
sym·bol·iza·tion
sym·bo·lo·pho·bia
sym·me·lus
pl sym·me·li
sym·met·ri·cal
or sym·met·ric
sym·me·try
pl sym·me·tries
sym·pa·thec·to·my
pl sym·pa·thec·to·mies
sym·pa·thet·ic
sym·pa·thet·i·cal·ly
sym·pa·thet·i·co·mi·met·ic
sym·pa·thet·i·co·to·nia

sym·pa·thet·i·co·ton·ic
sym·pa·thet·o·blast
sym·path·i·co·blast
sym·path·i·co·blas·to·ma
pl sym·path·i·co·blas·to·mas
or sym·path·i·co·blas·to·ma·ta

sym·path·i·co·go·ni·o·ma
pl sym·path·i·co·go·ni·o·mas
or sym·path·i·co·go·ni·o·ma·ta

sym·path·i·co·lyt·ic
sym·path·i·co·mi·met·ic
sym·path·i·co·to·nia
sym·path·i·co·ton·ic
sym·path·i·co·trop·ic
sym·pa·thin
sym·path·ism
sym·pa·thiz·er
sym·pa·tho·blast
sym·pa·tho·go·nia
sym·pa·tho·go·ni·o·ma
pl sym·pa·tho·go·ni·o·mas
or sym·pa·tho·go·ni·o·ma·ta

sym·pa·tho·lyt·ic
sym·pa·tho·mi·met·ic
sym·pa·thy
pl sym·pa·thies

sym·phal·an·gism
sym·phy·se·al
also sym·phys·i·al

sym·phys·i·on
sym·phy·si·ot·o·my
pl sym·phy·si·ot·o·mies

sym·phy·sis
pl sym·phy·ses

sym·phy·sis pu·bis
sym·phy·so·dac·tyl·ia
sym·plasm
sym·plast
sym·po·sium
pl sym·po·sia
or sym·po·siums

symp·tom
symp·tom·at·ic
symp·tom·at·i·cal·ly
symp·tom·at·o·log·i·cal
or symp·tom·at·o·log·ic

symp·tom·at·o·log·i·cal·ly
symp·tom·atol·o·gy
pl symp·tom·atol·o·gies

symp·tom·less
sym·pus
syn·aere·sis
var of syneresis

syn·aes·the·sia
var of synesthesia

syn·aes·thet·ic
var of synesthetic

syn·anas·to·mo·sis
pl syn·anas·to·mo·ses

sy·nan·che
syn·an·the·ma
pl syn·an·the·ma·ta
or syn·an·the·mas

syn·an·throp·ic
syn·an·thro·py
pl syn·an·thro·pies

syn·apse
pl syn·aps·es

syn·apse
syn·apsed
syn·aps·ing

syn·ap·sis
pl syn·ap·ses

syn·ap·tic
also syn·ap·ti·cal

syn·ap·ti·cal·ly
syn·ap·tol·o·gy
pl syn·ap·tol·o·gies

syn·ap·to·ne·mal com·plex
or syn·ap·ti·ne·mal com·plex

syn·ap·to·som·al
syn·ap·to·some

syn·ar·thro·dia
syn·ar·thro·di·al
syn·ar·thro·di·al·ly
syn·ar·thro·phy·sis
pl syn·ar·thro·phy·ses
syn·ar·thro·sis
pl syn·ar·thro·ses
syn·cary·on
var of synkaryon
syn·ceph·a·lus
pl syn·ceph·a·li
syn·chon·dro·sis
pl syn·chon·dro·ses
syn·chon·drot·o·my
pl syn·chon·drot·o·mies
syn·chro·nism
syn·chro·nous
syn·chro·ny
pl syn·chro·nies
syn·chro·tron
syn·chy·sis
syn·cli·nal
syn·clit·ic
syn·clo·nus
syn·co·pal
syn·co·pe
syn·cy·tial
syn·cy·tio·tro·pho·blast
syn·cy·tium
pl syn·cy·tia
syn·dac·tyl
or syn·dac·tyle
syn·dac·tyl·ia
syn·dac·tyl·ic
or syn·dac·ty·lous
syn·dac·ty·lism
syn·dac·ty·ly
pl syn·dac·ty·lies
syn·de·sis
syn·des·mi·tis
syn·des·mo·cho·ri·al
syn·des·mo·sis
pl syn·des·mo·ses
syn·des·mot·ic
syn·des·mot·omy
pl syn·des·mot·omies
syn·drome
syn·echia
pl syn·echiae
syn·eph·rine
syn·ere·sis
or syn·aere·sis
pl syn·ere·ses
or syn·aere·ses
syn·er·get·ic
syn·er·gia
syn·er·gic
also syn·er·gi·cal
syn·er·gi·cal·ly
syn·er·gism
syn·er·gist
syn·er·gis·tic
also syn·er·gis·ti·cal
syn·er·gis·ti·cal·ly
syn·er·gy
pl syn·er·gies
syn·es·the·sia
or syn·aes·the·sia
syn·es·thet·ic
or syn·aes·thet·ic
Syn·ga·mus
syn·ga·my
pl syn·ga·mies
syn·ge·ne·ic
syn·ge·ne·sio·trans·plan·ta·tion
syn·gen·e·sis
pl syn·gen·e·ses
syn·ge·net·ic
syn·gig·no·scism
syn·i·ze·sis
or syn·e·ze·sis
syn·kary·on
also syn·kari·on
or syn·cary·on
syn·ki·ne·sis
pl syn·ki·ne·ses
syn·ki·net·ic
syn·oph·rys
syn·op·to·phore
syn·or·chism
also syn·or·chi·dism
syn·os·tose
syn·os·tosed
syn·os·tos·ing
syn·os·to·sis
also syn·os·te·osis
pl syn·os·to·ses
also syn·os·te·oses
syn·os·tot·ic
syn·os·tot·i·cal·ly
syn·o·tia
syn·o·tus
syn·o·vec·to·my
pl syn·o·vec·to·mies

sy·no·via
sy·no·vi·al
sy·no·vi·al·ly
syn·ovi·oma
pl syn·ovi·omas
or syn·ovi·oma·ta
sy·no·vi·tis
syn·tac·tic
or syn·tac·ti·cal
syn·tac·tics
syn·tal·i·ty
pl syn·tal·i·ties
syn·tax·is
syn·tec·tic
also syn·tec·ti·cal
syn·thase
syn·ther·mal
syn·the·sis
pl syn·the·ses
syn·the·size
syn·the·sized
syn·the·siz·ing
syn·the·tase
syn·thet·ic
also syn·thet·i·cal
syn·thet·i·cal·ly
syn·ton·ic
syn·tro·phism
syn·tro·pho·blast
syn·tro·pho·blas·tic
syn·trop·ic
syn·tro·py
pl syn·tro·pies
Sy·pha·cia
syph·il·e·mia
syph·i·lid
syph·i·lis
syph·i·lit·ic
syph·i·li·za·tion
syph·i·lize
syph·i·lized
syph·i·liz·ing
syph·i·lo·derm
or syph·i·lo·der·ma
pl syph·i·lo·derms
or syph·i·lo·der·ma·ta
syph·i·log·ra·pher
syph·i·log·ra·phy
pl syph·i·log·ra·phies
syph·i·loid
syph·i·lol·o·gist
syph·i·lol·o·gy
pl syph·i·lol·o·gies
syph·i·lo·ma
pl syph·i·lo·mas
or syph·i·lo·ma·ta
syph·i·lom·a·tous
syph·i·lo·phobe
syph·i·lo·pho·bia
syph·i·lo·psy·cho·sis
pl syph·i·lo·psy·cho·ses
syph·i·lo·ther·a·py
pl syph·i·lo·ther·a·pies
syr·ing·ad·e·nous
sy·ringe
sy·ringed
sy·ring·ing
sy·rin·go·bul·bia
syr·in·go·ma
pl syr·in·go·mas
or syr·in·go·ma·ta
sy·rin·go·my·elia
sy·rin·go·my·el·ic
sy·rin·go·my·e·lo·cele
syr·inx
pl sy·rin·ges
or syr·inx·es
sys·sar·co·sis
pl sys·sar·co·ses
sys·tal·tic
sys·tem
sys·tem·at·ic
also sys·tem·at·i·cal
sys·tem·at·i·cal·ly
sys·tem·ati·za·tion
sys·tem·atize
sys·tem·atized
sys·tem·atiz·ing
sys·tem·ic
sys·tem·i·cal·ly
sys·to·le
sys·tol·ic
sys·trem·ma
sy·zy·gial
syz·y·gy
pl syz·y·gies

T

Ta·ban·i·dae
Ta·ba·nus
ta·bar·di·llo
ta·bel·la
pl ta·bel·lae
ta·bes
pl ta·bes
ta·bes·cent

ta·bes dor·sa·lis
ta·bet·ic
ta·bet·i·form
tab·id
ta·ble·spoon
ta·ble·spoon·ful
pl ta·ble·spoon·fuls
also ta·ble·spoons·ful

tab·let
ta·boo
also ta·bu
pl ta·boos
also ta·bus

ta·bo·pa·ral·y·sis
pl ta·bo·pa·ral·y·ses

ta·bo·pa·re·sis
pl ta·bo·pa·re·ses

tab·u·lar
tache noire
pl taches noires

ta·chet·ic
ta·chis·to·scope
ta·chis·to·scop·ic
ta·chis·to·scop·i·cal·ly
tach·o·gram
ta·chog·ra·phy
pl ta·chog·ra·phies

ta·chom·eter
tachy·aux·e·sis
pl tachy·aux·e·ses

tachy·car·dia
rapid heart action
(*see* bradycardia)

tachy·car·di·ac
tachy·lo·gia
ta·chym·e·ter
tachy·pha·gia
tachy·phy·lax·is
pl tachy·phy·lax·es

tachy·pnea
also tachy·pnoea

tachy·pne·ic
tachy·rhyth·mia
ta·chys·ter·ol
tachy·sys·tole
tac·tile
tac·til·i·ty
pl tac·til·i·ties

tac·tion
tac·toid
tac·tom·e·ter
tac·tu·al
tac·tu·al·ly
tae·di·um vi·tae
tae·nia
also te·nia
pl tae·ni·ae
or tae·nias
also te·nias
band of tissue

tae·nia
also te·nia
pl tae·nias
also te·nias
tapeworm

tae·nia·cide
also te·nia·cide

tae·nia·fuge
also te·nia·fuge

Tae·nia·rhyn·chus
tae·ni·a·sis
also te·ni·a·sis

tag·a·tose
tail·bone
ta·ko·sis
ta·lal·gia
tal·cum
tal·i·pes
tal·i·pom·a·nus
ta·lo·cal·ca·ne·al
ta·lo·na·vic·u·lar
tal·on·id
ta·lo·tib·i·al
ta·lus
pl ta·li

tam·bour
tam·pon
tam·pon·ade
or tam·pon·age

tan·nase
tan·nate
tan·nic
tan·nin
tan·ta·lum
tan·trum
ta·pe·tal
ta·pe·to·ret·i·nal
ta·pe·tum
pl ta·pe·ta

tape·worm
taph·e·pho·bia
tap·i·no·ceph·a·ly
pl tap·i·no·ceph·a·lies

tap·i·o·ca
ta·pir·oid
ta·pote·ment
tar·an·tism
ta·ran·tu·la
pl ta·ran·tu·las
also ta·ran·tu·lae

ta•rax•a•cum
tar•dive
tare
  tared
  tar•ing
tar•get
ta•ro
  pl ta•ros
tar•ry
  tar•ri•er
  tar•ri•est
tars•ad•e•ni•tis
tar•sal
tar•sa•le
  pl tar•sa•lia
tar•sal•gia
tar•sec•to•my
  pl tar•sec•to•mies
tar•si•tis
tar•so•ma•la•cia
tar•so•meta•tar•sal
tar•so•pha•lan•ge•al
tar•so•phy•ma
  pl tar•so•phy•mas
  or tar•so•phy•ma•ta
tar•so•plas•ty
  pl tar•so•plas•ties
tar•sor•rha•phy
  pl tar•sor•rha•phies
tar•sot•o•my
  pl tar•sot•o•mies
tar•sus
  pl tar•si
tar•tar
tar•tar•ic
tar•trate
tar•trat•ed
  also tar•tar•at•ed
tat•too
  also ta•too
  pl tat•toos
  also ta•toos
tau•rine
tau•ro•cho•late
tau•ro•cho•lic
tau•to•me•ni•al
tau•to•mer•ic
tau•tom•er•ism
tax•is
  pl tax•es
tax•on
  pl taxa
  also tax•ons
tax•o•nom•ic
  also tax•o•nom•i•cal
tax•o•nom•i•cal•ly
tax•on•o•mist
tax•on•o•my
  pl tax•on•o•mies
Tay-Sachs dis•ease
T cell
tear•gas
  verb
tear gas
  noun
teart
tea•spoon
tea•spoon•ful
  pl tea•spoon•fuls
  also tea•spoons•ful
tech•ne•tium
tech•ne•tron•ic
tech•nic
tech•ni•cal
tech•ni•cian
tech•nique
tech•nol•o•gist
tech•nol•o•gy
  pl tech•nol•o•gies
tec•ti•form
tec•to•ceph•a•ly
  pl tec•to•ceph•a•lies
tec•ton•ic
tec•to•ri•al
tec•to•ri•um
  pl tec•to•ria
tec•to•spi•nal
tec•tum
  pl tec•ta
teeth
  pl of tooth
teethe
  teethed
  teeth•ing
teeth•ridge
teg•men
  pl teg•mi•na
teg•men•tal
teg•men•tum
  or teg•u•men•tum
  pl teg•men•ta
  or teg•u•men•ta
teg•u•ment
teg•u•men•tal
teg•u•men•ta•ry
tei•chop•sia
te•la
  pl te•lae

tel·aes·the·sia
var of telesthesia

tel·aes·thet·ic
var of telesthetic

tel·al·gia

tel·an·gi·ec·ta·sia
or tel·an·gi·ec·ta·sis
pl tel·an·gi·ec·ta·sias
or tel·an·gi·ec·ta·ses

tel·an·gi·ec·tat·ic

tel·an·gi·o·ma
pl tel·an·gi·o·mas
or tel·an·gi·o·ma·ta

tel·an·gi·o·sis
pl tel·an·gi·o·ses
or tel·an·gi·o·sis·es

tele·car·dio·gram

tele·car·dio·phone

tele·den·dron

tele·di·a·stol·ic

te·leg·o·ny
pl te·leg·o·nies

tele·ki·ne·sis
pl tele·ki·ne·ses

tele·lec·tro·car·dio·gram

tele·me·ter

tele·met·ric

tele·met·ri·cal·ly

te·lem·e·try
pl te·lem·e·tries

tel·en·ce·phal·ic

tel·en·ceph·a·lon
pl tel·en·ceph·a·la

te·le·o·log·i·cal
or te·le·o·log·ic

te·le·ol·o·gy
pl te·le·ol·o·gies

tele·op·sia

te·leo·roent·gen·o·gram

tele·path·ic

tele·path·i·cal·ly

te·lep·a·thist

te·lep·a·thy
pl te·lep·a·thies

tele·ra·di·og·ra·phy
pl tele·ra·di·og·ra·phies

tel·er·gy
pl tel·er·gies

tele·roent·gen·o·gram

tele·roent·gen·og·ra·phy
pl tele·roent·gen·og·ra·phies

tel·es·the·sia
or tel·aes·the·sia

tel·es·thet·ic
or tel·aes·thet·ic

tele·sys·tol·ic

tele·ther·a·py
pl tele·ther·a·pies

tel·lu·rate

tel·lu·ric

tel·lu·ri·um

telo·cen·tric

telo·den·dri·on
pl telo·den·dria

telo·lec·i·thal

telo·mere

telo·phase

telo·phrag·ma
pl telo·phrag·ma·ta

Telo·spo·rid·ia

telo·spo·rid·i·an

tem·per·a·ment

tem·per·a·ture

tem·plate
or tem·plet

tem·ple

tem·po·ral

tem·po·ro·man·dib·u·lar

tem·po·ro·max·il·lary

tem·po·ro-oc·cip·i·tal

tem·po·ro·pa·ri·etal

te·na·cious

te·nac·i·ty
pl te·nac·i·ties

te·nac·u·lum
pl te·nac·u·la
or te·nac·u·lums

ten·den·cy
pl ten·den·cies

ten·der

ten·der·ness

ten·di·ni·tis
or ten·don·itis

ten·di·no·plas·ty
pl ten·di·no·plas·ties

ten·di·nous

ten·do
pl ten·di·nes

ten·dol·y·sis
pl ten·dol·y·ses

ten·do·mu·cin
ten·don
ten·don·itis
var of tendinitis

ten·do·plas·ty
pl ten·do·plas·ties

ten·do·vag·i·nal
ten·do·vag·i·ni·tis
te·nec·to·my
pl te·nec·to·mies

te·nes·mus
te·nia
var of taenia

te·nia·cide
var of taeniacide

te·nia·fuge
var of taeniafuge

te·ni·a·sis
var of taeniasis

ten·nis el·bow
te·no·de·sis
pl te·no·de·ses

ten·o·dyn·ia
te·nol·y·sis
pl te·nol·y·ses

te·no·myo·plas·ty
pl te·no·myo·plas·ties

te·no·my·ot·o·my
pl te·no·my·ot·o·mies

te·no·nec·to·my
pl te·no·nec·to·mies

te·no·ni·tis
Ten·on's cap·sule
te·non·to·myo·plas·ty
pl te·non·to·myo·plas·ties

te·non·to·my·ot·o·my
pl te·non·to·my·ot·o·mies

ten·o·phyte
teno·plas·tic
te·no·plas·ty
pl te·no·plas·ties

te·nor·rha·phy
pl te·nor·rha·phies

ten·os·to·sis
pl ten·os·to·ses
or ten·os·to·sis·es

teno·syn·o·vec·to·my
pl teno·syn·o·vec·to·mies

te·no·syn·o·vi·tis
ten·o·tome
te·not·o·mist
te·not·o·mize
te·not·o·mized
te·not·o·miz·ing
te·not·o·my
pl te·not·o·mies

teno·vag·i·ni·tis
ten·si·om·e·ter
ten·sion
ten·sor
ten·ta·cle
ten·to·ri·al
ten·to·ri·um
pl ten·to·ria

ten·to·ri·um ce·re·bel·li
te·pa
ter·as
pl tera·ta

te·rat·ic
ter·a·tism
ter·a·to·blas·to·ma
pl ter·a·to·blas·to·mas
or ter·a·to·blas·to·ma·ta

ter·a·to·car·ci·no·ma
pl ter·a·to·car·ci·no·mas
or ter·a·to·car·ci·no·ma·ta

te·rato·gen
ter·a·to·gen·e·sis
pl ter·a·to·gen·e·ses

ter·a·to·gen·et·ic
or ter·a·to·gen·ic

ter·a·toid
ter·a·to·log·i·cal
or ter·a·to·logic

ter·a·tol·o·gist
ter·a·tol·o·gy
pl ter·a·tol·o·gies

ter·a·to·ma
pl ter·a·to·mas
or ter·a·to·ma·ta

ter·a·to·pho·bia
ter·a·to·sis
ter·a·to·sper·mia
ter·bi·um
ter·e·bene
ter·e·bin·thi·nate
ter·e·bin·thine
ter·e·bra·che·sis
pl ter·e·bra·che·ses

teres
pl ter·e·tes

ter·mi·nal
ter·mi·nal·ly
ter·mi·na·tion
ter·mi·nol·o·gy
pl ter·mi·nol·o·gies

ter·mi·nus
pl ter·mi·ni
or ter·mi·nus·es

ter·na·ry
ter·pene
ter·pe·nic
ter·pin
ter·pin·e·ol
ter·pi·nol
ter·tian
ter·tia·ry
pl ter·tia·ries

ter·tip·a·ra
pl ter·tip·a·ras
or ter·tip·a·rae

tes·sel·lat·ed
also tes·se·lat·ed

test·cross
tes·ti·cle
tes·tic·u·lar
tes·tis
pl tes·tes

tes·toid
tes·tos·ter·one
test-tube
adj

test tube
noun

tet·a·nal
te·tan·ic
te·tan·i·cal·ly
te·tan·i·form
tet·a·nig·e·nous
tet·a·nil·la
tet·a·nism
tet·a·ni·za·tion
tet·a·nize
tet·a·nized
tet·a·niz·ing
tet·a·node
tet·a·noid
tet·a·no·ly·sin
tet·a·nom·e·ter
tet·a·no·spas·min
tet·a·nus
tet·a·ny
pl tet·a·nies

te·tar·ta·no·pia
te·tar·to·cone
also tet·ar·cone

te·tar·to·co·nid
also tet·ar·co·nid

tet·ra·ba·sic
tet·ra·ba·sic·i·ty
pl tet·ra·ba·sic·i·ties

tet·ra·ben·a·zine
tet·ra·bra·chi·us
tet·ra·bro·mo·phe·nol·phtha·lein
tet·ra·caine
tet·ra·chlo·ride
tet·ra·chlo·ro·eth·ane
also tet·ra·chlor·eth·ane

tet·ra·chlo·ro·eth·yl·ene
tet·ra·cy·cline
tet·rad
tet·ra·dac·ty·ly
te·trad·ic
tet·ra·eth·yl·am·mo·ni·um
tet·ra·eth·yl·thi·u·ram
te·trag·e·nous
tet·ra·hy·dro·can·nab·i·nol
tet·ra·hy·me·na
te·tral·o·gy
pl te·tral·o·gies

te·tral·o·gy of Fal·lot
tet·ra·mas·tia
Te·tram·er·es
tet·ra·meth·yl·am·mo·ni·um
tet·ra·meth·yl·ene·di·amine
tet·ra·nop·sia
tet·ra·pep·tide
tet·ra·ple·gia
tet·ra·ploid
tet·ra·pod
tet·ra·pus
tet·ra·pyr·role
tet·ra·sac·cha·ride
te·tras·ce·lus
tet·ra·so·mic
tet·ra·sti·chi·a·sis
tet·ra·tom·ic
tet·ra·vac·cine

tet·ra·va·lent
te·tro·do·tox·in
or tet·ra·odon·tox·in
tet·rose
te·trox·ide
tet·ter
Tex·as fe·ver
tex·is
tex·ti·form
tex·tur·al
tex·ture
T-group
thal·am·en·ce·phal·ic
thal·am·en·ceph·a·lon
pl thal·am·en·ceph·a·la
tha·lam·ic
tha·lam·i·cal·ly
thal·a·mo·cele
or thal·a·mo·coele
thal·a·mo·cor·ti·cal
thal·a·mo·len·tic·u·lar
thal·a·mo·teg·men·tal
thal·a·mot·o·my
pl thal·a·mot·o·mies
thal·a·mus
pl thal·a·mi
thal·as·se·mia
also thal·ass·ane·mia
thal·as·se·mic
tha·las·so·pho·bia
tha·las·so·ther·a·py
pl tha·las·so·ther·a·pies
tha·lid·o·mide
thal·li·um
Thal·loph·y·ta
thal·lo·phyte
thal·lo·phyt·ic
thal·lo·spore
thal·lo·tox·i·co·sis
pl thal·lo·tox·i·co·ses
thal·lus
pl thal·li
or thal·lus·es
tham·uria
than·a·to·bi·o·log·ic
than·a·to·gno·mon·ic
than·a·toid
than·a·tol·o·gy
pl than·a·tol·o·gies
than·a·to·ma·nia
than·a·to·phid·ia
than·a·to·pho·bia
than·a·top·sy
pl than·a·top·sies
Than·a·tos
the·ba·ic
the·ba·ine
the·be·sian ves·sel
also the·be·sian vein
or the·be·sian chan·nel
the·ca
pl the·cae
the·cal
or the·cate
the·ci·tis
thec·o·dont
the·co·ma
pl the·co·mas
or the·co·ma·ta
the·co·steg·no·sis
pl the·co·steg·no·ses
or the·co·steg·no·sis·es
thee·lin
thee·lol
thei·le·ria
pl thei·le·ri·ae
also thei·le·rias
thei·le·ri·a·sis
or thei·le·ri·o·sis
the·ine
the·lal·gia
the·lar·che
The·la·zia
thel·a·zi·a·sis
the·le·plas·ty
pl the·le·plas·ties
the·ler·e·thism
the·li·tis
the·li·um
pl the·lia
the·lon·cus
the·lor·rha·gia
the·lo·thism
thel·y·gen·ic
thel·y·to·cia
the·nar
theo·bro·ma oil
theo·bro·mine
theo·ma·nia

theo·pho·bia
the·oph·yl·line
the·o·ret·i·cal
also the·o·ret·ic
the·o·ret·i·cal·ly
the·o·ry
pl the·o·ries
ther·a·peu·sis
pl ther·a·peu·ses
ther·a·peu·tic
also ther·a·peu·ti·cal
ther·a·peu·ti·cal·ly
ther·a·peu·tics
ther·a·peu·tist
the·ra·pia
ther·a·pist
ther·a·py
pl ther·a·pies
ther·en·ceph·a·lous
the·ri·ac
the·ri·a·ca
the·ri·a·ca an·drom·a·chi
the·ri·at·rics
Ther·i·di·idae
the·ri·o·ma
pl the·ri·o·mas
or the·ri·o·ma·ta
ther·mae
ther·mal
ther·mal·ge·sia
ther·ma·tol·o·gy
pl ther·ma·tol·o·gies
therm·es·the·sia
therm·es·the·si·om·e·ter
ther·mic
therm·is·tor
ther·mo·an·al·ge·sia
ther·mo·an·es·the·sia
ther·mo·cau·tery
pl ther·mo·cau·ter·ies
ther·mo·chem·is·try
pl ther·mo·chem·is·tries
ther·mo·chro·ism
ther·mo·co·ag·u·la·tion
ther·mo·cou·ple
ther·mo·cur·rent
ther·mo·dif·fu·sion
ther·mo·di·lu·tion
ther·mo·du·ric
ther·mo·dy·nam·ics
ther·mo·ex·ci·to·ry
ther·mo·gen·e·sis
pl ther·mo·gen·e·ses
ther·mo·gen·ic
ther·mo·gram
ther·mo·graph
ther·mo·graph·ic
ther·mo·graph·i·cal·ly
ther·mog·ra·phy
pl ther·mog·ra·phies
ther·mo·hy·per·al·ge·sia
ther·mo·hy·per·es·the·sia
ther·mo·hyp·es·the·sia
ther·mo·in·hib·i·to·ry
ther·mo·la·bile
ther·mol·y·sis
pl ther·mol·y·ses
ther·mo·lyt·ic
ther·mo·mas·sage
ther·mom·e·ter
ther·mo·met·ric
ther·mom·e·try
pl ther·mom·e·tries
ther·mo·neu·ro·sis
pl ther·mo·neu·ro·ses
ther·moph·a·gy
pl ther·moph·a·gies
ther·mo·phile
also ther·mo·phil
ther·mo·phil·ic
or ther·moph·i·lous
ther·mo·pho·bia
ther·mo·phore
ther·mo·phyl·ic
ther·mo·pile
ther·mo·plas·tic
ther·mo·ple·gia
ther·mo·pol·yp·nea
ther·mo·re·cep·tor
ther·mo·reg·u·la·tion
ther·mo·reg·u·la·tor

ther·mo·reg·u·la·to·ry
ther·mo·scope
ther·mo·set
ther·mo·sta·ble
ther·mo·stat
ther·mo·stat·i·cal·ly
ther·mo·ste·re·sis
pl ther·mo·ste·re·ses

ther·mo·stro·muhr
ther·mo·sys·tal·tic
ther·mo·tac·tic
ther·mo·tax·is
pl ther·mo·tax·es

ther·mo·ther·a·py
pl ther·mo·ther·a·pies

ther·mo·to·nom·e·ter
ther·mo·tra·che·ot·o·my
pl ther·mo·tra·che·ot·o·mies

ther·mo·trop·ic
ther·mot·ro·pism
the·sau·ro·sis
pl the·sau·ro·ses
or the·sau·ro·sis·es

the·sis
pl the·ses

thia·ben·da·zole
thi·acet·azone
thi·ami·nase
thi·a·mine
also thi·a·min

thi·a·zide
thi·a·zol·sul·fone
thick-wind·ed
thigh·bone
thig·mes·the·sia
thig·mo·tax·is
pl thig·mo·tax·es

thig·mot·ro·pism
thi·mer·o·sal
thin-lay·er chro·ma·tog·ra·phy
thio·bac·te·ri·um
pl thio·bac·te·ria

thio·car·ba·mide
thio·chrome
thio·cy·a·nate
thio·di·phe·nyl·amine
thio·gua·nine
thi·one·ine
thi·on·ic
thio·pen·tal
thio·pen·tone
thio·phene
Thi·o·rid·a·zine
thio·sin·amine
thio·sul·fate
thio·te·pa
thio·ura·cil
thio·urea
third-de·gree burn
thixo·trop·ic
thix·ot·ro·py
pl thix·ot·ro·pies

Thom·as splint
Thom·sen's dis·ease
thon·zyl·amine
tho·ra·cec·to·my
pl tho·ra·cec·to·mies

tho·ra·cen·te·sis
pl tho·ra·cen·te·ses

tho·rac·ic
tho·ra·co·ce·los·chi·sis
pl tho·ra·co·ce·los·chi·ses
or tho·ra·co·ce·los·chi·sis·es

tho·ra·co·cen·te·sis
pl tho·ra·co·cen·te·ses

tho·ra·co·cyl·lo·sis
pl tho·ra·co·cyl·lo·ses
or tho·ra·co·cyl·lo·sis·es

tho·ra·co·dyn·ia
tho·ra·co·gas·tros·chi·sis
pl tho·ra·co·gas·tros·chi·ses
or tho·ra·co·gas·tros·chi·sis·es

tho·ra·co·lap·a·rot·o·my
pl tho·ra·co·lap·a·rot·o·mies

tho·ra·co·lum·bar
tho·ra·col·y·sis
pl tho·ra·col·y·ses

tho·ra·com·e·lus
pl tho·ra·com·e·li

tho·ra·cop·a·gus
pl tho·ra·cop·a·gus·es
or tho·ra·cop·a·gi

tho·ra·co·par·a·ceph·a·lus
pl tho·ra·co·par·a·ceph·a·li

tho·ra·co·plas·ty
pl tho·ra·co·plas·ties

tho·ra·cos·chi·sis
pl tho·ra·cos·chi·ses
or tho·ra·cos·chi·sis·es

tho·ra·co·scope
tho·ra·co·scop·ic
tho·ra·cos·co·py
pl tho·ra·cos·co·pies

tho·ra·cos·to·my
pl tho·ra·cos·to·mies

tho·ra·cot·o·my
pl tho·ra·cot·o·mies

tho·rax
pl tho·rax·es
or tho·ra·ces

tho·ri·um
thor·ough·pin
thread·worm
thready
thread·i·er
thread·i·est
threat·en
threat·ened
threat·en·ing
thre·o·nine
thre·ose
threp·sol·o·gy
pl threp·sol·o·gies

thresh·old
throb
throbbed
throb·bing

throm·base
throm·bas·the·nia
throm·bec·to·my
pl throm·bec·to·mies

throm·bi
pl of thrombus

throm·bin
throm·bo·an·gi·i·tis
pl throm·bo·an·gi·it·i·des

throm·bo·an·gi·i·tis ob·lit·er·ans
throm·bo·ar·ter·i·tis
throm·bo·blast
throm·boc·la·sis
pl throm·boc·la·ses

throm·bo·clas·tic
throm·bo·cyte
throm·bo·cy·the·mia
throm·bo·cyt·ic
throm·bo·cy·to·pe·nia
throm·bo·cy·to·pe·nic
throm·bo·cy·to·poi·e·sis
pl throm·bo·cy·to·poi·e·ses

throm·bo·cy·to·sis
pl throm·bo·cy·to·ses

throm·bo·em·bo·lec·to·my
pl throm·bo·em·bo·lec·to·mies

throm·bo·em·bol·ic
throm·bo·em·bo·lism
throm·bo·en·dar·ter·ec·to·my
pl throm·bo·en·dar·ter·ec·to·mies

throm·bo·en·do·car·di·tis
throm·bo·gen
throm·bo·gen·ic
throm·bo·ki·nase
throm·bo·lym·phan·gi·tis
pl throm·bo·lym·phan·git·i·des

throm·bol·y·sis
pl throm·bol·y·ses

throm·bo·lyt·ic
throm·bon
throm·bop·a·thy
pl throm·bop·a·thies

throm·bo·pe·nia
throm·bo·phil·ia
throm·bo·phle·bi·tis
pl throm·bo·phle·bit·i·des

throm·bo·plas·tic
throm·bo·plas·ti·cal·ly
throm·bo·plas·tin
throm·bo·plas·tin·o·gen
throm·bo·poi·e·sis
pl throm·bo·poi·e·ses

throm•bose
throm•bosed
throm•bos•ing
throm•bo•sis
pl throm•bo•ses

throm•bo•sta•sis
pl throm•bo•sta•ses

throm•bot•ic
throm•bus
pl throm•bi

throt•tle
throt•tled
throt•tling
thu•li•um
thumb•nail
thy•mec•to•mize
thy•mec•to•mized
thy•mec•to•miz•ing
thy•mec•to•my
pl thy•mec•to•mies

thy•mer•ga•sia
thy•mic
thy•mi•co•lym•phat•ic
thy•mi•dine
thy•mine
thy•mi•tis
thy•mo•cyte
thy•mol
thy•mo•ma
pl thy•mo•mas
or thy•mo•ma•ta

thy•mop•a•thy
pl thy•mop•a•thies

thy•mus
pl thy•mus•es
or thy•mi

thy•ro•ar•y•te•noid
thy•ro•cal•ci•to•nin
thy•ro•car•di•ac
thy•ro•cele
thy•ro•cer•vi•cal
thy•ro•chon•drot•o•my
pl thy•ro•chon•drot•o•mies

thy•ro•cri•cot•o•my
pl thy•ro•cri•cot•o•mies

thy•ro•epi•glot•tic
thy•ro•gen•ic
or thy•rog•e•nous

thy•ro•glob•u•lin
thy•ro•glos•sal
thy•ro•hy•al
thy•ro•hy•oid
also thy•ro•hy•oid•ean

thy•roid
thy•roi•dal
thy•roid•ec•to•mize
thy•roid•ec•to•mized
thy•roid•ec•to•miz•ing
thy•roid•ec•to•my
pl thy•roid•ec•to•mies

thy•roid•itis
thy•roid•ot•o•my
pl thy•roid•ot•o•mies

thy•roid-stim•u•lat•ing hor•mone
thy•ro•nine
thy•ro•para•thy•roid•ec•to•my
pl thy•ro•para•thy•roid•ec•to•mies

thy•ro•pri•val
thy•ro•pro•tein
thy•rop•to•sis
pl thy•rop•to•ses
or thy•rop•to•sis•es

thy•rot•o•my
pl thy•rot•o•mies

thy•ro•tox•ic
thy•ro•tox•ic•i•ty
pl thy•ro•tox•ic•i•ties

thy•ro•tox•i•co•sis
pl thy•ro•tox•i•co•ses

thy•ro•tox•in
thy•ro•tro•phic
or thy•ro•tro•pic

thy•ro•tro•phi•cal•ly
thy•ro•tro•phin
or thy•ro•tro•pin

thy•rox•ine
or thy•rox•in

tib•ia
pl tib•i•ae
also tib•i•as

tib•i•al
tib•i•a•lis
pl tib•i•a•les

tib•io•fib•u•la
pl tib•io•fib•u•lae
or tib•io•fib•u•las

tib·io·fib·u·lar
tib·io·tar·sal
tic dou·lou·reux
tick-borne
tid·al
tight·ness
ti·groid
ti·grol·y·sis
pl ti·grol·y·ses
tim·bre
also tim·ber
tinc·tion
tinc·to·ri·al
tinc·to·ri·al·ly
tinc·ture
tinc·tured
tinc·tur·ing
tin·ea
tin·ea bar·bae
tin·ea ca·pi·tis
tin·ea cor·po·ris
tin·ea cru·ris
tin·e·al
tin·ea pe·dis
tin·ea ver·si·col·or
tin·gle
tin·gled
tin·gling
tin·ni·tus
tint·o·met·ric
tint·om·e·try
pl tint·om·e·tries
ti·queur
ti·sane
Ti·se·li·us ap·pa·ra·tus
also Ti·se·li·us cell
tis·sue
tis·su·lar
ti·ta·ni·um
ti·ter
or ti·tre
tit·il·la·tion
ti·trant
ti·trate
ti·trat·ed
ti·trat·ing
ti·tra·tion
tit·u·ba·tion
T lym·pho·cyte
to·bac·co
pl to·bac·cos
also to·bac·coes
to·co·dy·na·mom·e·ter
or to·ko·dy·na·mom·e·ter
to·col·o·gy
also to·kol·o·gy
pl to·col·o·gies
also to·kol·o·gies
to·coph·er·ol
toe·drop
toe·nail
toi·let
tol·bu·ta·mide
tol·er·ance
tol·er·ant
tol·er·ate
tol·er·at·ed
tol·er·at·ing
tol·er·a·tion
to·lo·ni·um
tol·u·ene
to·lu·idine
tol·u·ol
tom·a·tine
to·men·tum
pl to·men·ta
Tomes's fi·ber
or Tomes's fi·bril
to·mo·gram
to·mo·graph
to·mo·graph·ic
to·mog·ra·phy
pl to·mog·ra·phies
to·mo·ma·nia
tone-deaf
tone-deaf·ness
tongue
tongue·less
tongue-tie
tongue-tied
tongue-ty·ing
or tongue-tie·ing
ton·ic
to·nic·i·ty
pl to·nic·i·ties
tono·clon·ic
tono·fi·bril
also tono·fi·bril·la
pl tono·fi·brils
also tono·fi·bril·lae
ton·o·gram
ton·o·graph
to·nog·ra·phy
pl to·nog·ra·phies
to·nom·e·ter
to·no·met·ric
to·nom·e·try
pl to·nom·e·tries
to·no·plast

ton·o·scope
ton·sil
ton·sil·lar
or ton·sil·lary
ton·sil·lec·to·my
pl ton·sil·lec·to·mies
ton·sil·li·tis
ton·sil·lo·lith
ton·sil·lo·tome
ton·sil·lot·o·my
pl ton·sil·lot·o·mies
to·nus
tooth
pl teeth
tooth·ache
top·ag·no·sis
pl top·ag·no·ses
to·pal·gia
to·pec·to·my
pl to·pec·to·mies
top·es·the·sia
to·pha·ceous
to·phus
pl to·phi
top·i·cal
top·i·cal·ly
top·og·no·sia
or top·og·no·sis
pl top·og·no·sias
or top·og·no·sis·es
to·po·graph·ic
to·pog·ra·phy
pl to·pog·ra·phies
to·pol·o·gy
pl to·pol·o·gies
topo·nar·co·sis
pl topo·nar·co·ses
topo·neu·ro·sis
pl topo·neu·ro·ses
top·onym
to·pon·y·my
also to·pon·o·my
pl to·pon·y·mies
also to·pon·o·mies
tor·cu·lar
tor·cu·lar He·ro·phi·li
to·rose
tor·por
torque
torqued
torqu·ing
tor·re·fac·tion
tor·re·fy
also tor·ri·fy
tor·re·fied
also tor·ri·fied
tor·re·fy·ing
also tor·ri·fy·ing
tor·sion
tor·so
pl tor·sos
or tor·si
also tor·soes
tor·ti·col·lis
tor·u·la
pl tor·u·lae
also tor·u·las
tor·u·lop·sis
pl tor·u·lop·ses
tor·u·lo·sis
tor·u·lus
pl tor·u·li
to·rus
pl to·ri
to·ti·po·ten·cy
pl to·ti·po·ten·cies
to·ti·po·tent
to·ti·po·ten·tial
to·ti·po·ten·ti·al·i·ty
pl to·ti·po·ten·ti·al·i·ties
tour·ni·quet
tox·a·phene
Tox·as·ca·ris
tox·emia
also tox·ae·mia
tox·emic
also tox·aemic
tox·ic
tox·i·cant
tox·ic·i·ty
pl tox·ic·i·ties
Tox·i·co·den·dron
tox·i·co·der·ma
pl tox·i·co·der·mas
or tox·i·co·der·ma·ta
tox·i·co·der·ma·ti·tis
pl tox·i·co·der·ma·ti·tis·es
or tox·i·co·der·ma·tit·i·des
tox·i·co·gen·ic
tox·i·coid
tox·i·co·log·i·cal
or tox·i·co·log·ic
tox·i·col·o·gist
tox·i·col·o·gy
pl tox·i·col·o·gies
tox·i·co·ma·nia
tox·i·co·path·ic

tox·i·co·pho·bia
tox·i·co·sis
pl tox·i·co·ses
tox·i·der·mi·tis
tox·if·er·ine
tox·if·er·ous
toxi·gen·ic
toxi·ge·nic·i·ty
pl toxi·ge·nic·i·ties
tox·in
tox·in–an·ti·tox·in
Tox·o·cara
tox·oid
tox·oph·o·rous
also tox·o·phor·ic
toxo·plas·ma
pl toxo·plas·mas
or toxo·plas·ma·ta
also toxo·plas·ma
toxo·plas·mic
toxo·plas·mo·sis
pl toxo·plas·mo·ses
tra·bec·u·la
pl tra·bec·u·lae
also tra·bec·u·las
tra·bec·u·lar
also tra·bec·u·late
or tra·bec·u·lat·ed
tra·bec·u·la·tion
trac·er
tra·chea
pl tra·che·ae
also tra·che·as
tra·che·al
tra·che·al·gia
tra·che·itis
trach·e·lec·to·my
pl trach·e·lec·to·mies

trach·e·lis·mus
trach·e·li·tis
trach·e·lo·dyn·ia
tra·che·lo·mas·toid
tra·che·lo·plas·ty
pl tra·che·lo·plas·ties
tra·che·lor·rha·phy
pl tra·che·lor·rha·phies
trach·e·lot·o·my
pl trach·e·lot·o·mies
tra·cheo·bron·chi·al
tra·cheo·bron·chi·tis
pl tra·cheo·bron·chit·i·des
tra·cheo·bron·chos·co·py
pl tra·cheo·bron·chos·co·pies
tra·cheo·esoph·a·ge·al
tra·che·oph·o·ny
pl tra·che·oph·o·nies
tra·cheo·plas·ty
pl tra·cheo·plas·ties
tra·cheo·py·o·sis
pl tra·cheo·py·o·ses
tra·che·or·rha·gia
tra·che·os·chi·sis
pl tra·che·os·chi·ses
also tra·che·os·chi·sis·es
tra·che·os·co·py
pl tra·che·os·co·pies

tra·cheo·ste·no·sis
pl tra·cheo·ste·no·ses
tra·che·os·to·my
pl tra·che·os·to·mies
tra·che·ot·o·mize
tra·che·ot·o·mized
tra·che·ot·o·miz·ing
tra·che·ot·o·my
pl tra·che·ot·o·mies
tra·cho·ma
tra·cho·ma·tous
tra·chy·chro·mat·ic
tra·chy·pho·nia
trac·tion
trac·tor
trac·tot·o·my
pl trac·tot·o·mies
trac·tus
pl trac·tus
trag·a·canth
tra·gal
trago·mas·chal·ia
tra·gus
pl tra·gi
train·sick
train·sick·ness
tran·quil·ize
or tran·quil·lize
tran·quil·ized
or tran·quil·lized
tran·quil·iz·ing
or tran·quil·liz·ing

tran·quil·iz·er
also tran·quil·liz·er

trans·ab·dom·i·nal
trans·acet·y·lase
trans·ac·tion
trans·am·i·nase
trans·am·i·nate
trans·am·i·nat·ed
trans·am·i·nat·ing
trans·am·i·na·tion
trans·an·i·ma·tion
trans·au·di·ent
trans·ca·lent
trans·cal·lo·sal
trans·con·dy·lar
trans·cor·ti·cal
tran·scribe
tran·scribed
tran·scrib·ing
tran·scrip·tion
trans·cu·ta·ne·ous
also trans·cu·ta·ne·al

trans·duce
trans·duced
trans·duc·ing
trans·duc·tion
tran·sect
tran·sec·tion
trans·fer·ase
trans·fer·ence
trans·fer·rin
trans·fer RNA
trans·fix
trans·fix·ion
trans·fo·ra·tion
trans·form
trans·for·ma·tion
trans·fuse
trans·fused
trans·fus·ing
trans·fu·sion
trans·fu·sion·al
tran·sient
trans·il·i·ac
trans·il·lu·mi·nate
trans·il·lu·mi·na·tion
trans·il·lu·mi·na·tor
trans·isth·mi·an
tran·sis·tor
trans·late
trans·lat·ed
trans·lat·ing
trans·la·tion
trans·lo·ca·tion
trans·lu·cen·cy
pl trans·lu·cen·cies

trans·lu·cent
trans·mem·brane
trans·meth·yl·ation
trans·mi·gra·tion
trans·mis·si·bil·i·ty
pl trans·mis·si·bil·i·ties
trans·mis·si·ble
trans·mis·sion
trans·mit
trans·mit·ted
trans·mit·ting
trans·mit·ta·ble
trans·mit·tance
trans·mit·ter
trans·mu·ral
trans·or·bit·al
trans·pep·ti·da·tion
trans·phos·phor·y·la·tion
tran·spir·able
tran·spi·ra·tion
tran·spire
trans·pired
trans·pir·ing
trans·pla·cen·tal
trans·plant
trans·plan·ta·tion
trans·port
trans·pose
trans·posed
trans·pos·ing
trans·po·si·tion
trans·seg·men·tal
trans·sex·u·al
trans·tho·rac·ic
trans·tho·rac·i·cal·ly
trans·tra·che·al
tran·sub·stan·ti·ate
tran·sub·stan·ti·at·ed

tran·sub·stan·ti·at·ing
tran·sub·stan·ti·a·tion
tran·su·date
tran·su·da·tion
tran·sude
tran·sud·ed
tran·sud·ing
trans·ure·thral
trans·vag·i·nal
trans·ver·sa·lis
trans·verse
trans·ver·sec·to·my
pl trans·ver·sec·to·mies
trans·ver·sion
trans·ver·sus
pl trans·ver·si
trans·ves·tism
also trans·ves·ti·tism
trans·ves·tite
tran·yl·cy·pro·mine
tra·pe·zi·al
tra·pe·zi·form
tra·pe·zi·um
pl tra·pe·zi·ums
or tra·pe·zia
tra·pe·zi·us
trap·e·zoid
trau·ma
pl trau·ma·ta
or trau·mas
trau·mat·ic
trau·mat·i·cal·ly
trau·ma·tism
trau·ma·ti·za·tion
trau·ma·tize
trau·ma·tized
trau·ma·tiz·ing
trau·ma·tol·o·gy
pl trau·ma·tol·o·gies
trau·ma·top·nea
tra·vail
trea·cle
treat·abil·i·ty
pl treat·abil·i·ties
treat·able
treat·ment
tre·ha·lase
tre·ha·lose
Treitz's mus·cle
or Treitz's lig·a·ment
Trem·a·to·da
trem·a·tode
trem·ble
trem·bled
trem·bling
trem·el·loid
trem·el·lose
tremo·pho·bia
trem·or
trem·u·lous
trem·u·lous·ly
trem·u·lous·ness
trench fe·ver
trench foot
trench mouth
Tren·de·len·burg po·si·tion
tre·pan
tre·panned
tre·pan·ning
trep·a·na·tion
treph·i·na·tion
tre·phine
tre·phined
tre·phin·ing
treph·o·cyte
treph·one
trep·i·dant
trep·i·da·tion
trepo·ne·ma
pl trepo·ne·ma·ta
or trepo·ne·mas
trepo·ne·ma·to·sis
pl trepo·ne·ma·to·ses
trepo·neme
trep·o·ne·mi·ci·dal
tre·pop·nea
trep·pe
tri·ac·e·tin
tri·ad
tri·age
tri·al
tri·am·cin·o·lone
tri·an·gle
tri·an·gu·la·ris
pl tri·an·gu·la·res
tri·at·o·ma
tri·atom·ic
tri·azine
tri·bade
tri·bad·ic
trib·a·dism

trib·a·dy
pl trib·a·dies

tri·ba·sic
tri·bo·lu·mi·nes·cence
tri·bro·mo·eth·a·nol
tri·bu·tyr·in
tri·car·box·yl·ic
tri·ceps
pl tri·ceps·es
also tri·ceps

tri·chi·a·sis
tri·chi·na
pl tri·chi·nae
also tri·chi·nas

trich·i·nel·la
pl trich·i·nel·lae

trich·i·nel·li·a·sis
pl trich·i·nel·li·a·ses

trich·i·ni·a·sis
pl trich·i·ni·a·ses

trich·i·niza·tion
trich·i·nize
trich·i·nized
trich·i·niz·ing
tri·chi·no·scope
trich·i·no·sis
pl trich·i·no·ses

tri·chi·nous
trich·i·on
tri·chlor·fon
tri·chlo·ride
tri·chlo·ro·ace·tic
also tri·chlor·ace·tic

tri·chlo·ro·eth·yl·ene
also tri·chlor·eth·yl·ene

tri·chlo·ro·meth·ane
tricho·bac·te·ria
tricho·be·zoar
tricho·ceph·a·li·a·sis
pl tricho·ceph·a·li·a·ses

Trich·o·ceph·a·lus
tricho·cyst
Trich·o·dec·tes
Trich·o·der·ma
tricho·ep·i·the·li·o·ma
pl tricho·ep·i·the·li·o·mas
or tricho·ep·i·the·li·o·ma·ta

tricho·es·the·sia
trich·o·gen
tri·chog·e·nous
also trich·o·gen·ic

tricho·glos·sia
tri·choid
tri·chol·o·gy
pl tri·chol·o·gies

tri·cho·ma
tri·cho·ma·to·sis
tri·chom·a·tous
tri·chome
tri·cho·mic
tricho·mo·na·cid·al

tricho·mo·na·cide
tricho·mon·ad
tricho·monad·al
or tricho·mo·nal

Tricho·mon·as
tricho·mo·ni·a·sis
pl tricho·mo·ni·a·ses

tricho·my·co·sis
pl tricho·my·co·ses

tricho·no·do·sis
pl tricho·no·do·ses
or tricho·no·do·sis·es

trich·op·a·thy
pl trich·op·a·thies

tricho·pho·bia
tricho·phy·tid
tricho·phy·to·be·zoar
tricho·phy·ton
pl tricho·phy·ta
also tricho·phy·tons

tricho·phyt·o·sis
tricho·pti·lo·sis
pl tricho·pti·lo·ses

trich·or·rhex·is
pl trich·or·rhex·es

tri·cho·sis
pl tri·cho·ses

Tricho·spo·ron
tricho·spo·ro·sis
pl tricho·spo·ro·ses
or tricho·spo·ro·sis·es

tricho·sta·sis
pl tricho·sta·ses

tricho·stron·gy·lo·sis

Tricho·stron·gy·lus
tricho·til·lo·ma·nia
tricho·til·lo·man·ic
tri·chot·o·my
pl tri·chot·o·mies
tri·chro·ic
tri·chro·ism
tri·chro·mat
tri·chro·mat·ic
tri·chro·ma·tism
tri·chro·ma·top·sia
tri·chrome
tri·chro·mic
trich·u·ri·a·sis
pl trich·u·ri·a·ses
Trich·u·ris
tri·cip·i·tal
tri·corn
tri·cor·nute
tri·cre·sol
tri·crot·ic
tri·cro·tism
tri·cus·pid
tri·cus·pi·date
also tri·cus·pi·da·ted
tri·dac·tyl
or tri·dac·ty·lous
also tri·dac·tyle
tri·dent
tri·den·tate
tri·der·mic
tri·eth·a·nol·amine
tri·eth·io·dide
tri·eth·yl·amine
tri·eth·yl·ene·mel·amine
tri·fa·cial
tri·fid
tri·fluo·per·a·zine
tri·fo·cal
tri·fo·li·o·sis
pl tri·fo·li·o·ses
tri·fo·li·um
tri·fur·cate
tri·fur·cat·ed
tri·fur·cat·ing
tri·fur·ca·tion
tri·gem·i·nal
tri·gem·i·nus
pl tri·gem·i·ni
tri·gem·i·ny
pl tri·gem·i·nies
tri·glyc·er·ide
tri·go·nal
tri·go·nal·ly
tri·gone
also tri·gon
trig·o·nel·line
tri·go·nid
tri·go·ni·tis
trigo·no·ceph·a·lous
or trigo·no·ce·phal·ic
trigo·no·ceph·a·ly
pl trigo·no·ceph·a·lies
tri·go·num
pl tri·go·nums
or tri·go·na
tri·go·num ha·ben·u·lae
tri·hy·brid
tri·io·do·thy·ro·nine
tri·lam·i·nar
also tri·lam·i·nate
tri·lo·bate
or tri·lo·bat·ed
or tri·lobed
tri·loc·u·lar
or tri·loc·u·late
tril·o·gy
pl tril·o·gies
tri·man·u·al
tri·mes·ter
tri·metha·di·one
tri·meth·yl·amine
tri·meth·yl·ene
tri·mor·phic
tri·mor·phous
tri·ni·tro·glyc·er·in
tri·ni·tro·phe·nol
tri·ni·tro·tol·u·ene
tri·nu·cle·ate
tri·nu·cle·o·tide
tri·ole·in
tri·ose
tri·ox·ide
tri·pal·mi·tin
trip·a·ra
pl trip·a·ras
or trip·a·rae
tri·par·tite
tri·pel·en·na·mine

tri·pep·tide
tri·pha·sic
tri·phe·nyl·meth·ane
tri·phos·pha·tase
tri·phos·phate
tri·phos·pho·pyr·i·dine nu·cle·o·tide
tri·ple·gia
trip·let
tri·plex
trip·lo·blas·tic
trip·loid
tri·plo·pia
tri·pod
trip·sis
tri·que·trous
tri·que·trum
  pl tri·que·tra

tri·ra·di·al
tri·ra·di·al·ly
tri·ra·di·us
  pl tri·ra·dii
  also tri·ra·di·us·es

tri·sac·cha·ride
tris·mus
tri·so·mic
tri·so·my
  pl tri·so·mies

tri·splanch·nic
tri·stea·rin
trit·an·ope
trit·an·opia
tri·ti·at·ed
trit·i·ca·le
tri·ti·ceous
tri·ti·ceum
  pl tri·ti·cei

trit·i·cum
tri·ti·um
trito·cone
tri·to·co·nid
trit·u·ra·ble
trit·u·rate
  trit·u·rat·ed
  trit·u·rat·ing
trit·u·ra·tion
tri·va·lence
  or tri·va·len·cy
  pl tri·va·lenc·es
  or tri·va·len·cies

tri·val·ent
tri·valve
tri·val·vu·lar
tro·car
  also tro·char

tro·chan·ter
tro·chan·ter·ic
tro·chan·tin
  also tro·chan·tine

tro·chan·tin·i·an
tro·che
troch·lea
troch·le·ar
troch·le·ar·i·form
troch·le·ar·is
trocho·ce·pha·lia
tro·choid
tro·choi·des
  pl tro·choi·des

tro·land
Trom·bic·u·la
Trom·bi·cu·li·dae
tro·pa·co·caine
tro·pane
tro·pate
tro·pe·ine
troph·ec·to·derm
troph·ede·ma
  pl troph·ede·mas
  or troph·ede·ma·ta

tro·phe·ma
troph·e·sy
  pl troph·e·sies

tro·phic
tro·phism
tro·pho·blast
tro·pho·blas·tic
tro·pho·cyte
tro·pho·derm
tro·pho·dy·nam·ics
tro·phol·o·gy
  pl tro·phol·o·gies

tro·pho·neu·ro·sis
  pl tro·pho·neu·ro·ses

tro·pho·neu·rot·ic
tro·pho·nu·cle·us
  pl tro·pho·nu·clei
  also tro·pho·nu·cle·us·es

tro·phop·a·thy
  pl tro·phop·a·thies

tro·pho·plast
tro·pho·spon·gia
  vascular spongy mucous membrane

tro·pho·spon·gi·um
intracellular canal system

tro·pho·tax·is
pl tro·pho·tax·es

tro·pho·trop·ic
tro·phot·ro·pism
tro·pho·zo·ite
tro·pia
trop·ic ac·id
trop·i·cal
tro·pine
tro·pism
tro·po·col·la·gen
tro·pom·e·ter
tropo·my·o·sin
trun·cal
trun·cate
trun·cat·ed
trun·cat·ing

trun·cus
pl trun·ci

trun·cus ar·te·ri·o·sus
try·pan blue
try·pano·ci·dal
try·pano·cide
try·pano·so·ma
pl try·pano·so·mas
or try·pano·so·ma·ta

try·pano·some
try·pano·so·mi·a·sis
pl try·pano·so·mi·a·ses

try·pan red
tryp·ars·amide
tryp·sin
tryp·sin·iza·tion
tryp·sin·o·gen
trypt·amine
tryp·tic
tryp·to·phan
or tryp·to·phane

tryp·to·pha·nase
tset·se
pl tset·se
or tset·ses

tsu·tsu·ga·mu·shi
tu·ba
tub·age
tub·al
tu·bec·to·my
pl tu·bec·to·mies

tu·ber
tu·ber ci·ne·re·um
tu·ber·cle
tu·ber·cled
tu·ber·cu·lar
tu·ber·cu·late
or tu·ber·cu·lat·ed

tu·ber·cu·la·tion
tu·ber·cu·lid
or tu·ber·cu·lide

tu·ber·cu·lin
tu·ber·cu·lo·cid·al
tu·ber·cu·lo·derm
also tu·ber·cu·lo·der·ma

tu·ber·cu·lo·fi·broid
tu·ber·cu·loid
tu·ber·cu·lo·ma
pl tu·ber·cu·lo·mas
also tu·ber·cu·lo·ma·ta

tu·ber·cu·lo·pho·bia
tu·ber·cu·lo·sis
pl tu·ber·cu·lo·ses

tu·ber·cu·lo·stat·ic
tu·ber·cu·lous
tu·ber·cu·lous·ly
tu·ber·cu·lum
pl tu·ber·cu·la

tu·ber·cu·lum ci·ne·re·um
tu·ber·os·i·tas
pl tu·ber·os·i·ta·tes

tu·ber·os·i·ty
pl tu·ber·os·i·ties

tu·ber·ous
also tu·ber·ose

tu·bo·cu·ra·rine
tu·bo·lig·a·men·tous
tubo-ovar·i·an
tu·bo·peri·to·ne·al
tu·bo·uter·ine
tu·bo·vag·i·nal
tu·bu·lar
tu·bule
tu·bu·lus
pl tu·bu·li

tu·la·re·mia
tu·la·re·mic
tulle gras

tu·me·fa·cient
tu·me·fac·tion
tu·me·fy
  tu·me·fied
  tu·me·fy·ing
tu·mer·ic
  var of turmeric

tu·mes·cence
tu·mes·cent
tu·mid
tu·mid·i·ty
tum·my
  pl tum·mies

tu·mor
  also tu·mour

tu·mor·al
tu·mor·i·gen·e·sis
  pl tu·mor·i·gen·e·ses

tu·mor·i·gen·ic
tu·mor·i·ge·nic·i·ty
  pl tu·mor·i·ge·nic·i·ties

tu·mor·ous
tu·mul·tus
Tun·ga
tung·sten
tu·nic
tu·ni·ca
  pl tu·ni·cae

tu·ni·ca al·bu·gi·nea
  pl tu·ni·cae al·bu·gi·ne·ae

tu·ni·cin
tun·ing fork
tun·nel

tu·ra·cin
tur·bid
tur·bi·dim·e·ter
tur·bi·di·met·ric
tur·bi·di·met·ri·cal·ly
tur·bi·dim·e·try
  pl tur·bi·dim·e·tries

tur·bid·i·ty
  pl tur·bid·i·ties

tur·bi·nal
tur·bi·nate
  also tur·bi·nat·ed

tur·bi·nec·to·my
  pl tur·bi·nec·to·mies

tur·bi·not·o·my
  pl tur·bi·not·o·mies

tur·ges·cence
tur·ges·cent
tur·gid
tur·gid·i·ty
  pl tur·gid·i·ties

tur·gid·ness
tur·gor
Türk cell
  or Türk's cell

tur·mer·ic
  or tu·mer·ic

Tur·ner's syn·drome
tur·pen·tine
tur·ri·ceph·a·ly
  pl tur·ri·ceph·a·lies

tus·sal
tus·sis
tus·sive

tween-brain
twee·zers
twen·ty-twen·ty
  or 20/20

twin
  twinned
  twin·ning
twin·born
twinge
  twinged
  twing·ing
    or twinge·ing

ty·lo·ma
  pl ty·lo·mas
  or ty·lo·ma·ta

ty·lo·sin
ty·lo·sis
  pl ty·lo·ses

ty·lot·ic
tym·pa·nal
tym·pan·ic
tym·pa·nism
tym·pa·ni·tes
  also tym·pa·ni·tis *abdominal distension with gas (see* tympanitis)

tym·pa·nit·ic
tym·pa·ni·tis
  inflammation of the middle ear (see tympanites)

tym·pa·no·mas·toid
tym·pa·no·mas·toid·i·tis
  pl tym·pa·no·mas·toid·it·i·des

tym·pa·no·plas·ty
pl tym·pa·no·plas·ties

tym·pa·no·sta·pe·di·al

tym·pa·not·o·my
pl tym·pa·not·o·mies

tym·pa·nous

tym·pa·num
pl tym·pa·na
also tym·pa·nums

tym·pa·ny
pl tym·pa·nies

typh·lec·to·my
pl typh·lec·to·mies

typh·li·tis

typh·lo·di·cli·di·tis

typh·lo·em·py·ema
pl typh·lo·em·py·ema·ta
or typh·lo·em·py·emas

typh·lo·li·thi·a·sis
pl typh·lo·li·thi·a·ses

typh·lo·meg·a·ly
pl typh·lo·meg·a·lies

typh·lo·pto·sis
pl typh·lo·pto·ses

typh·lo·sis

typh·los·to·my
pl typh·los·to·mies

ty·phoid

ty·phoi·dal

ty·pho·pneu·mo·nia

ty·phous

ty·phus

typ·i·cal

ty·ra·mine

ty·ro·ci·dine
or ty·ro·ci·din

Ty·rode so·lu·tion
or Ty·rode's so·lu·tion

ty·rog·e·nous

ty·roid

ty·ros·i·nase

ty·ro·sine

ty·ro·sin·emia

tyro·sin·osis

tyro·sin·uria

ty·ro·thri·cin

U

uber·ous

uber·ty
pl uber·ties

ubi·qui·none

ud·der

ul·cer
ul·cered
ul·cer·ing

ul·cer·ate
ul·cer·at·ed
ul·cer·at·ing

ul·cer·ation

ul·cer·ative

ul·cero·gen·ic

ul·cero·mem·bra·nous

ul·cer·ous

ul·cus
pl ul·cera

ule·gy·ria

uler·y·the·ma

ulet·ic

ul·na
pl ul·nae
or ul·nas

ul·nad

ul·nar

uloid

ulo·sis
pl ulo·ses
or ulo·sis·es

ulot·ic

ulot·o·my
pl ulot·o·mies

ulot·ri·chous

ul·ti·mo·gen·i·ture

ul·ti·mum mor·i·ens

ul·tra·brachy·ce·phal·ic

ul·tra·cen·tri·fu·ga·tion

ul·tra·cen·tri·fuge

ul·tra·fil·ter

ul·tra·fil·tra·tion

ul·tra·mi·cro·scope

ul·tra·mi·cro·scop·ic

ul·tra·mi·cro·scop·i·cal·ly

ul·tra·mi·cros·co·py
pl ul·tra·mi·cros·co·pies

ul·tra·mi·cro·tome
ul·tra·son·ic
ul·tra·sono·gram
ul·tra·so·nog·ra·phy
pl ul·tra·so·nog·ra·phies
ul·tra·sound
ul·tra·struc·tur·al
ul·tra·struc·tur·al·ly
ul·tra·struc·ture
ul·tra·thin
ul·tra·vi·o·let
um·bil·i·cal
um·bil·i·cate
or um·bil·i·cat·ed
um·bil·i·ca·tion
um·bil·i·cus
pl um·bil·i·ci
or um·bil·i·cus·es
um·bo
pl um·bo·nes
or um·bos
um·bo·nate
un·anes·the·tized
un·bal·ance
un·bal·anced
un·bal·anc·ing
un·cal
un·cia
pl un·ci·ae
un·ci·form
un·ci·nal
un·ci·nar·ia
un·ci·na·ri·a·sis
pl un·ci·na·ri·a·ses
un·ci·nate
un·ci·na·tum
pl un·ci·na·ta
or un·ci·na·tums
un·cir·cum·cised
un·com·pli·cat·ed
un·con·di·tion·al
un·con·di·tioned
un·con·scious
un·con·scious·ly
un·con·scious·ness
un·co·or·di·nat·ed
unc·tion
unc·tu·ous
unc·tu·ous·ly
un·cus
pl un·ci
un·dec·y·len·ate
un·dec·y·le·nic
un·der·achiev·er
un·der·arm
un·der·cut
un·der·de·vel·oped
un·der·de·vel·op·ment
un·der·lip
un·der·nour·ished
un·der·nu·tri·tion
un·der·sexed
un·der·shot
un·der·slung
un·der·toe
un·der·weight
un·de·scend·ed
un·di·ag·nosed
un·dif·fer·en·ti·at·ed
un·di·gest·ed
un·dine
un·du·lant
un·du·late
or un·du·lat·ed
un·du·la·tion
un·en·cap·su·lat·ed
un·erupt·ed
un·gual
also un·gui·nal
un·guent
Un·guic·u·la·ta
un·guic·u·late
also un·guic·u·lat·ed
un·guis
pl un·gues
un·gu·la
pl un·gu·lae
Un·gu·la·ta
un·gu·late
un·gu·li·grade
un·healthy
un·health·i·er
un·health·i·est
uni·al·gal
uni·ar·tic·u·lar
uni·ax·i·al
uni·ax·i·al·ly
uni·bas·al
uni·cam·er·al
uni·cam·er·al·ly
uni·cel·lu·lar

uni·cel·lu·lar·i·ty
pl uni·cel·lu·lar·i·ties
uni·cen·tral
uni·cen·tric
uni·cor·nous
uni·cus·pid
also uni·cus·pi·date
uni·di·rec·tion·al
uni·fac·to·ri·al
uni·fi·lar
uni·fla·gel·late
uni·glan·du·lar
uni·grav·i·da
pl uni·grav·i·das
or uni·grav·i·dae
uni·lat·er·al
uni·lat·er·al·ly
uni·lo·bar
uni·loc·u·lar
un·im·paired
un·in·hib·it·ed
uni·nu·cle·ate
also uni·nu·cle·ar
uni·oc·u·lar
uni·oval
or uni·ovu·lar
unip·a·ra
pl unip·a·ras
or unip·a·rae
uni·pa·ren·tal
unip·a·rous
uni·po·lar
uni·po·lar·i·ty
pl uni·po·lar·i·ties
unip·o·tent
uni·po·ten·tial
uni·sep·tate

uni·sex·u·al
uni·tary
uni·va·lent
un·linked
un·med·ul·lat·ed
un·my·elin·at·ed
un·of·fi·cial
un·or·ga·nized
un·paired
un·phys·i·o·log·ic
also un·phys·i·o·log·i·cal
un·pig·ment·ed
un·re·ac·tive
un·re·duced
un·re·spon·sive
un·rest
un·sat·u·rat·ed
un·sex
un·sound
un·spec·i·fied
un·sta·ble
un·stained
un·stri·at·ed
un·treat·ed
un·vac·ci·nat·ed
un·well
up·set
up·set
up·set·ting
up·take
ura·chal
ura·chus
ura·cil
ura·cra·sia
ura·gogue
ura·mil

ura·nin
ura·ni·um
ura·no·plas·ty
pl ura·no·plas·ties
ura·no·ple·gia
ura·nos·chi·sis
pl ura·nos·chi·ses
also ura·nos·chi·sis·es
ura·no·staph·y·lo·plas·ty
pl ura·no·staph·y·lo·plas·ties
ura·no·staph·y·lor·rha·phy
pl ura·no·staph·y·lor·rha·phies
ura·ro·ma
urate
ura·te·mia
urat·ic
ura·tu·ria
ur·cei·form
ur·ce·o·late
urea
ure·al
ure·am·e·ter
ure·am·e·try
pl ure·am·e·tries
ure·ase
ure·de·ma
pl ure·de·mas
or ure·de·ma·ta
ure·ide
ure·mia
or urae·mia
ure·mic
or urae·mic

ure·mi·gen·ic
ure·om·e·ter
ureo·tel·ic
ureo·te·lism
ure·si·es·the·sia
ure·sis
ure·ter
ure·ter·al
or ure·ter·ic
ure·ter·ec·ta·sis
or ure·ter·ec·ta·sia
ure·ter·ec·to·my
pl ure·ter·ec·to·mies
ure·ter·ic
ure·ter·itis
ure·tero·cele
ure·tero·co·los·to·my
pl ure·tero·co·los·to·mies
ure·tero·cys·tos·to·my
pl ure·tero·cys·tos·to·mies
ure·tero·en·ter·ic
ure·tero·en·ter·os·to·my
pl ure·tero·en·ter·os·to·mies
ure·ter·og·ra·phy
pl ure·ter·og·ra·phies
ure·tero·hy·dro·ne·phro·sis
pl ure·tero·hy·dro·ne·phro·ses
ure·tero·il·e·os·to·my
pl ure·tero·il·e·os·to·mies
ure·tero·in·tes·ti·nal
ure·tero·lith
ure·tero·li·thi·a·sis
pl ure·tero·li·thi·a·ses
ure·tero·li·thot·o·my
pl ure·tero·li·thot·o·mies
ure·ter·ol·y·sis
pl ure·ter·ol·y·ses
ure·tero·neo·cys·tos·to·my
pl ure·tero·neo·cys·tos·to·mies
ure·tero·neo·py·elos·to·my
pl ure·tero·neo·py·elos·to·mies
ure·tero·ne·phrec·to·my
pl ure·tero·ne·phrec·to·mies
ure·ter·op·a·thy
pl ure·ter·op·a·thies
ure·tero·pel·vic
ure·tero·plas·ty
pl ure·tero·plas·ties
ure·tero·py·eli·tis
ure·tero·py·elog·ra·phy
pl ure·tero·py·elog·ra·phies
ure·tero·py·elo·ne·os·to·my
pl ure·tero·py·elo·ne·os·to·mies
ure·tero·py·elo·ne·phri·tis
pl ure·tero·py·elo·ne·phrit·i·des
ure·tero·py·elo·ne·phros·to·my
pl ure·tero·py·elo·ne·phros·to·mies
ure·tero·py·elo·plas·ty
pl ure·tero·py·elo·plas·ties
ure·tero·py·elos·to·my
pl ure·tero·py·elos·to·mies
ure·ter·or·rha·gia
ure·ter·or·rha·phy
pl ure·ter·or·rha·phies
ure·tero·sig·moid·os·to·my
pl ure·tero·sig·moid·os·to·mies
ure·ter·os·to·my
pl ure·ter·os·to·mies
ure·ter·ot·o·my
pl ure·ter·ot·o·mies
ure·tero·vag·i·nal
ure·tero·ves·i·cal
ure·thane
or ure·than
ure·thra
pl ure·thras
or ure·thrae
ure·thral
ure·threc·to·my
pl ure·threc·to·mies

ure·thri·tis
pl ure·thrit·i·des
ure·thro·bul·bar
ure·thro·cele
ure·thro·cys·ti·tis
pl ure·thro·cys·tit·i·des
ure·thro·gram
ure·thro·graph
ure·throm·e·ter
ure·thro·per·i·ne·al
ure·thro·plas·ty
pl ure·thro·plas·ties
ure·thro·pros·tat·ic
ure·thro·rec·tal
ure·thror·rha·phy
pl ure·thror·rha·phies
ure·thror·rhea
ure·thro·scope
ure·thro·scop·ic
ure·thros·co·py
pl ure·thros·co·pies
ure·thro·spasm
ure·thro·ste·no·sis
pl ure·thro·ste·no·ses
ure·thros·to·my
pl ure·thros·to·mies
ure·thro·tome
ure·throt·o·my
pl ure·throt·o·mies
ure·thro·vag·i·nal
ur·gency
pl ur·gen·cies
ur·hi·dro·sis
pl ur·hi·dro·ses
uric·ac·i·de·mia
uric·ac·i·du·ria
uri·case
uri·ce·mia
uri·col·y·sis
pl uri·col·y·ses
uri·co·lyt·ic
uri·cos·uria
uri·co·su·ric
uri·co·tel·ic
uri·co·te·lism
uri·nal
uri·nal·y·sis
pl uri·nal·y·ses
uri·nary
uri·nate
uri·nat·ed
uri·nat·ing
uri·na·tion
urine
uri·nif·er·ous
uri·nip·a·rous
uri·no·gen·i·tal
uri·no·ma
pl uri·no·mas
or uri·no·ma·ta
uri·nom·e·ter
uri·nom·e·try
pl uri·nom·e·tries
urin·ous
uro·bi·lin
uro·bi·li·ne·mia
uro·bi·lin·o·gen
uro·bi·lin·o·gen·uria
uro·chrome
uro·chro·mo·gen
uro·cris·ia
uro·cy·ano·gen
uro·cy·a·no·sis
pl uro·cy·a·no·ses
uro·er·y·thrin
uro·gas·trone
uro·gen·i·tal
urog·e·nous
uro·glau·cin
uro·gram
urog·ra·phy
pl urog·ra·phies
uro·he·ma·tin
uro·ki·nase
uro·lith
uro·li·thi·a·sis
pl uro·li·thi·a·ses
uro·lith·ic
uro·log·ic
or uro·log·i·cal
urol·o·gist
urol·o·gy
pl urol·o·gies
uro·lu·tein
urom·e·ter
uro·nos·co·py
pl uro·nos·co·pies
urop·a·thy
pl urop·a·thies
uro·pep·sin
uro·phe·in
uro·poi·e·sis
pl uro·poi·e·ses
uro·poi·et·ic
uro·por·phy·rin
uro·ru·bin

uros·che·sis
pl uros·che·ses

uros·cop·ic
uros·co·py
pl uros·co·pies

uro·sep·sis
pl uro·sep·ses

uro·tox·ic
uro·tox·ic·i·ty
pl uro·tox·ic·i·ties

uro·xan·thin
ur·ti·cant
ur·ti·car·ia
ur·ti·car·i·al
ur·ti·car·io·gen·ic
ur·ti·cate
ur·ti·cat·ed
ur·ti·cat·ing
ur·ti·ca·tion
uru·shi·ol
us·tu·la·tion
uta
uter·al·gia
uter·ine
uter·i·tis
utero·ab·dom·i·nal
utero·cer·vi·cal
utero·ges·ta·tion
uter·og·ra·phy
pl uter·og·ra·phies

uter·om·e·ter
utero-ovar·i·an
utero·pel·vic
utero·pexy
pl utero·pex·ies

utero·plas·ty
pl utero·plas·ties

utero·sa·cral
utero·sal·pin·gog·ra·phy
pl utero·sal·pin·gog·ra·phies

uter·ot·o·my
pl uter·ot·o·mies

utero·ton·ic
utero·tub·al
utero·vag·i·nal
utero·ves·i·cal
uter·us
pl uteri
also uter·us·es

utri·cle
utric·u·lar
utric·u·li·tis
utric·u·lo·sac·cu·lar
utric·u·lus
pl utric·u·li

uvea
uve·al
uve·itis
pl uve·it·i·des

uveo·par·ot·id
uveo·par·oti·tis
uveo·scle·ri·tis
uvio·re·sis·tant
uvu·la
pl uvu·las
or uvu·lae

uvu·lar
uvu·lar·ly
uvu·lec·to·my
pl uvu·lec·to·mies

uvu·li·tis
uvu·lop·to·sis
pl uvu·lop·to·ses

uvu·lo·tome
uvu·lot·o·my
pl uvu·lot·o·mies

V

vac·ci·na·ble
vac·ci·nal
vac·ci·nate
vac·ci·nat·ed
vac·ci·nat·ing
vac·ci·na·tion
vac·ci·na·tor
vac·cine
vac·ci·nee
vac·cin·ia
vac·cin·i·al
vac·cin·iform
vac·ci·noid
vac·ci·no·ther·a·py
pl vac·ci·no·ther·a·pies

vac·u·o·lar
vac·u·o·late
vac·u·o·lat·ed
vac·u·o·lat·ing
vac·u·o·la·tion
vac·u·ole
vac·u·ol·iza·tion
vac·u·um
pl vac·u·ums
or vac·ua

va·gal

va·gi·na
pl va·gi·nae
or va·gi·nas

vag·i·nal
vag·i·nal·itis
vag·i·nal·ly
va·gi·na·pexy
pl va·gi·na·pex·ies

vag·i·nate
or vag·i·nat·ed

va·gi·na ten·di·
nis
vag·i·nec·to·my
pl vag·i·nec·to·mies

vag·i·nis·mus
vag·i·ni·tis
vag·i·no·cele
vag·i·no·dyn·ia
vag·i·no·fix·a·tion
vag·i·no·la·bi·al
vag·i·no·my·co·sis
pl vag·i·no·my·co·ses

vag·i·no·per·i·ne·
ot·o·my
pl vag·i·no·per·i·ne·
ot·o·mies

vag·i·no·plas·ty
pl vag·i·no·plas·ties

vag·i·no·scope
vag·i·nos·co·py
pl vag·i·nos·co·pies

vag·i·not·o·my
pl vag·i·not·o·mies

va·gi·tus
va·gi·tus uter·in·
us

va·got·o·mize
va·got·o·mized
va·got·o·miz·ing
va·got·o·my
pl va·got·o·mies

va·go·to·nia
also va·goto·ny
pl va·go·to·nias
also va·goto·nies

va·go·ton·ic
va·go·tro·pic
va·go·va·gal
va·grant
va·gus
pl va·gi

va·lence
va·len·cy
pl va·len·cies

va·lent
val·er·ate
va·le·ric ac·id
also va·le·ri·an·ic ac·
id

val·e·tu·di·nar·i·
an
val·e·tu·di·nar·i·
an·ism
val·gus
va·line
val·in·o·my·cin
val·late
val·lec·u·la
pl val·lec·u·lae

Val·sal·va ma·
neu·ver
val·va
pl val·vae

valve
valve of Bau·hin
valve of Ger·lach
valve of Has·ner
valve of Hei·ster
valve of Hous·ton
valve of Kerck·
ring
valve of The·be·
si·us
valve of Vieus·
sens
val·vi·form
val·vot·o·my
pl val·vot·o·mies

val·vu·la
pl val·vu·lae

val·vu·la co·li
val·vu·la con·ni·
vens
pl val·vu·lae con·ni·
ven·tes

val·vu·lar
val·vu·la spi·ra·lis
pl val·vu·lae spi·ra·
les

val·vu·li·tis
val·vu·lo·plas·ty
pl val·vu·lo·plas·ties

val·vu·lo·tome
val·vu·lot·o·my
pl val·vu·lot·o·mies

vam·pire
vam·pir·ism
van·a·date
va·na·di·um
va·na·di·um·ism

van·co·my·cin
van den Bergh test
van Hoorne's ca·nal
va·nil·la
vanil·late
va·nil·lic
van·il·lin
va·nil·lism
Van Slyke meth·od
va·por
va·por·iza·tion
va·por·ize
va·por·ized
va·por·iz·ing
va·por·iz·er
va·po·ther·a·py
pl va·po·ther·a·pies
Va·quez's dis·ease
vari·abil·i·ty
pl vari·abil·i·ties
vari·able
vari·ance
vari·ant
vari·a·tion
var·i·ca·tion
var·i·ce·al
var·i·cel·la
var·i·cel·li·form
var·i·co·bleph·a·ron
var·i·co·cele
var·i·co·ce·lec·to·my
pl var·i·co·ce·lec·to·mies
var·i·cog·ra·phy
pl var·i·cog·ra·phies
vari·coid
var·i·com·phal·lus
var·i·co·phle·bi·tis
pl var·i·co·phle·bit·i·des
var·i·cose
also var·i·cosed
var·i·co·sis
pl var·i·co·ses
var·i·cos·i·ty
pl var·i·cos·i·ties
var·i·cot·o·my
pl var·i·cot·o·mies
va·ric·u·la
va·ri·o·la
va·ri·o·lar
var·i·o·late
var·i·o·lat·ed
var·i·o·lat·ing
va·ri·o·la vac·cin·ia
va·ri·o·loid
va·ri·o·lous
va·ri·o·lo·vac·cine
var·ix
pl var·i·ces
Va·ro·li·an
var·us
vas
pl va·sa
vas ab·er·rans
pl va·sa ab·er·ran·tia
va·sa bre·via
va·sa ef·fer·en·tia
vasal
va·sa va·so·rum
vas·cu·lar
vas·cu·lar·i·ty
pl vas·cu·lar·i·ties
vas·cu·lar·iza·tion
vas·cu·lar·ize
vas·cu·lar·ized
vas·cu·lar·iz·ing
vas·cu·la·ture
vas·cu·li·tis
pl vas·cu·li·ti·des
vas def·er·ens
pl va·sa def·er·en·tia
va·sec·to·mize
va·sec·to·mized
va·sec·to·miz·ing
va·sec·to·my
pl va·sec·to·mies
vas·i·fac·tion
vasi·fac·tive
or vaso·fac·tive
va·si·form
vas·i·tis
va·so·ac·tive
va·so·ac·tiv·i·ty
pl va·so·ac·tiv·i·ties
va·so·con·stric·tion

va·so·con·stric·tive
va·so·con·stric·tor
va·so·de·pres·sor
va·so·di·la·ta·tion
va·so·di·la·tion
va·so·di·la·tor
va·so·for·ma·tive
va·so·gan·gli·on
pl va·so·gan·glia
or va·so·gan·gli·ons
va·sog·ra·phy
pl va·sog·ra·phies
va·so·in·hib·i·tor
va·so·in·hib·i·to·ry
va·so·li·ga·tion
va·so·mo·tion
va·so·mo·tor
va·so·neu·ro·sis
pl va·so·neu·ro·ses
va·so·pres·sin
va·so·pres·sor
va·so·re·flex
va·so·sec·tion
va·so·spasm
va·so·spas·tic
va·so·to·cin
va·so·ton·ic
va·so·va·gal
vas·tus ex·ter·nus
vas·tus in·ter·me·di·us
vas·tus in·ter·nus
vas·tus lat·er·alis
vas·tus me·di·alis
Va·ter's am·pul·la
Va·ter's cor·pus·cle
vec·tor
vec·tor·car·dio·gram
vec·tor·car·dio·graph·ic
vec·tor·car·di·og·ra·phy
pl vec·tor·car·di·og·ra·phies
vec·to·ri·al
ve·gan
ve·gan·ism
veg·e·ta·ble
veg·e·tal
veg·e·tar·i·an
veg·e·tar·i·an·ism
veg·e·ta·tion
veg·e·ta·tive
ve·hi·cle
vein
ve·la·men
pl ve·lam·i·na
vel·a·men·tous
vel·a·men·tum
pl vel·a·men·ta
ve·lar
ve·li·form
vel·li·cate
vel·li·cat·ed
vel·li·cat·ing
vel·li·ca·tion
ve·loc·i·ty
pl ve·loc·i·ties
Vel·peau's ban·dage
ve·lum
pl ve·la
ve·na
pl ve·nae
ve·na ca·va
pl ve·nae ca·vae
ve·na ca·val
ve·na co·mes
pl ve·nae com·i·tes
ve·nae vor·ti·co·sae
ve·na·tion
ve·nec·to·my
pl ve·nec·to·mies
ven·e·nate
ven·e·nat·ed
ven·e·nat·ing
ven·e·na·tion
ven·e·nif·er·ous
ve·ne·re·al
ve·ne·re·o·log·i·cal
ve·ne·re·ol·o·gist
ve·ne·re·ol·o·gy
or ven·er·ol·o·gy
pl ve·ne·re·ol·o·gies
or ven·er·ol·o·gies
ven·ery
pl ven·eries
vene·sec·tion
or veni·sec·tion
vene·su·ture
ven·in
ve·ni·punc·ture
also ve·ne·punc·ture

veno·cly·sis
pl veno·cly·ses

ve·no·fi·bro·sis
pl ve·no·fi·bro·ses

veno·gram

veno·graph·ic

ve·nog·ra·phy
pl ve·nog·ra·phies

ven·om

ven·o·mo·sal·i·vary

ve·no·mo·tor

ven·om·ous

ve·no·per·i·to·ne·os·to·my
pl ve·no·per·i·to·ne·os·to·mies

ve·no·pres·sor

ve·no·scle·ro·sis
pl ve·no·scle·ro·ses

ve·nose

ve·nos·i·ty
pl ve·nos·i·ties

ve·no·sta·sis
pl ve·no·sta·ses

ve·not·o·my
pl ve·not·o·mies

ve·nous

ve·no·ve·nos·to·my
pl ve·no·ve·nos·to·mies

ven·ter

ven·ti·late
ven·ti·lat·ed
ven·ti·lat·ing

ven·ti·la·tion

ven·trad

ven·tral

ven·tra·lis

ven·tri·cle

ven·tri·co·lum·na
pl ven·tri·co·lum·nae

ven·tri·cor·nu
pl ven·tri·cor·nua

ven·tri·cose

ven·tric·u·lar

ven·tric·u·lar·is

ven·tric·u·li·tis

ven·tric·u·lo·cis·ter·nos·to·my
pl ven·tric·u·lo·cis·ter·nos·to·mies

ven·tric·u·lo·gram

ven·tric·u·log·ra·phy
pl ven·tric·u·log·ra·phies

ven·tric·u·lo·punc·ture

ven·tric·u·los·co·py
pl ven·tric·u·los·co·pies

ven·tric·u·los·to·my
pl ven·tric·u·los·to·mies

ven·tric·u·lo·sub·arach·noid

ven·tric·u·lot·o·my
pl ven·tric·u·lot·o·mies

ven·tric·u·lus
pl ven·tric·u·li

ven·tri·duc·tion

ven·tri·me·sal

ven·tro·fix·a·tion

ven·tro·hys·ter·o·pexy
pl ven·tro·hys·ter·o·pexies

ven·tro·lat·er·al

ven·tro·lat·er·al·ly

ven·tro·me·di·al
also ven·tro·me·di·an

ven·tro·me·di·al·ly

ven·tros·co·py
pl ven·tros·co·pies

ven·tro·sus·pen·sion

ven·tro·ves·i·co·fix·a·tion

ven·u·la

ven·u·lar

ven·ule

ve·ra·trine

ve·ra·trum

ver·bal

ver·bal·ly

ver·big·er·a·tion

ver·bile

ver·bo·ma·nia

ver·di·gris

ver·do·per·ox·i·dase

ver·gence

ver·mi·ci·dal

ver•mi•cide
ver•mic•u•lar
ver•mic•u•la•tion
ver•mi•cule
ver•mic•u•lose
ver•mi•form
ver•mif•u•gal
ver•mi•fuge
ver•mil•ion
or ver•mil•lion

ver•mil•ion•ec•to•my
pl ver•mil•ion•ec•to•mies

ver•min
pl ver•min

ver•mi•na•tion
ver•min•osis
pl ver•min•oses

ver•min•ous
ver•min•ous•ly
ver•mis
pl ver•mes

ver•mix
ver•nal
ver•ni•er
ver•nix
or ver•nix ca•se•o•sa

ver•no•nia
ver•ru•ca
pl ver•ru•cae

ver•ru•ca acu•mi•na•ta
ver•ru•ca plan•tar•is
ver•ru•ca se•nil•is
ver•ru•ca vul•ga•ris
ver•ru•ci•form
ver•ru•cose
ver•ru•co•sis
pl ver•ru•co•ses

ver•ru•cous
ver•ru•ga
ver•ru•ga per•u•a•na
also ver•ru•ga pe•ru•vi•ana

ver•si•col•or
or ver•si•col•ored

ver•sion
ver•te•bra
pl ver•te•brae
or ver•te•bras

ver•te•bral
ver•te•bral•ly
Ver•te•bra•ta
ver•te•brate
ver•te•brat•ed
ver•te•brec•to•my
pl ver•te•brec•to•mies

ver•te•bro•chon•dral
ver•te•bro•cos•tal
ver•te•bro•sa•cral
ver•te•bro•ster•nal
ver•tex
pl ver•tex•es
or ver•ti•ces

ver•ti•cal
ver•ti•cal•ly
ver•ti•cil
ver•ti•cil•late
ver•tig•i•nous
ver•ti•go
pl ver•ti•goes
or ver•ti•gos
or ver•tig•i•nes

ver•u•mon•ta•ni•tis
ver•u•mon•ta•num
ve•si•ca
pl ve•si•cae

ves•i•cal
adjective (*see* vesicle)

ves•i•cant
ves•i•cate
ves•i•cat•ed
ves•i•cat•ing
ves•i•ca•tion
ves•i•ca•to•ry
pl ves•i•ca•to•ries

ves•i•cle
noun (*see* vesical)

ves•i•co•cele
ves•i•co•cer•vi•cal
ves•i•co•pros•tat•ic
ves•i•cot•o•my
pl ves•i•cot•o•mies

ves•i•co•uter•ine
ves•i•co•vag•i•nal
ve•sic•u•la
pl ve•sic•u•lae
also ve•sic•u•las

ve•sic•u•lar
ve•sic•u•late
ve•sic•u•la•tion

ve•sic•u•lec•to•my
pl ve•sic•u•lec•to•mies
ve•sic•u•li•tis
ve•sic•u•lo•cav•ern•ous
ve•sic•u•log•ra•phy
pl ve•sic•u•log•ra•phies
ve•sic•u•lo•pap•u•lar
ve•sic•u•lo•pus•tu•lar
ve•sic•u•lot•o•my
pl ve•sic•u•lot•o•mies
ves•sel
ves•tib•u•lar
ves•ti•bule
ves•tib•u•lo•spi•nal
ves•tib•u•lot•o•my
pl ves•tib•u•lot•o•mies
ves•tib•u•lo-ure•thral
ves•tib•u•lum
pl ves•tib•u•la
ves•tige
ves•ti•gial
ves•ti•gial•ly
ves•tig•i•um
pl ves•tig•ia
ve•ta
vet•er•i•nar•i•an
vet•er•i•nary
pl vet•er•i•nar•ies
via
pl vias *or* vi•ae

vi•a•bil•i•ty
pl vi•a•bil•i•ties
vi•a•ble
vi•a•bly
vi•al
vi•bex
pl vi•bi•ces
vi•brate
vi•brat•ed
vi•brat•ing
vi•bra•tion
vi•bra•tor
vi•bra•to•ry
vib•rio
vib•ri•on
vib•ri•o•sis
pl vib•ri•o•ses
vi•bris•sa
pl vi•bris•sae
vi•bur•num
vi•car•i•ous
vi•ci•a•nose
vi•cious
Vid•i•an ar•tery
Vid•i•an nerve
vig•il
vig•il•am•bu•lism
vig•i•lance
vig•or
vil•lose
vil•lo•si•tis
vil•los•i•ty
pl vil•los•i•ties
vil•lous
vil•lous•ly
vil•lus
pl vil•li

vil•lus•ec•to•my
pl vil•lus•ec•to•mies
vin•blas•tine
Vin•ca
vin•ca•leu•ko•blas•tine
Vin•cent's an•gi•na
Vin•cent's in•fec•tion
also Vin•cent's sto•ma•ti•tis
vin•cris•tine
vin•cu•lum
pl vin•cu•lums *or* vin•cu•la
vin•e•gar
vi•nic
vi•nous
vi•nyl•ben•zene
vi•nyl ether
vi•o•la•ceous
vio•my•cin
vi•os•ter•ol
vi•per
Vi•per•i•dae
vi•ral
Vir•chow's node
vi•re•mia
also vi•rae•mia
vi•re•mic
vi•res
pl of vis
vir•gin
vir•gin•al
vir•gin•i•ty
pl vir•gin•i•ties

vir·gin·ium
vi·ri·cid·al
vi·ri·cide
vir·ile
vir·i·les·cence
vir·il·ism
vi·ril·i·ty
pl vi·ril·i·ties
vir·il·iza·tion
vir·il·ize
vir·il·ized
vir·il·iz·ing
vi·ri·on
vi·rip·o·tent
vi·ro·log·i·cal
or vi·ro·log·ic
vi·ro·log·i·cal·ly
vi·rol·o·gist
vi·rol·o·gy
pl vi·rol·o·gies
vi·ro·sis
pl vi·ro·ses
vir·tu·al
vi·ru·cid·al
vi·ru·cide
vir·u·lence
or vir·u·len·cy
pl vir·u·lenc·es
or vir·u·len·cies
vir·u·lent
vir·u·lent·ly
vir·u·lif·er·ous
vi·rus
vi·ru·stat·ic
vis
pl vi·res
vis a ter·go
pl vi·res a ter·go

vis·cera
pl of viscus
vis·cer·al
vis·cer·al·gia
vis·cero·gen·ic
vis·cero·in·hib·i·to·ry
vis·cero·meg·a·ly
pl vis·cero·meg·a·lies
vis·cero·mo·tor
vis·cero·pa·ri·etal
vis·cer·op·to·sis
pl vis·cer·op·to·ses
vis·cer·op·tot·ic
vis·cero·sen·so·ry
vis·cero·tome
vis·cer·o·to·nia
vis·cer·o·ton·ic
vis·cer·o·trop·ic
vis·cer·ot·ro·pism
vis·cid
vis·cid·i·ty
pl vis·cid·i·ties
vis·cid·ly
vis·com·e·ter
vis·com·e·try
pl vis·com·e·tries
vis·co·sim·e·ter
vis·co·sim·e·try
pl vis·co·sim·e·tries
vis·cos·i·ty
pl vis·cos·i·ties
vis·cous
vis·cus
pl vis·cera

vi·sion
vi·su·al
vi·su·al·iza·tion
vi·su·al·ize
vi·su·al·ized
vi·su·al·iz·ing
vi·su·al·iz·er
vi·suo·au·di·to·ry
vis·u·og·no·sis
pl vis·u·og·no·ses
vi·suo·psy·chic
vi·suo·sen·so·ry
vi·tal
vi·tal·ism
vi·tal·ist
vi·tal·is·tic
vi·tal·i·ty
pl vi·tal·i·ties
vi·tals
vi·tal signs
vi·ta·mer
vi·ta·min
vi·ta·min·iza·tion
vi·ta·min·ize
vi·ta·min·ized
vi·ta·min·iz·ing
vi·ta·min·ol·o·gy
pl vi·ta·min·ol·o·gies
vi·tel·lin
vi·tel·line
vi·tel·lo·gen·e·sis
pl vi·tel·lo·gen·e·ses
vi·tel·lo·lu·tein
vi·tel·lo·ru·bin
vi·tel·lus
vi·ti·a·tion

vit·i·lig·i·nous
vit·i·li·go
vit·reo·den·tine
vit·re·ous
vit·re·um
vi·tri·na
vit·ri·ol
vit·ri·ol·ic
vi·var·i·um
pl vi·var·ia
or vi·var·i·ums
vi·vax ma·lar·ia
viv·i·dif·fu·sion
viv·i·fi·ca·tion
vi·vi·par·i·ty
pl vi·vi·par·i·ties
vi·vip·a·rous
vivi·sect
vivi·sec·tion
vivi·sec·tion·al
vivi·sec·tion·ist
vivi·sec·tor
Vlem·inckx' so·lu·tion
also Vlem·inckx' lo·tion
vo·cal
vo·ces
pl of vox
Vo·ges-Pros·kauer re·ac·tion
or Vo·ges-Pros·kauer test
vola
vo·lar
vol·a·tile
vol·a·til·iza·tion
vol·a·til·ize
vol·a·til·ized
vol·a·til·iz·ing
vo·le·mic
vo·li·tion
vo·li·tion·al
Volk·mann's ca·nal
vol·ley
pl vol·leys
also vol·lies
vol·sel·lum
pl vol·sel·la
volt·age
vol·ta·ic
vol·ta·ism
vol·ta·me·ter
volt-am·me·ter
volt-am·pere
volt·me·ter
vol·u·me·nom·e·ter
vol·un·tary
vo·lute
vo·lu·tin
vol·vox
vol·vu·lus
vo·mer
vo·mer·ine
vom·ero·bas·i·lar
vom·ero·na·sal
vom·i·ca
pl vom·i·cae
vom·it
vom·i·tive
vom·i·tu·ri·tion
vom·i·tus
vor·tex
pl vor·ti·ces
also vor·tex·es
vor·ti·cel·la
pl vor·ti·cel·lae
or vor·ti·cel·las
vor·ti·cose
vox
pl vo·ces
voy·eur
voy·eur·ism
voy·eur·is·tic
vul·ca·ni·za·tion
vul·ca·nize
vul·ca·nized
vul·ca·niz·ing
vul·ga·ris
vul·ner·a·bil·i·ty
pl vul·ner·a·bil·i·ties
vul·ner·a·ble
vul·ner·ary
pl vul·ner·ar·ies
vul·sel·la
vul·sel·lum
pl vul·sel·la
vul·va
pl vul·vae
vul·val
vul·var
vul·vec·to·my
pl vul·vec·to·mies
vul·vi·tis
vul·vo·cru·ral
vul·vo·vag·i·nal
vul·vo·vag·i·ni·tis

W

wad·ding
wad·dle
  wad·dled
  wad·dling
wa·fer
waist·line
wake·ful·ness
Wal·dey·er's ton·sil·lar ring
Wal·dey·er's zon·al lay·er
Wal·le·ri·an de·gen·er·a·tion
wall·eye
wall·eyed
wap·per-jawed
war·ble
War·burg ap·pa·ra·tus
war·fa·rin
warm-blood·ed
warm-blood·ed·ness
warty
  war·ti·er
  war·ti·est
Was·ser·mann re·ac·tion
wast·er
wa·ter·borne
Wa·ter·house-Frid·er·ich·sen syn·drome
wa·ter·shed
wa·ter tooth·pick
  also wa·ter pick

Wat·son-Crick mod·el
Wat·so·ni·us
watt·age
wat·tle
watt·me·ter
wave·length
wean·ling
wea·sand
We·ber-Fech·ner law
We·ber's cor·pus·cle
  or We·ber's pouch

We·ber's law
Wechs·ler-Belle·vue test
Wei·gert's meth·od
weight·less·ness
Weil-Fe·lix re·ac·tion
  or Weil-Felix test

Weil's dis·ease
Weis·man·ni·an
Welch ba·cil·lus
well·born
well-bred
Werl·hof's dis·ease
Wer·nicke's cen·ter
Wert·heim's op·er·a·tion
Wes·ter·gren meth·od
weth·er
Whar·ton's duct
Whar·ton's jel·ly
wheel·chair
wheeze
  wheezed
  wheez·ing
whelk
whelp
whip·lash
whip·worm
whirl·pool
whis·per
  whis·pered
  whis·per·ing
white·comb
white·head
Whit·field's oint·ment
whit·low
whoop·ing cough
Wi·dal's re·ac·tion
  or Wi·dal re·ac·tion

wig·gler
Wil·der·muth's au·ri·cle
  or Wil·der·muth's ear

Wil·lis's ar·tery
Wil·lis's cir·cle
Wil·lis's cords
  or Wil·lis's tra·bec·u·lae

Wilms's tu•mor
Wil•son's dis•ease
wind•age
wind-bro•ken
wind•burn
wind•chill
wind•gall
wind•pipe
wind puff
or wind-puff
wind suck•ing
Wins•low's fo•ra•men
win•ter•green
wish ful•fill•ment
wish•ful think•ing
with•draw•al
with•ers
wit•zel•sucht
wob•bles
wohl•fahr•tia
Wolff•ian body
Wolff•ian duct
wol•fram
wolfs•bane
Wol•las•ton dou•blet
womb
Wool•ner's tu•ber•cle
or Wool•ner's point
or Wool•ner's tip
wool•sort•er's dis•ease
word-as•so•ci•a•tion test
word sal•ad
work-up
also work•up
Wor•mi•an bone
worm•seed
Woulff bot•tle
Wright's stain
wrin•kle
Wris•berg's car•ti•lage
Wris•berg's gan•gli•on
Wris•berg's nerve
wrist•drop
writ•er's cramp
wry•neck
Wuch•er•e•ria
wuch•er•e•ri•a•sis

X

xan•thate
xan•the•las•ma
xan•thene
xan•thic
xan•thin
a plant pigment
xan•thine
a nitrogenous base esp. of animal tissues
xan•tho•chro•mat•ic
xan•tho•chro•mia
xan•tho•chro•mic
xan•tho•cy•a•nop•sia
xan•tho•gran•u•lo•ma
pl xan•tho•gran•u•lo•mas
or xan•tho•gran•u•lo•ma•ta
xan•tho•ma
pl xan•tho•mas
or xan•tho•ma•ta
xan•tho•ma•to•sis
pl xan•tho•ma•to•ses
xan•thoma•tous
xan•thone
xan•tho•phyll
xan•tho•pro•te•ic
xan•tho•pro•tein
xan•thop•sia
xan•thop•sin
xan•thop•ter•in
xan•tho•sine
xan•tho•sis
pl xan•tho•ses
xan•thous
xanth•uren•ic
X-dis•ease
xe•nic
xe•ni•cal•ly
xe•no•bi•ol•o•gy
pl xe•no•bi•ol•o•gies
xe•no•di•ag•no•sis
pl xe•no•di•ag•no•ses
xe•no•di•ag•nos•tic
xe•no•ge•ne•ic
xe•no•graft
xen•o•me•nia
xe•non
xe•no•pho•bia

xen·oph·thal·mia
Xeno·psyl·la
Xen·o·pus
xe·ran·tic
xe·ro·der·ma
xe·ro·me·nia
xe·ro·myc·te·ria
xe·roph·a·gy
also xe·ro·pha·gia
pl xe·roph·a·gies
also xe·ro·pha·gias

xe·roph·thal·mia
xe·roph·thal·mic
xe·ro·ra·di·og·ra·phy
pl xe·ro·ra·di·og·ra·phies

xe·ro·sis
pl xe·ro·ses

xe·ro·sto·mia
xe·ro·tes
xe·rot·ic
xi·phi·ster·nal
xi·phi·ster·num
pl xi·phi·ster·na

xipho·cos·tal
xiph·o·dyn·ia
xi·phoid
also xi·phoi·dal

xiph·oid·itis
xi·phop·a·gus
X-ir·ra·di·ate
X-ir·ra·di·a·tion
X-ra·di·a·tion
x-ray
verb

X ray
noun

xy·lene
xy·lo·ke·tose
xy·lol
xy·lose
xy·lu·lose
xys·ma
xys·ter

Y

yaw·ey
yaws
yer·ba ma·té
yilt
var of gilt

yo·gurt
or yo·ghurt

yo·him·bine
yoke
yoked
yok·ing
yolk
yolk sac
yolk stalk
yper·ite
yt·ter·bi·um
yt·tri·um

Z

Zan·thox·y·lum
ze·atin
zea·xan·thin
Zee·man ef·fect
ze·in
Zen·ker's fluid
ze·o·lite
ze·ro
pl ze·ros
also ze·roes

Zim·mer·mann re·ac·tion
or Zim·mer·mann test

zinc
zinced
or zincked

zinc·ing
or zinck·ing

zinc·if·er·ous
zinc·oid
Zinn's lig·a·ment
zir·co·ni·um
zo·ac·an·tho·sis
pl zo·ac·an·tho·ses

zo·an·thro·py
pl zo·an·thro·pies

zo·et·ic
zoe·trope
also zoo·trope

zo·ic
Zöll·ner's lines
zo·na
pl zo·nae
or zo·nas

zon·al
zon·al·ly
zo·na pel·lu·ci·da
pl zo·nae pel·lu·ci·dae

zo·na ra·di·a·ta
pl zo·nae ra·di·a·tae

zo·na·ry
zon·ate
also zon·at·ed

zon·es·the·sia
zo·nif·u·gal
zo·nip·e·tal
zonu·la
pl zonu·lae
or zonu·las
zo·nu·lar
zon·ule
zon·ule of Zinn
zo·nu·li·tis
zo·nu·ly·sis
pl zo·nu·ly·ses
zoo·der·mic
zoo·eras·tia
zoo·gen·ic
zo·og·e·nous
also zo·o·ge·ne·ous
zoo·geo·graph·ic
also zoo·geo·graph·i·cal
zoo·geo·graph·i·cal·ly
zoo·ge·og·ra·phy
pl zoo·ge·og·ra·phies
zo·og·o·ny
pl zo·og·o·nies
zoo·graft
zo·og·ra·phy
pl zo·og·ra·phies
zo·oid
zoo·lag·nia
Zo·o·mas·ti·gi·na
zo·on·o·my
pl zo·on·o·mies
zoo·no·sis
pl zoo·no·ses
zoo·not·ic
zoo·par·a·site
zoo·par·a·sit·ic
zoo·path·ol·o·gy
pl zoo·path·ol·o·gies
zo·oph·a·gous
zoo·phile
zoo·phil·ia
also zo·oph·i·lism
zoo·phil·ic
zo·oph·i·list
zo·oph·i·lous
zoo·pho·bia
zoo·plas·ty
pl zoo·plas·ties
zo·op·sia
zoo·spore
zo·os·ter·ol
zoo·tech·nics
zoo·ther·a·py
pl zoo·ther·a·pies
zoo·troph·ic
zos·ter
zos·ter·i·form
zos·ter·oid
Z-plas·ty
zyg·apoph·y·sis
pl zyg·apoph·y·ses
zyg·i·on
pl zyg·ia
also zyg·i·ons
zy·goc·i·ty
pl zy·goc·i·ties
zy·go·dac·ty·ly
pl zyo·go·dac·ty·lies
zy·go·ma
pl zy·go·ma·ta
also zy·go·mas
zy·go·mat·ic
zy·go·mat·i·co·au·ric·u·la·ris
pl zy·go·mat·i·co·au·ric·u·la·res
zy·go·mat·i·co·fa·cial
zy·go·mat·i·co·max·il·lary
zy·go·mat·i·co-or·bit·al
zy·go·mat·i·co·tem·po·ral
zy·go·mat·i·cus
zy·go·max·il·la·ry
Zy·go·my·ce·tes
zy·go·my·ce·tous
zy·go·sis
pl zy·go·ses
zy·gos·i·ty
pl zy·gos·i·ties
zy·go·sperm
zy·go·spore
zy·go·style
zy·gote
zy·go·tene
zy·got·ic
zy·got·i·cal·ly
zy·mase
zy·mo·gen
zy·mo·gen·ic
zy·mog·e·nous
zy·mo·hy·drol·y·sis
pl zy·mo·hy·drol·y·ses
zy·moid

zy•mol•o•gy
pl zy•mol•o•gies

zy•mol•y•sis
pl zy•mol•y•ses

Zy•mo•ne•ma

zy•mo•plas•tic

zy•mo•pro•tein

zy•mo•san

zy•mo•scope

zy•mo•sis
pl zy•mo•ses

zy•mos•then•ic

zy•mot•ic

zy•mot•i•cal•ly

ABBREVIATIONS

Most of the abbreviations included in this list have been normalized to one form. Chemical symbols (as **Na**) are included when they can be placed in alphabetical sequence readily without causing confusion. There is considerable variation in the use of periods, in typeface, and in capitalization (as in cgs, c.g.s., C.G.S., *C.G.S.*).

a about, absent, absolute, absorbency, absorbent, accommodation, acetum, acid, acidity, actin, active, activity, allergist, allergy, alpha, ampere, angstrom unit, anode, answer, ante, anterior, aqua, area, argon, artery, asymmetric, asymmetry, atria
Å angstrom unit
AA achievement age, Alcoholics Anonymous
AAF ascorbic acid factor
AAL anterior axillary line
A&P anterior and posterior, auscultation and percussion
A&W alive and well
ab abort, abortion, about
AB aid to blind, Bachelor of Arts
ABC atomic, biological, and chemical
abd abdomen, abdominal
abdom abdomen, abdominal
abs absent, absolute
ABS acute brain syndrome
abt about
ac acute, alternating current
Ac actinium
acc acceleration, according
ACh acetylcholine
AChE acetylcholinesterase
ACS antireticular cytotoxic serum
act active
ACTH adrenocorticotrophic hormone
AD average deviation
ADC aid to dependent children
add adduction, adductor
ADH antidiuretic hormone
adj adjunct
ADL activities of daily living
adm administration, administrator, admission, admit
ADP adenosine diphosphate
ae *or* **aet** *or* **aetat** [L *aetatis*] of age, aged
AF audio frequency, auricular fibrillation
AFB acid-fast bacillus
Ag [L *argentum*] silver
agglut agglutination
agt agent
AHF antihemolytic factor, antihemophilic factor
AHG antihemophilic globulin, antihuman globulin
AI artificial insemination
AID artificial insemination by donor
AIH artificial insemination by husband
AJ ankle jerk
AK above knee
Al aluminum
alb albumin
alc alcohol
ALG antilymphocyte globulin, antilymphocytic globulin
alk alkaline
ALS amyotrophic lateral sclerosis, antilymphocyte serum, antilymphocytic serum
alt alternate, altitude
alv alveolar
Am americium
am ammeter, amperemeter, amplitude modulation
AM [L *ante meridiem*] before noon, [ML *Artium Magister*] Master of Arts
AMA against medical advice, American Medical Association
amb ambulance, ambulatory
AMI acute myocardial infarction
amp amperage, ampere, ampule, amputation
amt amount

ANA American Nurses Association
anal analysis, analytic, analyze
anat anatomic, anatomical, anatomy
anh anhydrous
anhyd anhydrous
ans answer
ANS autonomic nervous system
ap apothecaries
AP action potential, alkaline phosphatase, anterior pituitary, anteroposterior, aortic pressure
APC aspirin, phenacetin, and caffeine
app appendix
appl applied
approx approximate, approximately
appt appointment
AQ accomplishment quotient, achievement quotient
Ar argon
ARD acute respiratory disease
as astigmatism
As arsenic
AS aortic stenosis, arteriosclerosis
ASA [*a*cetyl*s*alicylic *a*cid] aspirin
ASAP as soon as possible
ASCVD arteriosclerotic cardiovascular disease
ASHD arteriosclerotic heart disease
assn association
asst assistant
as tol as tolerated
at airtight
At astatine
AT achievement test
atm atmosphere, atmospheric
ATP adenosine triphosphate
at wt atomic weight
Au [L *aurum*] gold
au angstrom unit, antitoxin unit
aux auxiliary
av average, avoirdupois
AV arteriovenous, atrioventricular
avdp avoirdupois
ax axis
Az [F *azote*] nitrogen
b bacillus, balnium, barometric, bath, Baumé scale, behavior, Benoist scale, born, brother
B boron
Ba barium
BA bronchial asthma, buccoaxial
bact bacteria, bacterial, bacteriological, bacteriology, bacterium
BaE *or* **BAE** barium enema
bal balance
BAL [*B*ritish *A*nti-*L*ewisite] dimercaprol
B&O belladonna and opium
bar barometer, barometric
baso basophil
BBB bundle branch block
BBT basal body temperature
BCG [*B*acillus *C*almette-*G*uérin] tuberculosis vaccine, ballistocardiogram, bromcresyl green
BE barium enema, below elbow
Be beryllium
Bé Baumé
BFP biological false-positive
BH bill of health
BHC benzene hexachloride
BHL biological half-life
Bi bismuth
bili bilirubin
biol biologic, biological, biologist, biology
BJ biceps jerk
Bk berkelium
BK below knee
bld blood
BM Bachelor of Medicine, basal metabolism, bowel movement
BMR basal metabolic rate
BO body odor
BOD biochemical oxygen demand, biological oxygen demand
bot botanical, botany, bottle
BP blood pressure, boiling point, British Pharmacopoeia
Br bromine
BRP bathroom privileges
BS bowel sounds, breath sounds
BST blood serological test
BT bedtime, brain tumor
BTU British thermal unit

BUN blood urea nitrogen
BW blood Wassermann, body weight
Bx biopsy

c calorie, cathode, centimeter, cervical, clonus, closure, cobalt, cocaine, coefficient, contact, contraction, coulomb, cylinder
C carbon, Celsius, centigrade, complement
Ca calcium
CA cancer, carcinoma, cardiac arrest, chronological age
CAC cardiac accelerator center
CAD coronary artery disease
CAI confused artificial insemination
cal small calorie
Cal large calorie
canc canceled
cap capacity, capsule
CAT children's apperception test
cath cathartic, catheter
cav cavity
Cb columbium
CB [L *Chirurgiae Baccalaureus*] Bachelor of Surgery
CBC complete blood count
CBD closed bladder drainage, common bile duct
CBF cerebral blood flow
CBR chemical, bacteriological, and radiological
CBS chronic brain syndrome
CBW chemical and biological warfare
cc cubic centimeter
CC chief complaint, commission certified, critical condition, current complaint
CCA chick cell agglutination, chimpanzee corzya agent
CCI chronic coronary insufficiency
CCK cholecystokinin
CCT chocolate coated tablet
CCTe cathodal closure tetanus
CCU coronary care unit
Cd cadmium
CD communicable disease, constant drainage, contagious disease, convulsive disorder, curative dose
CDC calculated date of confinement
Ce cerium
CE cardiac enlargement
Cel celsius
cen central
Ceph floc cephalin flocculation
CER conditioned emotional response
cert certificate, certified
cerv cervical
CES central excitatory state
cf [L *confer*] compare
Cf californium
CF chest and left leg, complement fixation, cystic fibrosis
CFT complement fixation test
CG center of gravity, chorionic gonadotropin
cgs centimeter gram-second
ch child, chronic
ChB [L *Chirurgiae Baccalaureus*] Bachelor of Surgery
CHD childhood disease
ChE cholinesterase
chem chemical, chemist, chemistry
CHF congestive heart failure
chg change
chl chloroform
CHO carbohydrate
chol cholesterol
chr chronic
CI chemotherapeutic index
CICU coronary intensive care unit
cir *or* **circ** circular
circ circulation
cl centiliter, clavicle, clinic, closure
Cl chloride, chlorine
CL chest and left arm, corpus luteum, critical list
clin clinical
CLL chronic lymphocytic leukemia
CLO cod liver oil
cm centimeter
Cm curium
CM [L *Chirurgiae Magister*] Master of Surgery, circular muscle

CMV cytomegalovirus
CNS central nervous system
Co cobalt, coenzyme
CO carbon monoxide, cardiac output
c/o complains of
coag coagulate, coagulation
coag time coagulation time
COC cathodal opening contraction
COCl cathodal opening clonus
COD chemical oxygen demand
coeff *or* **coef** coefficient
COH carbohydrate
col colony, color
coll collect, collection, colloidal, collyrium
comp comparative, compare, composition, compound
compl completed, complications
conc concentrated, concentration
cond condition
cond ref conditioned reflex
cond resp conditioned response
conf conference
cong congenital
const constant
cont containing, contents, continue, continued
conv convalescent
coord coordination
COPE chronic obstructive pulmonary emphysema
cor corrected
CoR congo red
cort cortex, cortical
CP capillary pressure, cerebral palsy, chemically pure, compare, constant pressure, cor pulmonale
CPC chronic passive congestion
cpd compound
CPE cytopathogenic effects
CPI constitutional psychopathic inferiority
CPK creatine phosphokinase
CPM counts per minute
CPZ chlorpromazine
Cr chromium, creatinine
CR cardiorespiratory, chest and right arm, clot retraction, conditioned reflex, conditioned response
CRD chronic respiratory disease
crit critical
CRO cathode ray oscilloscope
CrP creatine phosphate
CRP C-reactive protein
CRT cathode-ray tube, complex reaction time
cryst crystalline, crystallized
cs cesarean section, case, conditioned stimulus, consciousness, corticosteroid, current strength
Cs cesium
CSF cerebrospinal fluid
CSM cerebrospinal meningitis
CT circulation time, coated tablet, compressed tablet, corrective therapist
CTa catamenia (menstruation)
CTC chlortetracycline
ctr center
CTU centrigrade thermal unit
cu cubic
Cu copper
CU clinical unit
CUC chronic ulcerative colitis
cult culture
cur curative, current
CV cardiovascular
CVA cerebrovascular accident
CVP central venous pressure
CVR cardiovascular renal, cardiovascular respiratory, cerebrovascular resistance
CVS clean voided specimen
CW crutch walking
Cy cyanogen
cyl cylinder, cylindrical
cytol cytological, cytology

d date, daughter, day, dead, deceased, deciduous, degree, density, developed, deviation, dexter, diameter, died, diopter, disease, divorced, dorsal, dose, duration
D deuterium
da daughter, day
DA delayed action
DAH disordered action of the heart
D&C dilatation and curettage
DAT delayed action tablet, differential aptitude test

dau daughter
dbl double
DBP diastolic blood pressure
DBT dry bulb temperature
DC Dental Corps, diagnostic center, direct current, distocervical, doctor of chiropractic
DCc double concave
DCR direct critical response
DDS doctor of dental science, doctor of dental surgery
DDT dichlorodiphenyltrichloroethane
dec deceased, decompose
decd deceased, dead
def defecation, deficient, definite
deg degeneration, degree
del delusion
dent dental, dentist, dentistry
depr depression
derm dermatology
detn detention
devel development
dg decigram
DHEW Department of Health, Education and Welfare
DHO deuterium hydrogen oxide
DI deterioration index, diabetes insipidus
dia diameter, diathermy
diab diabetic
diag diagnosis, diagnostic, diagonal, diagram
diam diameter
diath diathermy
diff difference, differential blood count
dil dilute
dilat dilatation
dim diminished
DIP distal interphalangeal
diph diphtheria
dis disabled, disease
disc discontinue, discontinued
disch discharge, discharged
disp dispensary
dissd dissolved
div divide, division, divorced
DJD degenerative joint disease
dkg dekagram
dkl dekaliter
dkm dekameter
dl deciliter
DL danger list
DLE disseminated lupus erythematosus
dm decimeter
DM diabetes mellitus, diastolic murmur
DMD [L *dentariae medicinae doctor*] doctor of dental medicine
DMF decayed, missing, and filled teeth
DMSO dimethylsulfoxide
DMT dimethyltryptamine
DNA deoxyribonucleic acid
DNB dinitrobenzene
DO diamine oxidase, doctor of optometry, doctor of osteopathy
DOA dead on arrival
DOB date of birth
doc document
DOE dyspnea on exertion
dom domestic, dominant
DOPA dihydroxyphenylalanine
dos dosage
doz dozen
DP deep pulse, diphosgene, doctor of pharmacy, doctor of podiatry
DPA diphenylamine
DPH department of public health, doctor of public health
DPN diphosphopyridine nucleotide
DPT diphtheria-pertussis-tetanus (vaccines)
DQ deterioration quotient
dr dram, dressing
Dr doctor
DR delivery room
DS dead air space, dilute strength, dioptric strength
DSC doctor of surgical chiropody
DSD dry sterile dressing
DT delirium tremens, distance test, duration of tetany
DTMA desoxycorticosterone trimethylacetate
DTN diphtheria toxin normal
DTP diphtheria, tetanus, and pertussis
DU diagnosis undetermined
dup duplicate
DV dilute volume

DVM doctor of veterinary medicine
DW distilled water
dwt pennyweight
Dx diagnosis
Dy dysprosium

E emmetropia, enema, enzyme, experimenter, eye
ea each
EA educational age
ECF extracellular fluid
ECG electrocardiogram
ECT electroconvulsive therapy
ED effective dose, erythema dose
EDC expected date of confinement
EDN electrodessication
EDR electrodermal response
EDTA ethylenediaminetetraacetic acid
EEG electroencephalogram, electroencephalograph
EENT eye, ear, nose and throat
e.g. [L *exempli gratia*] for example
Eh standard oxidation-reduction potential
EHBF extrahepatic blood flow
EHL effective half-life
EJ elbow jerk
EKG electrocardiogram, electrocardiograph
elec electric, electrical, electricity
elix elixir
EM electron microscope
emb embryo, embryology
EMF electromotive force
EMG electromyogram, electromyography
EMIC emergency maternity and infant care
emul emulsion
enl enlarged
ENT ear, nose and throat
EOA examination, opinion and advice
EOG electrooculogram, electrooculograph
EOM extraocular movement, extraocular muscle
eos *or* **eosin** eosinophil
epil epilepsy, epileptic
epith epithelial, epithelium
eq equal, equivalent
Er erbium
ER emergency room, endoplasmic reticulum, equivalent roentgen, extended release
ERG electroretinogram
ERPF effective renal plasma flow
Es Einsteinium
ESF erythropoietic stimulating factor
esp especial, especially
ESP extrasensory perception
ESR electron spin resonance, erythrocyte sedimentation rate
EST electroshock therapy
ET educational therapy
et al [L *et alibi*] and elsewhere, [L *et alii*] and others
etc [L *et cetera*] and so forth
et seq [L *et sequens*] and the following one, [L *et sequentes* or *et sequentia*] and the following ones
Eu europium
ex examined, example, exercise
exam examination
exc except, exception
exp experiment, experimental, expired
expt experiment
exptl experimental
ext external, extract, extremity

f failure, family, farad, father, female, feminine, fibrous, focal length, foot, formula, function, [L *filius*] son, [L *frater*] brother
F fluorine
F Fahrenheit
FA fatty acid, filterable agent, first aid, folic acid
FACP fellow American College of Physicians
FACS fellow American College of Surgeons
FAD flavin adenine dinucleotide
Fah *or* **Fahr** Fahrenheit
fam family
FAMA fellow American Medical Association

FD fan douche, fatal dose, focal distance
FDA Food and Drug Administration
Fe iron
fem female, feminine, femur
ff following
FF fat free, filtration fraction, force fluid
FHS fetal heart sounds
FHT fetal heart tone
fib fibrillation
fig figure
fl fluid
FL focal length
fl oz fluid ounce
Fm fermium
FMD foot and mouth disease
FMN *or* **FM** flavin mononucleotide
fp freezing point
fpm feet per minute
fps feet per second
fr from
FR flocculation reaction
Fr francium
FRCP fellow Royal College of Physicians
FRCS fellow Royal College of Surgeons
freq frequency
fsd focus-to-skin distance (X ray)
FSH follicle-stimulating hormone
ft feet, foot
FUO fever of undetermined origin
Fx fracture

g gauge, gender, gingival, glucose, grain, gram
Ga gallium
GA gastric analysis
GABA gamma aminobutyric acid
gal galactose, gallon
galv galvanic, galvanism, galvanized
gang *or* **gangl** ganglion, ganglionic
G-A-S general adaptation syndrome
GB gallbladder, [code name] sarin
GBS gallbladder series
GC gonococcus
Gd gadolinium
Ge germanium
GE gastroenterology
gen general, genus
GFR glomerular filtration rate
GH growth hormone
GHRF growth hormone releasing factor
GI gastrointestinal, globin insulin, growth-inhibiting
GL greatest length
GLC gas-liquid chromatography
gm gram
GM and S General Medicine and Surgery
GOE gas, oxygen and ether (anesthesia)
GOR general operating room
gp group
GP general paralysis, general paresis, general practitioner
GpTh group therapy
gr gamma roentgen, grain, gravity
grad gradient, graduated
GRAS generally recognized as safe
grav gravid, gravity
GSH glutathione (reduced form)
GSSG glutathione (oxidized form)
GSW gunshot wound
GTH gonadotrophic hormone
GU genitourinary
guid guidance
GV gentian violet
gyn gynecologic, gynecological, gynecologist, gynecology

h height, hour, horizontal
H flagella, heroin, hydrogen, hypodermic
HA headache
HAD hospital administration
Hb hemoglobin
HB heart block
HBP high blood pressure
HC home care, hydrocortisone
HCG human chorionic gonadotropin
hct hematocrit

HCVD hypersensitive cardiovascular disease
HD Hansen's disease, hearing distance
HDLW distance at which a watch is heard with left ear
HDRW distance at which a watch is heard with right ear
He helium
HE virus human enteric virus
HEENT head, eyes, ears, nose, throat
hemi hemiplegia
HEW Department of Health, Education and Welfare
hf half
Hf hafnium
hg hectogram, hemoglobin
Hg [NL *hydrargyrum*] mercury
HGH human growth hormone
HH hard of hearing
HHb reduced hemoglobin
HI hemagglutination inhibition
HIC heart information center
HID headache, insomnia, depression
HIF Health Information Foundation
hl hectoliter
HL half-life
hm hectometer
HM hand movements
HMC heroin, morphine, and cocaine
HMD hyaline membrane disease
HMG human menopausal gonadotrophin
HMO heart minute output
HN head nurse
Ho holmium
HOP high oxygen pressure
hor horizontal
hosp hospital
HP high potency, high pressure, hot pack, hot pad, hydrostatic pressure
HPF high power field
HPG human pituitary gonadotrophin
HPI history of present illness
HPN hypertension
hr hour
HR heart rate
HS heart sounds, house surgeon
HSA human serum albumin
ht height
HT hydrotherapy, hypodermic tablet
HV hyperventilation
HVD hypertensive vascular disease
HVL half-value layer
Hx history, hypoxanthine
Hy hypermetropia
hyd hydraulics, hydrostatics
hyg hygiene
hyp hyperresonance, hypertrophy
hys hysteria

i incisor (deciduous), insoluble, optically inactive
I incisor (permanent), iodine, internal medicine
IA impedance angle, intraarterial
IAA indoleacetic acid
IAFI infantile amaurotic familial idiocy
I and D incision and drainage
I and O intake and output
ib *or* **ibid** [L *ibidem*] in the same place
IC inspiratory capacity, inspiratory center, intensive care, intercostal, interstitial cell, intracerebral, intracutaneous
ICF intracellular fluid
ICN International Council of Nurses
ICPMM incisors, canines, premolars, molars
ICT inflammation of connective tissue, insulin coma therapy
ICU intensive care unit
id [L *idem*] same
ID identification, inside diameter, intradermal
i.e. [L *id est*] that is
IE [G *immunitäts Einheit*] immunizing unit
IF interstitial fluid
Ig immunoglobulin
IH infectious hepatitis
IHSA iodinated human serum albumin

IHSS idiopathic hypertrophic subaortic stenosis
Il illinium
IM intramuscular, intramuscularly
immunol immunology
imp important, impression
in inch
In indium
inc incomplete, inconclusive, increase
incl including, inclusive
incr increase, increased, increment
incur incurable
ind independent
IND investigational new drug
indic indication, indicative
inf infant, infantile, infected, infection, inferior, infusion
Inf infirmary
infl influence
ing inguinal
INH isoniazid
INI intranuclear inclusion
inj injection, injury
INPRONS information processing in the central nervous system
ins insurance
insol insoluble
insp inspiration
inst institute
instr instructor
int intermittent, intern, internal
inv inversion
invol involuntary
IO intraocular
IOP intraocular pressure
IP International Pharmacopoeia interphalangeal, intraperitoneal
IPH interphalangeal
IPPB intermittent positive pressure breathing
IPPF International Planned Parenthood Federation
IPPR intermittent positive pressure respiration
IPSP inhibitory postsynaptic potential
IQ intelligence quotient
Ir iridium
IR infrared, internal resistance
IRI immunoreactive insulin
is island
ISC interstitial cell
ISF interstitial fluid
isom isometric
ISP distance between iliac spines
IST insulin shock therapy
ITP idiopathic thrombocytopenic purpura
ITT insulin tolerance test
IU immunizing unit, international unit
IUCD intrauterine contraceptive device
IUD intrauterine device
IV intravenous, intravenously, intraventricular
IVC inferior vena cava
IVCD intraventricular conduction defect
IVD intervertebral disc
IVP intravenous pyelogram
IVT intravenous transfusion
IZS insulin zinc suspension

J joint
JAI juvenile amaurotic idiocy
JAMA Journal of the American Medical Association
jct junction
JJ jaw jerk
JND just noticeable difference
jour journal
jt *or* **jnt** joint
juv juvenile

K absolute zero, constant, kelvin, [NL *kalium*] potassium
ka [G *kathode*] cathode
kc kilocycle
KC cathodal closing
kcal kilocalorie
KCC cathodal closing contraction
KCT cathodal closing tetanus
KD cathodal duration
KDT cathodal duration tetanus
kg kilogram
KI Krönig's isthmus
KJ knee jerk
KK knee kick
kl kiloliter
km kilometer

KOC cathodal opening contraction
Kr krypton
KS ketosteroid
KUB kidney, ureter and bladder

L left, lethal, lewisite, licensed, light, liter, lower, lumen
La lanthanum
LA left angle, left atrium, left auricle
lab laboratory
lab proc laboratory procedure
lac laceration
LAD lactic acid dehydrogenase
L and A light and accommodation (pupil reaction)
L and B left and below
L and W living and well
lap laparotomy
LAP leukocyte alkaline phosphatase
laryngol laryngologist, laryngology
lat lateral, latitude
LATS long-acting thyroid stimulator
lb pound
LB low back
LBD left border dullness
LBH length, breadth, height
LBP low back pain, low blood pressure
LCCS low cervical cesarean section
LCM left costal margin, lymphocytic choriomeningitis
LD lethal dose
LDH lactate dehydrogenase, lactic dehydrogenase
LE left eye, lower extremity, lupus erythematosus
LES local excitatory state
Leu leucine
LF limit of flocculation, low frequency
LGV lymphogranuloma venereum
LH left hand, luteinizing hormone
LHS left heart strain
Li lithium
LIF left iliac fossa
lig ligament
lin linear
liq liquid, liquor
LKS liver, kidney, spleen
LLBCD left lower border of cardiac dullness
LLE lower left extremity
LLL left lower lobe (lung)
LLQ left lower quadrant (abdomen)
lm lumen
LM longitudinal muscle
LMD local medical doctor
LMP last menstrual period
LNMP last normal menstrual period
LOA leave of absence
loc cit [L *loco citato*] in the place cited
log logarithm
LOM limitation of motion
LOP leave on pass
LP latent period, low pressure, lumbar puncture
LPF leukocytosis-promoting factor
LPN licensed practical nurse
LQ lower quadrant
Lr lawrencium
LR latency relaxation
LRF liver residue factor
LSB left sternal border
LSD lysergic acid diethylamide
LSK liver, spleen, kidneys
lt left, light
LTB laryngeal tracheal bronchitis
ltd limited
LTH luteotropic hormone
Lu lutetium
LUE left upper extremity
LUL left upper lobe (lung)
LUQ left upper quadrant (abdomen)
lv leave
LV left ventricle
LVH left ventricular hypertrophy
LVN licensed vocational nurse
lym *or* **lymph** lymphocyte

m macerate, male, malignant, married, masculine, mass, mature, mean, melts at, memory, [L *mentum*] chin, [L *meridies*] noon, metabolite,

meter, micrococcus, minute, molar, molecular weight, morphine, mother, murmur, muscle, [L *mutitas*] dullness, myopia
ma milliampere
MA menstrual age, mental age, mentum anterior
MABP mean arterial blood pressure
mac macerate
MAC maximum allowable concentration
MAF minimum audible field
mag magnification, [L *magnus*] large
MAO monoamine oxidase
MAOI monoamine oxidase inhibitor
MAP minimum audible pressure
masc masculine
MAT manual arts therapist
max maximum
MBP mean blood pressure
MCAT medical college admissions test
MCB membranous cytoplasmic bodies
MCD mean corpuscular diameter
mcg microgram
MCH mean corpuscular hemoglobin
MCHC mean corpuscular hemoglobin concentration
MCL midclavicular line
MCV mean corpuscular volume
md median
Md mendelevium
MD medical department, [NL *medicinae doctor*] doctor of medicine, mentally deficient, mitral disease, muscular dystrophy
MDH malic dehydrogenase
MDR minimum daily requirement
MDS master of dental surgery
Me methyl
ME medical examiner, middle ear
meas measure, measurement
MeB methylene blue
med medial, median, medical, medicinal, medicine, medium
MED minimal effective dose
MEF maximal expiratory flow
meg megacycle
mem member
memb membrane
MEP mean effective pressure, motor end plate
mEq milliequivalent
Met methionine
MFD minimum fatal dose
MFG modified heat degraded gelatin
MFT muscle function test
mg milligram
Mg magnesium
MH marital history, menstrual history, mental health
MHA Mental Health Association
MHB maximum hospital benefit
MHD minimum hemolytic dose
MI mitral insufficiency, myocardial infarction
mid middle
MID minimum infective dose
min minim, minimal, minimum, minute
MIO minimal identifiable odor
misc miscellaneous
mit insuf mitral insufficiency
mixt mixture
mks meter-kilogram-second
ml midline, milliliter
MLD minimum lethal dose
mm millimeter
mM millimole
MM mucous membrane
MMPI Minnesota Multiphasic Personality Inventory
MMT manual muscle test
Mn manganese
mo month
Mo molybdenum
MO mineral oil
mod moderate
mol molecular, molecule
MOM milk of magnesia
mon *or* **mono** monocyte, mononucleosis
morph morphological, morphology
mOsm milliosmol
mp melting point
MP mentum posterior, mesiopulpal,

metacarpophalangeal
MPC maximum permissible concentration
MPH master of public health
MPI multiphasic personality inventory
MPN most probable number
mr milliroentgen
MR mentally retarded, metabolic rate, methyl red
MRD minimum reacting dose
mrhm milliroentgen per hour at one meter
MRL medical record librarian
mRNA messenger RNA
MRU minimal reproductive units
MS master of science, master of sugery, mitral stenosis, morphine sulfate, multiple sclerosis
msec millisecond
MSG monosodium glutamate
MSH melanocyte-stimulating hormone
MSL midsternal line
MSN master of science in nursing
MSRPP multidimensional scale for rating psychiatric patients
MST mean survival time
MSW master of social welfare, master of social work
MT medical technologist medical technology, metatarsal
MTT mean transit time
MTX methotrexate
musc muscle
mv millivolt
Mv mendelevium
MVV maximum voluntary ventilation
MW molecular weight
my myopia
myco mycobacterium

N nasal, nerve, neurology, neuter, neutron dosage unit, nitrogen, nonmalignant, normal, number
Na sodium
NA numerical aperture, nurse's aide
NAD nicotinamide-adenine dinucleotide, no appreciable disease
NADP nicotinamide-adenine dinucleotide phosphate
NAMH National Association for Mental Health
N and T nose and throat
N and V nausea and vomiting
nat native, natural
Nb niobium
NB newborn, [L *nota bene*] note well
NBM nothing by mouth
NCA National Council on Alcoholism
NCI National Cancer Institute
Nd neodymium
ND neutral density
NDA National Dental Association
Ne neon
NE not enlarged
neg negative
neurol neurological, neurology
NF National Formulary
NFIP National Foundation for Infantile Paralysis
NG no good
Ni nickel
NIH National Institutes of Health
NIMH National Institute of Mental Health
nl [L *non licet*] it is not permitted
NM neuromuscular, nitrogen mustard
NMI no middle initial
NMN nicotinamide mononucleotide
NMR nuclear magnetic resonance
nn nerves
NND new and nonofficial drugs
NNR new and nonofficial remedies
no number
No nobelium
NO nitric oxide
NOP not otherwise provided for
NOPHN National Organization for Public Health Nursing
norm normal

NOS not otherwise specified
Np neptunium
np neuropsychiatric, neuropsychiatry, nucleoplasmic, nucleoprotein, nursing procedure
NPO [L *non per os*] nothing by mouth
NPT normal pressure and temperature
nr near
NR neutral red, no refill, normal range
NS nervous system, neurosurgery, normal saline, normal serum
NSFTD normal spontaneous full-term delivery
NSPB National Society for the Prevention of Blindness
NSR normal sinus rhythm
NSU nonspecific urethritis
NT no test
NTA National Tuberculosis Association
NTP normal termperature and pressure
nuc nucleated
nucl nucleus
Nv naked vision
NYD not yet diagnosed

O occiput, oral, orally, oxygen
OA occiput anterior, old age, osteoarthritis
O and C onset and course
OASP organic acid soluble phosphorus
ob [L *obiit*] he died, obstetrical, obstetrician, obstetrics
OBG *or* **OB-GYN** obstetrician-gynecologist, obstetrics-gynecology
obs observed, observer, observation
obstet obstetrical, obstetrics
OC oxygen consumed
occas occasionally
occup occupation, occupational
od doctor of optometry, occupational disease, optical density, outside diameter, overdose
OF occipital-frontal
off official
OHD organic heart disease
OHI ocular hypertension indicator
oint ointment
OJ orange juice
ol oleum
OM otitis media
ONP operating nursing procedure
OOB out of bed
OOLR ophthalmology, otology, laryngology, rhinology
OP occiput posterior, operation, osmotic pressure, other than psychotic, outpatient
OPC outpatient clinic
op cit [L *opere citato*] in the work cited
OPD outpatient department, outpatient dispensary
oph *or* **ophth** ophthalmic, ophthalmologic, ophthalmologist, ophthalmology, ophthalmoscope, ophthalmoscopy
opt optical, optician, optics, optional
OR operating room
O-R oxidation-reduction
ord orderly
org organic
orig origin, original
Os osmium
OT objective test, occupational therapy
OTC over-the-counter, oxytetracycline
oz ounce

P parental, part, percentile, pharmacopeia, phosphorus, pint, plasma, pole, population, position, positive, posterior, postpartum, presbyopia, pressure, psychiatry, pulse, pupil
Pa protactinium
PA paralysis agitans, pernicious anemia, posterior anterior, psychoanalyst, pulmonary artery
PABA para-aminobenzoic acid
PAC phenacetin, aspirin, caffeine

PAD phenacetin, aspirin, deoxyephedrine
palp palpable
P and A percussion and auscultation
P and N psychiatry and neurology
pap papilla
PAP primary atypical pneumonia
PAR postanesthetic recovery
PARU postanesthetic recovery unit
PAS para-aminosalicylic acid
PASA para-aminosalicylic acid
pat patent
path pathological, pathologist, pathology
Pb [L *plumbum*] lead, presbyopia
PB pressure breathing
PBI protein-bound iodine
PC phosphocreatine, present complaint
PCT plasmacrit test
PCV packed cell volume
Pd palladium
PD interpupillary distance, doctor of pharmacy, papilla diameter, paralyzing dose, pediatrics
PDA patent ductus arteriosus
PDB paradichlorobenzene
PDC private diagnostic clinic
pdr powder
Pe pressure on expiration
PE physical examination, probable error, pulmonary embolism
penic penicillin
PEP phosphoenolpyruvate
per period, periodic, person
perf perforated, perforation
perm permanent
perp perpendicular
pers personal
Pg pregnant
PG postgraduate, prostaglandin
pga pteroylglutamic acid
PGR psychogalvanic response
pH negative logarithm of the effective hydrogen-ion concentration or hydrogen-ion activity in gram equivalents per liter
Ph pharmacopoeia
PH past history, previous history, public health
PHA phytohemagglutinin
pharm pharmaceutical, pharmacist, pharmacy
PhC pharmaceutical chemist
PhD doctor of philosophy
PHK cells postmortem human kidney cells
PHS Public Health Service
phys physical, physician
physiol physiological, physiologist, physiology
PI present illness, proactive inhibition, protamine insulin
PID pelvic inflammatory disease
PIE pulmonary infiltration with eosinophilia
PIP proximal interphalangeal
PITR plasma iron turnover rate
pK dissociation constant
PK psychokinesis
PKU phenylketonuria
pl place, plate
PL light perception
Pm promethium
PM physical medicine, [L *post meridiem*] after noon, postmortem, presystolic murmur
PM and R physical medicine and rehabilitation
PMA test primary mental abilities test
PMB polymorphonuclear basophilic (leukocytes)
PMD private medical doctor
PME polymorphonuclear eosinophilic (leukocytes)
PMH past medical history
PMI past medical illness, point of maximum impulse, point of maximum intensity, previous medical illness
PMN polymorphonuclear neutrophilic (leukocytes)
PMP previous menstrual period
PMS postmenopausal syndrome, pregnant mare's serum
PN peripheral nerve, practical nurse, psychiatry-neurology, psychoneurotic
PNC penicillin

PND paroxysmal nocturnal dyspnea, postnasal drip
PNH paroxysmal nocturnal hemoglobinuria
PNPR positive-negative pressure respiration
PNS peripheral nervous system
pnx pneumothorax
Po polonium
PO phone order, postoperative
POA primary optic atrophy
poly polymorphonuclear leukocyte
pop population
POp postoperative
poplit popliteal
pos position, positive
post posterior, postmortem
post-op postoperative
pot potential, potion
PP postpartum, postprandial
PPC progressive patient care
PPCF plasma prothrombin conversion factor
PPD purified protein derivative
PPF pellagra preventive factor
PPLO [*p*leuro*p*neumonia-*l*ike *o*rganism] mycoplasma
ppm parts per million
ppt precipitate
Pr praseodymium, presbyopia, propyl
PR percentile rank, pressoreceptor, proctologist
PRA plasma renin activity
prac practice
pract practical
PRD partial reaction of degeneration
PRE progressive resistive exercise
pref preference
preg pregnant
prelim preliminary
pre-op preoperative
prep prepare, preparation
prev preventative, prevention, previous
prin principal
priv private
proc procedure, proceedings, process
Proct proctologist, proctology
prod product, production
prog prognosis
proj project
pros prostate
prosth prosthesis
prot protein
prox proximal
Ps prescription
PS plastic surgery, pulmonary stenosis, serum from a pregnant woman
PsAn psychoanalysis, psychoanalyst, psychoanalytic, psychoanalytical
PSE point of subjective equality
PSL potassium, sodium chloride, sodium lactate
PSMA progressive spinal muscular atrophy
P sol partly soluble
psych *or* **psychol** psychology
pt part, patient, pint, point
Pt platinum
PT physical therapy
PTA plasma thromboplastin antecedent, prior to admission
PTC phenylthiocarbamide, plasma thromboplastin component
PTF plasma thromboplastin factor
PTH parathyroid hormone
PTU propylthiouracil
Pu plutonium
PU pregnancy urine
pub public, published, publisher
pulm pulmonary
PUO pyrexia of undetermined origin
PV plasma volume
pva polyvinyl alcohol
PVC premature ventricular contraction
PVD peripheral vascular disease
PVM pneumonia virus of mice
PVP polyvinylpyrrolidone
pvt private
Px past history, physical examination, pneumothorax, prognosis
Pyr pyridine
PZI protamine zinc insulin

Q quantity, quartile
QNS quantity not sufficient

QRS segment of electrocardiograph
qt quart
qual qualitative, quality
quant quantitative, quantity
quar quarter, quarterly
qv [L *quod vide*] which see

R radioactive mineral, rectal, resistance, resistant, respiration, response, review, right, roentgen, roentgenologist, roentgenology
Ra radium
RA rheumatoid arthritis, right atrium, right auricle
rac racemic
rad radical, radius
RAIU radioactive iodine uptake
R and D research and development
R and R rate and rhythm (of pulse)
RAS reticular activating system
Rb rubidium
RBC red blood cells, red blood count
RBD right border of dullness
RBE relative biological effectiveness
RBF renal blood flow
RC red cell, respiration ceased, respiratory center
RCM right costal margin
RCO aliphatic acyl radical
RCT Rorschach Content Test
RD reaction of degeneration, retinal detachment
RdA reading age
RdQ reading quotient
RDS respiratory distress syndrome
Re rhenium
RE reticuloendothelium, right eye
readm readmission
rec record, recreation, recurrent
recond recondition
reconstr reconstruction
recryst recrystallize
rect rectified
ref reference
reg region, registered, regular
regen regenerate, regeneration
reg umb umbilical region
rehab *or* **rehabil** rehabilitation
rel relative
REL rate of energy loss
rem [*r*oentgen *e*quivalent *m*an] dosage of ionizing radiation equivalent in effect to one roentgen of X-ray or gamma-ray dosage
REM rapid eye movement
rep repeat, report
REP retrograde pyelogram
res research, reserve, residence, resident
RES reticuloendothelial system
resp respiration, respiratory, responsible
ret retired
retic reticulocyte
rev reverse, review, revolution
RF rheumatic fever, rheumatoid factor
RFR refraction
RGE relative gas expansion
rh rhonchi
Rh rhesus (blood factor), rhodium
RH relative humidity, right hand
RHC respirations have ceased
RHD relative hepatic dullness, rheumatic heart disease
rheum rheumatic, rheumatism
RHF right heart failure
Rhin rhinologist, rhinology
RI refractive index, respiratory illness, retroactive inhibition
RICM right intercostal margin
RIF right iliac fossa
RISA radioactive iodinated serum albumin
rl fine rales
Rl medium rales
RL coarse rales, reduction level
RLE right lower extremity
RLF retrolental fibroplasia
RLL right lower lobe (lung)
RLQ right lower quadrant (abdomen)
RLR right lateral rectus
RM respiratory movement
RML right mediolateral, right middle lobe
Rn radon
RN registered nurse

RNA ribonucleic acid
RNase *or* **RNAase** ribonuclease
Rnt roentgenologist, roentgenology
RO routine order
R/O rule out
ROM range of motion
rot rotation
RPF relaxed pelvic floor, renal plasma flow
RPM revolutions per minute
RPS renal pressor substance, revolutions per second
rpt report
RPT registered physical therapist
RQ recovery quotient, respiratory quotient
RR radiation response, recovery room
RR and E round, regular and equal (eye pupils)
RS reinforcing stimulus, review of symptoms
rt right
RT radiotherapy, reaction time, reading test, recreational therapy, registered technician
Ru ruthenium
RU Roentgen unit
RUE right upper extremity
RUL right upper lobe (lung)
rupt rupture
RUQ right upper quadrant (abdomen)
RV residual volume, retroversion, right ventricle
RVH right ventricular hypertrophy
Rx prescription, therapy, treatment

S sacral, scruple, second, section, sensation, sign, single, singular, son, stimulus, subject, sulfur, surgeon
Sa samarium
SA surface area
S-A sinoatrial
SAD sugar, acetone, diacetic acid
SAH subarachnoid hemorrhage
sanit sanitary, sanitation
sapon saponification
sat satellite, saturated
sat sol saturated solution
Sb [L *stibium*] antimony, strabismus
SB [NL *Scientiae Baccalaureus*] bachelor of science, Stanford-Binet (intelligence test)
sc science, scientific, subcutaneous
Sc scandium, scapula
SCB strictly confined to bed
sci science, scientific
SCU special care unit
SCV smooth, capsulated, virulent
SDA specific dynamic action, succinic dehydrogenase activity
sds sounds
Se selenium
SE saline enema, sanitary engineer
sec second, secondary, section
SEC soft elastic capsules
sed sedimentation
SED skin erythemal dose
sed rate sedimentation rate
sem semen, seminal
sem ves seminal vesicle
sep separate, separated, separation
ser serial, series, service
serv services
SF spinal fluid
SFC spinal fluid count
sg specific gravity
sh short, shoulder
SH serum hepatitis, social history, somatotrophic hormone
Si silicon
SI saturation index, soluble insulin, [F *Systèmes International d'Unités*] International System of Units
sib sibling
SIC surgical intensive care
SID sudden infant death
SIG sigmoidoscopy
sing singular
SK streptokinase
sl slightly
SL small lymphocyte
SLDH serum lactate dehydrogenase
SLE Saint Louis encephalitis,

systemic lupus erythematosus
sm small
Sm samarium
SM [NL *scientiae magister*] master of science, streptomycin
SMR somnolent metabolic rate, submucous resection
Sn [LL *stannum*] tin
SN student nurse
SNDO Standard Nomenclature of Diseases and Operations
SNM Society of Nuclear Medicine
SNS sympathetic nervous system
SOB shortness of breath
soc social
sol soluble, solution
soln solution
S-O-R stimulus-organism-response
sp species, specific, spinal
SP sacrum to pubis
S/P status post
SPCA serum prothrombin conversion accelerator, Society for the Prevention of Cruelty to Animals
SPCC Society for the Prevention of Cruelty to Children
spec special, specific, specimen
sp fl spinal fluid
sp gr specific gravity
spir spiral
spon spontaneous
SPR Society for Psychical Research
sq square
Sr strontium
SR sedimentation rate, sigma reaction, sinus rhythm, stomach rumble
SRN state registered nurse
sRNA [soluble *RNA*] transfer RNA
SRS slow reacting substance
SS saline soak, soapsuds, sterile solution
SSD source skin distance
SSE soap solution enema
sss [L *stratum super stratum*] layer upon layer
st stimulus
ST sedimentation time, slight trace, standardized test, surface tension, survival time
sta station
staph staphylococcus
std standard
STD skin test dose, standard test dose
STH somatotrophic hormone
STP standard temperature and pressure, standard temperature and pulse
strep streptococcus
struct structure
STS serum test for syphilis
STU skin test unit
SU sensation unit
subsp subspecies
substd substandard
sup superior, supination, [L *supra*] above
supp suppository
surg surgeon, surgery, surgical
sv single vibrations
SV simian virus, sinus venosus, stroke volume
SVC superior vena cava
SWR serum Wassermann reaction
Sx symptoms
syst system, systolic

T temperature, temporal, tension, thoracic, time, topical, total, trace, transverse
Ta tantalum
TA toxin-antitoxin, transaldolase, tuberculin alkaline
tab tablet
TAB typhoid, paratyphoid A, and paratyphoid B (vaccine)
TAH total abdominal hysterectomy
TAM toxoid-antitoxin mixture
T and A tonsillectomy and adenoidectomy, tonsillitis and adenoiditis, tonsils and adenoids
TAT tetanus antitoxin, thematic apperception test, toxin-antitoxin
Tb terbium
TB thymol blue, tubercle bacillus, tuberculosis

TBG thyroxine-binding globulin
TBLC term birth, living child
Tc technetium
TC tetracycline, tissue culture
TCA trichloroacetic acid
TCP tricresyl phosphate
TD typhoid dysentery
Te tellurium, tetanus
TE trial and error
tech technical
TED threshold erythema dose
temp temperature, temporal, temporary
TEPA triethylenephosphoramide
TEPP tetraethyl pyrophosphate
term terminal
tert tertiary
TF tactile fremitus, tuberculin filtrate, tuning fork
TG type genus
TGE transmissible gastroenteritis, tryptone glucose extract
TGT thromboplastin generation test
Th thoracic, thorax, thorium
TH thyroid hormone
THC tetrahydrocannabinol
Ti titanium
TI transverse diameter between ischia, tricuspid insufficiency
TIA transient ischemic attack
tinct tincture
TJ triceps jerk
Tl thallium
TL terminal limen, tubal ligation
TLC thin-layer chromatography, total lung capacity
Tm thulium
TM transport mechanism
TMV tobacco mosaic virus
Tn normal intraocular tension
TNT trinitrotoluene
TO target organ, telephone order, oral temperature
TP total protein, tuberculin precipitation
TPC thromboplastic plasma component
TPN triphosphopyridine nucleotide
TPP thiamine pyrophosphate
TPR temperature-pulse-respiration, total peripheral resistance
tr tincture, trace, traction, tremor
TR rectal temperature, therapeutic radiology, tuberculin R, turbidity reducing
trans transaction, transverse
TRF thyrotropin releasing factor
trg training
TRI total response index
tRNA transfer RNA
TS terminal sensation, test solution, thoracic surgery, tricuspid stenosis, triple strength, tubular sound
TSD target skin distance
TSH thyroid-stimulating hormone
TT transit time, tuberculin tested
TTH thyrotrophic hormone
TU toxic unit, transmission unit
TV tetrazolium violet, tidal volume, total volume, tuberculin volutin

U unit, uranium, urology
U and C urethral and cervical
UBA undenatured bacterial antigen
UBI ultraviolet blood irradiation
UCHD usual childhood diseases
UCL urea clearance test
UCR unconditioned response
UCS unconditioned stimulus
UCV uncontrolled variable
UD urethral discharge, uridine diphosphate
UDC usual diseases of childhood
UFA unesterified fatty acid
UHF ultrahigh frequency
UIBC unsaturated iron binding capacity
umb umbilical, umbilicus
UQ upper quadrant
UR unconditioned response
URI upper respiratory infection
urol urological, urologist, urology
US unconditioned stimulus

USD United States Dispensatory
USP United States Pharmacopoeia
UTI urinary tract infection
UTP uridine triphosphate
UV ultraviolet

V valve, vanadium, vein, vertex, [L *vide*] see, virulence, vision, visual acuity, volt, volume
va volt-ampere
VA visual acuity
vac vacuum
vacc vaccination
vag vaginal
V and T volume and tension (of pulse)
var variation, variety
VAR visual-aural range
vasc vascular
VAT ventricular activation time
VC color vision, vital capacity
VCC vasoconstrictor center
VCG vector cardiogram
VCS vasoconstrictor substance
VD venereal disease
VDA visual discriminatory acuity
VDC vasodilator center
VDG venereal disease-gonorrhoea
VDH valvular disease of the heart
VDM vasodepressor material
VDRL venereal disease research laboratory
VDS vasodilator substance, venereal disease-syphilis
VE vesicular exanthema
vel velocity
Vet veteran, veterinary
VF visual field, vocal fremitus
VG ventricular gallop, very good
VH veterans hospital
VHF very high frequency
VI volume index
VIC vasoinhibitory center
VIG vaccinia immune globulin
VL vision-left
VLF very low frequency
VM vasomotor, vestibular membrane, voltmeter
VNA Visiting Nurses Association
VO verbal order
vol volar, volume, volumetric, voluntary, volunteer
VP vapor pressure, venous pressure
VPB ventricular premature beats
vps vibrations per second
VR variable ratio, vision-right, vocal resonance
VRI virus respiratory infection
VS vesicular sound, vesicular stomatitis, veterinary surgeon, vital sign, volumetric solution
VU volume unit
VV vulva and vagina
VW vessel wall

W tungsten, water, watt, weight, wide, width
WAIS Wechsler's Adult Intelligence Scale
Wass Wassermann test
WB whole blood
WBC white blood cells
WC wheelchair
WD wet dressing
WHO World Health Organization
wk week
WL waiting list, wavelength
WO written order, water-in-oil
WP wet pack
WR Wassermann reaction
ws water soluble
wt weight

Xe xenon

Y young, yttrium
Yb ytterbium
yd yard
y/o years old
yr year
ys yellow spot (on retina)

Z zero, zone
Zn zinc
zool zoological, zoology
ZPG zero population growth
Zr zirconium

LATIN WORDS AND ABBREVIATIONS USED IN WRITING PRESCRIPTIONS

Form Used on Prescription	Complete Latin Word or Phrase	English Meaning
aa *or* āā	ana	of
a.c.	ante cibum *or* ante cibos	before meals
ad	ad	to (a specified amount)
add.	adde	add
	addatur	let it be added
	addantur	let them be added
ad lib.	ad libitum	at pleasure
admov.	admove	add
	admoveatur	let there be added
	admoveantur	let them be added
Adv.	adversum	against
agit.	agita	shake
aq.	aqua	water
aq. bull.	aqua bulliens	boiling water
aq. dest.	aqua destillata	distilled water
aq. ferv.	aqua fervens	hot water
Bib.	bibe	drink
b.i.d.	bis in die	twice a day
c *or* c̄	cum	with
Cap.	capiat	let him take
caps.	capsula	capsule
Chart.	charta	paper
Cib.	cibus	food
coch. mag.	cochleare magnum	tablespoonful or a large spoonful (about 1/2 oz)
coch. parv.	cochleare parvum	teaspoonful
Collut.	collutorium	mouthwash
Comp.	compositus	compounded
cong.	congius	gallon
D.	da	give
	detur	let it be given
	dentur	let them be given
de d. in d.	de die in diem	from day to day
Deglut.	deglutiatur	swallow
Dieb. alt.	diebus alternis	every other day
Dieb. tert.	diebus tertiis	every third day
dil.	dilue	dilute
Div.	divide	divide
d.t.d.	detur talis doses	let such a dose be given
	dentur tales doses	let such doses be given
	datus talis dosis	such a dose is given
elix.	elixir	elixir
et	et	and

ext.	extractum	extract
f. *or* ft.	fac	make
	fiat	let it be made
	fiant	let them be made
fl. *or* fld.	fluidus	fluid
Gm.	gramma	gram
gr.	granum *pl* grana	grain
gtt.	gutta *pl* guttae	drop
h.	hora	hour
h.s.	hora somni	at bedtime
liq.	liquor	solution
m.	minimum	minim
M.	misce	mix
mist.	mistura	mixture
m. dict. *or* mor. dict.	more dicto	in the manner directed
noct.	nocte	at night
non rep. *or* non repet.	non repetatur	do not refill
O.	octarius	pint
O.D.	oculus dexter	right eye
	oculo dextro	in the right eye
O.L.	oculus laevus	left eye
omn. hor.	omni hora	every hour
omn. noct.	omni nocte	every night
O.S.	oculus sinister	left eye
	oculo sinistro	in the left eye
p. ae.	partes aequales	equal parts
p.c.	post cibum *or* post cibos	after meals
pil	pilula *pl* pilulae	pill
p.r.n.	pro re nata	as needed
pulv.	pulvis	powder
q.d.	quaque die	every day
q.h.	quaque hora	every hour
q.i.d.	quater in die	four times a day
q.s.	quantum sufficit	as much as is needed
S. *or* Sig.	signa	write on label
s. *or* s̄	sine	without
s.a.	secundem artem	according to art
si op. sit	si opus sit	if necessary
sol.	solutio	solution
solv.	solve	dissolve
s.o.s.	si opus sit	if necessary
ss. *or* $\overline{ss}$	semis	one half
stat.	statim	at once
s.v.r.	spiritus vini rectificatus	rectified spirit of wine
syr.	syrupus	syrup
tab.	tabella *pl* tabellae	medicated tablet
tal.	talis *pl* tales	such a one
t.i.d.	ter in die	three times a day
tinct. *or* tr.	tinctura	tincture
ung.	unguentum	ointment
ut dict.	ut dictum	as directed
vin.	vinum	wine

WEIGHTS AND MEASURES

Unit	Abbr or Symbol	Equivalents in Other Units of Same System	Equivalent in Indicated System
		length	
	English system		*metric system*
mile	mi	5280 feet 320 rods 1760 yards	1.609 kilometers
rod	rd	5.50 yards 16.5 feet	5.029 meters
yard	yd	3 feet 36 inches	0.914 meters
foot	ft *or* ′	12 inches 0.333 yards	30.480 centimeters
inch	in *or* ″	0.083 feet 0.027 yards	2.540 centimeters
	metric system		*English system*
myriameter	myr	1×10^4 meters	6.2137 miles
kilometer	km	1000 meters	0.62137 miles
hectometer	hm	100 meters	109.36 yards
dekameter	dkm	10 meters	32.808 feet
meter	m	1 meter	39.370 inches
decimeter	dm	0.1 meters	3.9370 inches
centimeter	cm	0.01 meters	0.39370 inches
millimeter	mm	0.001 meters	0.039370 inches
micron	μ	1×10^{-6} meters	3.9370×10^{-5} inches
		weight	
	avoirdupois weight		*metric system*
ton	tn		
short ton		20 short hundredweight 2000 pounds	0.907 metric tons
long ton		20 long hundredweight 2240 pounds	1.016 metric tons
hundredweight	cwt		
short hundredweight		100 pounds 0.05 short tons	45.359 kilograms
long hundredweight		112 pounds 0.05 long tons	50.802 kilograms
pound	lb *or* lb av	16 ounces 7000 grains	0.453 kilograms
ounce	oz *or* oz av	16 drams 437.5 grains	28.349 grams

dram	dr *or* dr av	27.343 grains 0.0625 ounces	1.771 grams
grain	gr	0.036 drams 0.002285 ounces	0.0648 grams

	troy weight		*metric system*
pound	lb t	12 ounces 240 pennyweight 5760 grains	0.373 kilograms
ounce	oz t	20 pennyweight 480 grains	31.103 grams
pennyweight	dwt *also* pwt	24 grains 0.05 ounces	1.555 grams
grain	gr	0.042 pennyweight 0.002083 ounces	0.0648 grams

	apothecaries' weight		*metric system*
pound	lb ap	12 ounces 5760 grains	0.373 kilograms
ounce	oz ap *or* ℥	8 drams 480 grains	31.103 grams
dram	dr ap *or* ʒ	3 scruples 60 grains	3.887 grams
scruple	s ap *or* ℈	20 grains 0.333 drams	1.295 grams
grain	gr	0.05 scruples 0.002083 ounces 0.0166 drams	0.0648 grams

	metric system		*apothecaries' weight*
metric ton	MT *or* t	1×10^6 grams	2679.2 lbs
quintal	q	1×10^5 grams	267.92 lbs
kilogram	kg	1000 grams	2.6792 lbs
hectogram	hg	100 grams	3.2151 oz
dekagram	dag	10 grams	0.32151 oz
gram	g *or* gm	1 gram	0.032151 oz
decigram	dg	0.10 grams	1.5432 grains
centigram	cg	0.01 grams	0.15432 grains
milligram	mg	0.001 grams	0.015432 grains
microgram	μg	1×10^{-6} grams	1.5432×10^{-5} grains

capacity

	apothecaries' measure		*metric system*
gallon	gal	4 quarts (231 cubic inches)	3.785 liters
quart	qt	2 pints (57.75 cubic inches)	0.946 liters

pint	pt	4 gills (28.875 cubic inches)	0.473 liters
gill	gi	4 fluidounces (7.218 cubic inches)	118.291 milliliters
fluidounce	fl oz *or* f ℥	8 fluidrams (1.804 cubic inches)	29.573 milliliters
fluidram	fl dr *or* f ʒ	60 minims (0.225 cubic inches)	3.696 milliliters
minim	min *or* ♍	1/60 fluidram (0.003759 cubic inch)	0.061610 milliliters

	metric system		*apothecaries' measure*
kiloliter	kl	1000 liters	264.18 gals
hectoliter	hl	100 liters	26.418 gals
dekaliter	dal	10 liters	2.6418 gals
liter	l	1 liter	1.0567 qts
deciliter	dl	0.10 liters	3.3815 fl oz
centiliter	cl	0.01 liters	2.7052 fl dr
milliliter	ml	0.001 liters	16.231 minims
microliter	μl	1×10^{-6} liters	0.016231 minims

SIGNS AND SYMBOLS

apothecaries' measures

℥	ounce
f℥	fluidounce
*f*ʒ	fluidram
♏, ♍, ♏, *or* min	minim

apothecaries' weights

℔	pound
℥	ounce (as ℥ i *or* ℥ j, one ounce; ℥ ss, half an ounce; ℥ iss *or* jss, one ounce and a half; ℥ ij, two ounces)
ʒ	dram
℈	scruple

genetics

○	an individual, specif., a female—used chiefly in inheritance charts
□	an individual, specif., a male—used chiefly in inheritance charts
♀	female
♂ *or* ♁	male
×	crossed with; hybrid
+	wild type
F_1	offspring of the first generation
F_2	offspring of the second generation
F_3, F_4, F_5, etc.	offspring of the third, fourth, fifth, etc., generation
N	the haploid or gametic number of chromosomes
2N	the diploid or somatic number of chromosomes

mathematics

+	plus; positive ⟨$a + b = c$⟩—used also to indicate omitted figures or an approximation
−	minus; negative
±	plus or minus ⟨the square root of $4a^2$ is $\pm 2a$⟩
×	multiplied by; times ⟨$6 \times 4 = 24$⟩—also indicated by placing a dot between the factors ⟨$6 \cdot 4 = 24$⟩ or by writing factors other than numerals without signs
÷ *or* :	divided by ⟨$24 \div 6 = 4$⟩—also indicated by writing the divisor under the dividend with a line between ⟨$\frac{24}{6} = 4$⟩ or by writing the divisor after the dividend with an oblique line between ⟨3/8⟩
=	equals ⟨$6 + 2 = 8$⟩
>	is greater than ⟨$6 > 5$⟩
<	is less than ⟨$3 < 4$⟩
:	is to; the ratio of
∞	infinity
√ *or* √	root—used without a figure to indicate a square root ⟨as in $\sqrt{4} = 2$⟩ or with an index above the sign to indicate another degree ⟨as in $\sqrt[3]{3}$, $\sqrt[5]{7}$⟩; also denoted by a fractional index at the right of a number whose denominator expresses the degree of the root ⟨$3^{1/3} = \sqrt[3]{3}$⟩

miscellaneous

℞	take—used on prescriptions; prescription; treatment
☠	poison